Manual of Minor Oral Surgery for the General Dentist

Manual of Minor Oral Surgery for the General Dentist

Pushkar Mehra, BDS, DMD

Chairman, Department of Oral and Maxillofacial Surgery
Associate Dean for Hospital Affairs
Boston University Henry M. Goldman School of Dental Medicine;
Chief of Service, Oral and Maxillofacial Surgery, Boston Medical Center;
Chief of Service, Oral and Maxillofacial Surgery, Beth Israel Deaconess Medical Center
Boston, MA, USA

Richard D'Innocenzo, DMD, MD

Clinical Associate Professor and Director of Pre-doctoral Education
Department of Oral & Maxillofacial Surgery;
Vice Chairman, Dentistry and Oral & Maxillofacial Surgery, Boston Medical Center
Boston, MA, USA

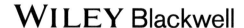

Contents

Contributors

Louay Abrass, DMD
Clinical Assistant Professor
Department of Endodontics
Boston University Henry M. Goldman School of Dental Medicine
Boston, MA, USA

Omar Abubaker, DMD, PhD
Professor and S. Elmer Bear Chair
Department of Oral and Maxillofacial Surgery
Medical College of Virginia School of Dentistry
Richmond, VA, USA

Hussam Batal, DMD
Assistant Professor
Department of Oral and Maxillofacial Surgery
Boston University Henry M. Goldman School of Dental Medicine
Boston, MA, USA

Dale A. Baur, DDS
Associate Professor and Chair
Department of Oral and Maxillofacial Surgery
Case Western Reserve University School of Dental Medicine
and University Hospitals/Case Medical Center
Cleveland, OH, USA

Jeffrey Bennett, DMD
Professor and Chair
Department of Oral Surgery and Hospital Dentistry
Indiana University School of Dentistry
Indianapolis, IN, USA

George Blakey, DDS
Clinical Associate Professor and Residency Program Director
Department of Oral and Maxillofacial Surgery
University of North Carolina School of Dentistry
Chapel Hill, NC, USA

Thomas C. Bourland, DDS, MS
Clinical Adjunct Faculty
Department of Oral and Maxillofacial Surgery
Texas A & M Baylor College of Dentistry
Dallas, TX, USA
Private Practice of Oral and Maxillofacial Surgery
Dallas, TX, USA

Frederico Brugnami, DDS
Private Practice of Periodontology and Implantology
Rome, Italy

Andrew Bushey, DMD, MD
Formerly, Resident, Department of Oral and Maxillofacial Surgery
Case Western Reserve University School of Dental Medicine/
Case Medical Center
Cleveland, OH, USA
Currently in Private Practice of Oral and Maxillofacial Surgery

Alfonso Caiazzo, DDS
Visiting Clinical Assistant Professor
Department of Oral and Maxillofacial Surgery
Boston University Henry M. Goldman School of Dental Medicine
Boston, MA, USA
Currently in Private Practice of Oral Surgery and Implantology, Salerno, Italy

Serge Dibart, DMD
Professor and Chair
Department of Periodontology and Oral Biology
Boston University Henry M. Goldman School of Dental Medicine
Boston, MA, USA

Thomas R. Flynn, DMD
Formerly, Associate Professor and Director of Pre-doctoral Education
Department of Oral and Maxillofacial Surgery
Harvard School of Dental Medicine
Boston, MA, USA
Currently in Private Practice of Oral and Maxillofacial Surgery, Reno, NV, USA

Marianela Gonzalez, DDS
Assistant Professor, Director of Undergraduate Studies
Department of Oral and Maxillofacial Surgery
Texas A & M Baylor College of Dentistry
Dallas, TX, USA

Cesar A. Guerrero, DDS
Division of Oral and Maxillofacial Surgery
Department of Surgery
University of Texas Medical Branch
Galveston, TX, USA

Pamela Hughes, DDS
Associate Professor and Chair
Department of Oral and Maxillofacial Surgery
Oregon Health & Science University
Portland, OR, USA

Jason Jamali, DDS, MD
Clinical Assistant Professor
Department of Oral and Maxillofacial Surgery
University of Illinois at Chicago
Chicago, IL, USA

Diana Jee-Hyun Lyu, DMD
Formerly, Intern, Department of Oral and Maxillofacial
Surgery
Case Western Reserve University School of Dental Medicine/
Case Medical Center
Cleveland, OH, USA
Currently, Resident, Department of Oral and Maxillofacial
Surgery, University of Minnesota School of Dentistry
Minneapolis, MN, USA

Antonia Kolokythas, DDS, MSc
Assistant Professor and Associate Program Director and
Director of Research
Department of Oral and Maxillofacial Surgery
University of Illinois at Chicago
Chicago, IL, USA

Kyle Kramer, DDS, MS
Assistant Clinic Professor of Dental Anesthesiology
Department of Oral Surgery and Hospital Dentistry
Indiana University School of Dentistry
Indianapolis, IN, USA

Din Lam, DMD, MD
Private Practice of Oral and Maxillofacial Surgery
Charlotte, NC, USA

Patrick J. Louis, DDS, MD
Professor and Residency Program Director
Department of Oral and Maxillofacial Surgery
University of Alabama at Birmingham
Birmingham, AL, USA

David W. Lui, DMD, MD
Assistant Professor
Department of Oral and Maxillofacial Surgery
Medical College of Virginia School of Dentistry
Richmond, VA, USA

Michael Miloro, DMD, MD, FACS
Professor, Department Head and Program Director
Department of Oral and Maxillofacial Surgery
University of Illinois at Chicago
Chicago, IL, USA

Daniel Oreadi, DDS
Assistant Professor
Department of Oral and Maxillofacial Surgery
Tufts University School of Dental Medicine
Boston, MA, USA

David C. Stanton, DMD, MD, FACS
Associate Professor
Department of Oral and Maxillofacial Surgery
and Pharmacology
University of Pennsylvania School of Dental Medicine
Philadelphia, PA, USA

Preface

This handbook is a guide and update for the general dentists who enjoy performing minor oral surgery in their office. It is meant to aid such "surgery-minded dentists" perform procedures more quickly, smoothly, easily, and safely. The easy to read and concise format also make it an indispensable tool for dental students as it allows them to develop an understanding of basic oral surgery principles with detailed emphasis on case selection, step-by-step operative techniques, and the prevention and/or management of complications.

The experience of dentists in minor oral surgery is quite varied and while some have had extensive experience and training through general practice residencies, military or other postgraduate programs, or a mentoring experience with an experienced practitioner, others have had only minimal instruction and training. Use of this handbook will diminish some of this discrepancy between experienced and inexperienced generalists and provide the necessary, contemporary knowledge base for the interested clinician.

The book presents a review of minor surgical procedures and relevant principles in several clinical surgical areas following the current standards of care. It is assumed that the reader possesses fundamental knowledge and skills in oral anatomy, patient/operator positioning for surgery, the care of soft and hard tissue during surgery, and basic patient management techniques. Therefore, the authors, all of whom are recognized leaders in their field, have skipped directly to the crux of each procedure. Within these pages, the authors share many pearls gleaned from years of experience and training to increase the readers' confidence and competence. Many procedures covered in this book are often performed by specialists and many a times, patients would be better served by being referred to specialists. This book will help readers also more clearly understand the scope of each surgical procedure and more accurately define their own capabilities and comfort zones.

CHAPTER 1

Patient Evaluation and History Taking

Dale A. Baur, Andrew Bushey, and Diana Jee-Hyun Lyu

Department of Oral and Maxillofacial Surgery, Case Western Reserve University School of Dental Medicine and University Hospitals/Case Medical Center, Cleveland, OH, USA

Introduction

The initial physical examination and evaluation of a patient is a critical component in the provision of care prior to any surgical procedure. A thorough patient assessment, including a physical exam and medical history, is necessary prior to even simple surgical events. The information gathered during this encounter can provide the clinician with information necessary to make treatment modifications and assess and stratify risks and potential complications associated with the treatment. Disregarding the importance of this exam can result in serious morbidity and even death. Prior to initiating any surgical procedure, an accurate dental diagnosis must be formulated based on the patient's chief complaint, history of present illness, a clinical dental examination, and appropriate and recent diagnostic imaging, such as a panoramic radiograph.

Medical history

The medical history of a patient is the most important information that a clinician can acquire and should be emphasized during the initial exam. With a thorough medical history, a skilled clinician can decide whether the patient is capable of undergoing a procedure and if any modifications should be made prior to the treatment. The dentist should be able to reliably predict how preexisting medical conditions might interfere with the patient's ability to respond successfully to a surgical insult and subsequently heal. A careful and systematic approach must be used to evaluate all surgical patients. Only in this way can potential complications be managed or avoided. The medical history should be updated annually, but it should also be reviewed at each appointment to be assured there are no significant changes and/or additions.

A detailed questionnaire that covers all common medical problems aids in the collection of information to formulate the patient's medical history (Figure 1.1). However, the dentist should review this questionnaire and ask focused questions as needed to clarify and expound on the past medical history. Any inconsistencies or discrepancies in the written or verbal history must be investigated. The dentist must formulate a thorough timeline of the patient's medical history, surgical history, social history (smoking, drinking, and illicit drug habits), family history, current and previous medications, and allergies. If lingering questions remain after reviewing the history with the patient, consultation with the patient's primary care physician should be considered. If the patient is unable to accurately review their medical history due to cognitive issues, then the caregiver and/or family must be prepared to provide the medical history. The use of any anticoagulants, corticosteroids, hypertension medication, and other medications should be thoroughly reviewed.[1] Female patients should be asked whether there is any possibility that they are pregnant; if there is uncertainty, urine beta-HCG is easy to obtain to provide a definitive answer. Allergies that should be addressed are those to medications and other items used in a dental office, such as latex. The medical history should emphasize the major organ systems, specifically the cardiovascular system, central nervous system, pulmonary system, endocrine system, along with the hepatic and renal systems.

Manual of Minor Oral Surgery for the General Dentist, Second Edition. Edited by Pushkar Mehra and Richard D'Innocenzo.

© 2016 John Wiley & Sons, Inc. Published 2016 by John Wiley & Sons, Inc.

Medical History

Patient's Name _____ Date of Birth _____

Physician's Name _____ Phone number _____

Please answer the following questions as completely as possible

1. Do you consider yourself to be in good health?   YES   NO
2. Are you now or have you been under a physician's care within the past year?   YES   NO
   If yes, specify the condition being treated: _____
3. Do you take any medication, including birth control pills?   YES   NO
   Please specify name and purpose of medication: _____
   _____
   _____

4. Do you have or have you ever had any heart or blood problems?   YES   NO
5. Have you ever been told that you have a heart murmur?   YES   NO
6. Do you require antibiotic medication before treatment for a heart condition?   YES   NO
7. Do you now have or have you ever had high blood pressure?   YES NO
8. Have you ever been diagnosed as being HIV positive or having AIDS?   YES NO
9. Have you ever had hepatitis or liver disease?   YES   NO
10. Have you ever had rheumatic fever, ___ asthma, ___ blood disorder, ____
    diabetes ___; rheumatism ____; arthritis ____; tuberculosis ___; venereal disease ___; heart attack ___;
    kidney disease ___; immune system disorder ___; any other diseases ___
    If so, specify: _____
11. Do you bleed easily?   YES   NO
12. Have you ever had any severe or unusual reaction to, or are you allergic to, any drugs, including the following:
    Penicillin____   Ibuprofen_____
    Aspirin_____   Codeine_____
    Acetaminophen____   Barbiturates_____

    Are you taking any of the following medications?
    Antibiotics _____   Digitalis or heart medication_____
    Anticoagulants (Blood thinners)_____   Nitroglycerin_____
    Aspirin _____   Antihistamine_____
    Tranquilizers _____   Oral contraceptives_____
    Insulin_____
13. Do you faint easily?   YES   NO
14. Have you ever had a reaction to dental treatment or local anesthetic?   YES   NO
15. Are you allergic to any local anesthetic?   YES   NO
16. Do you have any other allergies?   YES   NO
    If yes, please describe: _____
    _____
    _____
17. Have you ever had a nervous breakdown or undergone psychiatric treatment?   YES   NO
18. Have you ever had an addiction problem with alcohol or drugs?   YES   NO
19. Women: Are you or could you be pregnant   YES   NO
    Are you breast feeding now?   YES   NO
20. Are you in pain now?   YES   NO
21. When did you last see a dentist? _____
22. Who was your last dentist? _____
23. Are your teeth affecting your general health?   YES   NO
24. Do you have or have you had bleeding or sensitive gums?   YES   NO
25. Have you ever taken Fen Phen or similar appetite-suppressant drugs?   YES   NO
26. Do you smoke? If yes, how many cigarettes a day   YES   NO
27. Do you drink alcohol? If yes, how often   YES   NO

I hereby certify that the answers to the forgoing questions are accurate to the best of my ability. Since a change in my medical condition or in medications I take can affect dental treatment, I understand the importance of and agree to take the responsibility for notifying the dentist of any changes at any subsequent appointment.

Signature _____ Date _____
(Patient, legal guardian, or authorized agent of patient)

Figure 1.1 Medical history questionnaire. Source: Reprinted with permission from OMS National Insurance Company.

Cardiovascular system

As our population ages, the dentist is likely to see more patients with some aspects of cardiovascular disease. Hypertension is very common, and many patients are undiagnosed. Current studies note that nearly one-third of the US population has hypertension—defined as a systolic blood pressure higher than 139 mmHg or a diastolic blood pressure higher than 89 mmHg. Another one-quarter of the U.S. population has prehypertension—defined by a systolic blood pressure between 120 and 139 mmHg and a diastolic blood pressure between 80 and 89 mmHg.[2] For patients with a history of cardiovascular disease, vital signs should be monitored regularly during surgery (Table 1.1).

Systolic and diastolic blood pressures taken at multiple times remain the best means to diagnose and classify hypertension. When the blood pressure reading is mild to moderately high, the patient should be referred to their primary care physician for evaluation and to initiate hypertensive therapy. The patient should be monitored on each subsequent visit before treatment. If needed, the dentist can consider using some type of anxiety control protocol. When severe hypertension exists, which is defined as systolic blood pressure greater than 200 mmHg or diastolic pressure above 110 mmHg,[2] defer treatment and urgently refer the patient to their primary care physician or an emergency department.

Congestive heart failure (CHF) becomes more common with advanced age. This condition is typically characterized by dyspnea, orthopnea, fatigue, and lower extremity edema. Uncontrolled or new onset symptoms of CHF necessitate deferring surgical treatment until the patient has been medically optimized.

Coronary artery disease (CAD) also has an increasing prevalence as our population ages. Progressive narrowing of the coronary arteries leads to an imbalance in myocardial oxygen demand and supply. Oxygen demand can be further increased by exertion, stress, or anxiety during surgical procedures. When myocardial ischemic occurs, it can produce substernal chest pain, which may radiate to the arms, neck, or jaw. Other symptoms include diaphoresis, dyspnea, and nausea/vomiting. The dental practitioner is likely to see patients with a variety of presentations of CAD, including angina, history of myocardial infarction, coronary artery stent placement, coronary artery bypass grafting, etc. In these cases, the functional status of a patient is a very reliable predictor of risk for dentoalveolar surgery. The functional assessment of common daily activities is quantified in metabolic equivalents (METs). A MET is defined as the resting metabolic rate (the amount of oxygen consumed at rest) which is approximately 3.5 ml O_2/kg/min. Therefore, an activity with 2 METS requires twice the resting metabolism (Table 1.2).[3] Patients who are able to perform moderate activity (4 or more METs, e.g. walk around the block at 3–4 mph, light housework), are generally good candidates for dentoalveolar procedures without further cardiac work-up. Of course, any patient with signs of unstable CAD (new onset or altered frequency/intensity chest pain, decompensated CHF), elective surgery should be deferred until the patient is stabilized.

Table 1.1 Blood pressure classification

BP Classification	Systolic BP (mmHg)	Diastolic BP (mmHg)
Normal	<120	<80
Prehypertensive	120–139	80–89
Stage 1 hypertension	140–159	90–99
Stage 2 hypertension	≥160	≥100

Table 1.2 Table of METS for daily activities*

Activity	METS
Light intensity activities	*<3*
Sleeping	0.9
Writing, desk work, typing	1.8
Light house chores (washing dishes, cooking, making the bed)	2–2.5
Walking 2.5 mph	2.9
Moderate intensity activities	*3–6*
Walking 3.0 mph	3.3
Bicycling <10 mph	4.0
Gardening and yard work	3.5–4.4
Vigorous intensity activities	*>6*
Jogging	8.8–11.2
Basketball	11.1

*A MET is defined as the resting metabolic rate (the amount of oxygen consumed at rest) which is approximately 3.5 ml O_2/kg/min. Therefore, an activity with 2 METs requires twice the resting metabolism.

Dysrhythmias are often associated with CHF and CAD. Atrial fibrillation (AF) has become the default rhythm of the elderly, being the most common sustained arrhythmia. These patients are typically anticoagulated by a number of different medications. The dentist must be familiar with the medications as well as the mechanism of action. For minor procedures, anticoagulated patients often can be maintained on their anticoagulation protocol and undergo surgery without incident. Appropriate labs should be ordered as needed to check the anticoagulation status. However, if the dentist feels the anticoagulation protocol needs to be modified or discontinued prior to surgery, consultation with the prescribing physician is mandatory.

Patients with dysrhythmias will often have pacemakers and/or implanted defibrillators. There is no reported contraindication to treating patients with pacemakers, and no evidence exists showing the need for antibiotic prophylaxis in patients with pacemakers. The dentist must keep in mind that certain electrical equipment can interfere with the pacemaker (e.g. electrocautery), so precautions must be observed.

Cardiac conditions that require Subacute Bacterial Endocarditis (SBE) prophylaxis will be covered elsewhere in the text.

If any uncertainty exists regarding safely performing dentoalveolar surgery on a patient with a history of cardiovascular disease, the dentist should consider referring the patient to an oral and maxillofacial surgeon and/or performing the procedure in more controlled environment such as a hospital operating room.

Pulmonary system

Pulmonary disease is also becoming more common in our aging population. As aging occurs, there is a decrease in total capacity, expiratory reserve volume, and functional reserve volume. There is also a decrease in alveolar gas exchange surface.

Asthma is one of the most common pulmonary diseases that a dentist will encounter. True asthma involves the episodic narrowing of bronchioles with an overlying component of inflammation. Asthma is manifested by wheezing and dyspnea due to chemical irritation, respiratory infections, immunologic reactions, stress, or a combination of these factors. As part of the patient evaluation, the dentist should inquire about precipitating factors, frequency and severity of attacks, medications used, and response to medications. The severity of attacks can be gauged by the need for emergency room visits, hospital admissions, and past intubations. Asthmatic patients should be questioned specifically about an aspirin allergy because of the relatively high frequency of non-steroidal anti-inflammatory drug (NSAID) allergy in asthmatic patients. The asthmatic patient will often have a variety of prescription medications including beta-2 agonist inhalers, inhaled or systemic steroids, and leukotriene inhibitors. Prior to performing dentoalveolar surgery, the dentist needs to have an understanding of the mechanism of action of these medications. Management of the asthmatic patient involves recognition of the role of anxiety in bronchospasm initiation and of the potential adrenal suppression in patients receiving corticosteroid therapy. Elective oral surgery should be deferred if a respiratory tract infection or wheezing is present. In a patient whose asthma appears to be poorly controlled, pulmonary function testing as well as a medical consult would be prudent.

Chronic obstructive pulmonary disease (COPD) is the fourth leading cause of death in the United States. Airways lose their elastic properties, and become obstructed because of mucosal edema, excessive secretions, and bronchospasm. Patients with COPD frequently become dyspneic during mild-to-moderate exertion, and will report a chronic cough that produces large amounts of thick sputum. These patients are prone to frequent exacerbations due to respiratory infections.

The disease spectrum of COPD ranges from mild symptoms to those patient who require supplemental oxygen via nasal cannula. It is important for the dentist to keep in mind that these patients maintain their respiratory drive by hypoxemia, not hypercarbia, as in a normal individual.

COPD patients should have elective surgery deferred during periods of poor control or exacerbations. Patients on chronic steroid use should be considered for perioperative steroid supplementation. In those patients who smoke cigarettes, smoking cessations is ideal 4–8 weeks before surgery for maximum effect. However, smoking cessation for 72 hours will decrease carbon monoxide levels, although secretions may temporarily increase. Once again, if any questions remain about the patient's suitability for surgery, blood gas determinations, pulmonary function testing, and a medical consult should be obtained.

Table 1.3 Mini-Mental State Examination. Tool used to assess mental status based on 11 questions testing different areas of cognitive function totaling 30 points

Section	Question	Score
	ORIENTATION	
Temporal orientation (5 points)	What is the approximate time?	1 point
	What day of the week is it?	1 point
	What is the date today?	1 point
	What is the month?	1 point
	What is the year?	1 point
Spatial orientation (5 points)	Where are we now?	1 point
	What is this place?	1 point
	What is the address here?	1 point
	In which town are we?	1 point
	In which state are we?	1 point
	REGISTRATION	
Registration	Name three objects—1 second to say each, then ask the patient to recall all three. Repeat until the patient has learned all three. Count and record trial.	3 points
Attention and calculation	Serial 7s (stop after five correct)	1 point for each correct (5 points)
Remote memory	Ask for the 3 objects repeated above	3 points
	LANGUAGE	
Naming two objects	Watch and pen	2 points
Repeat	"No ifs, ands or buts."	1 point
Stage command	Follow a 3-stage command. "Take a piece of paper in your right hand, fold it in half, and put it on the floor."	3 points
Writing a complete sentence	Write a sentence that makes sense	1 point
Reading and obey	Close your eyes	1 point
Copy the diagram	Copy two pentagons with an intersection	1 point
Total score		30 points

Score	Results	Dementia
30–29	Normal	
28–26	Borderline cognitive dysfunction	
25–18	Marked cognitive dysfunction	Can be diagnosed
<17	Severe dysfunction	Severe dementia

Central nervous system

With age, cerebral atrophy occurs resulting in memory decline and in extreme cases, dementia. If any patient shows signs of cognitive decline, a baseline mental status exam can be performed to better assess the patient (Table 1.3).[3,4]

Patients who have a history of a cerebrovascular accident (CVA) are always susceptible to future events. Depending on the etiology of the CVA, these patients may be placed on anticoagulants and antihypertensives. If such a patient requires surgery, consultation with the patient's physician is desirable to optimize the patient for surgery. The patient's baseline neurologic status should be assessed and documented preoperatively.

Patients with a history of seizure disorders are fairly common. Prior to considering dentoalveolar surgery in these patients, the seizure disorder must be fully characterized. Useful questions to ask include frequency of seizures, the last seizure occurrence, and what medications are being used to control the seizure. The blood levels of some seizure medications, such as sodium valproate and carbamazepine, should be obtained to insure the levels are in the therapeutic range. If medication levels are sub-therapeutic, an appropriate dosing adjustment will be necessary.

Hepatic and renal systems

As with the other organ systems, renal function declines with age. After age 30, 1% of renal function is lost per year with a progressive loss of renal blood flow and a gradual loss of functioning glomeruli. This can result in prolonged elimination half-lives for medications and the reduced ability to excrete drugs and metabolites. Drugs that depend on renal metabolism or excretion should be avoided or used in modified doses to prevent systemic toxicity in renal patients. Appropriate drug doses should be calculated based on the patient's creatinine clearance levels. Nephrotoxic drugs, such as NSAIDs, should also be avoided in patients with renal failure.

Renal dialysis patients require special considerations prior to surgery. Dialysis treatment typically requires the presence of an arteriovenous shunt, which allows easy vascular access. The dentist should not use the shunt for venous access and avoid taking blood pressures on this arm. Elective procedures should be performed the day after a dialysis treatment. This allows the heparin used during dialysis to be eliminated and the patient to be in the best physiologic status with respect to intravascular volume, electrolytes, and metabolic by-products.

After renal or other solid organ transplantation, the patient will be on a variety of immune modulating medications. Odontogenic infections may rapidly progress and become life-threatening in these immunocompromised patients, and should be treated aggressively by the dentist. Prophylactic antibiotics used prior to dentoalveolar surgery in these patients is recommended.

The patient who suffers from hepatic damage, usually from infectious disease or alcohol abuse, will need special consideration prior to dental work. The patient may be prone to bleeding because many coagulation factors produced in the liver are reduced. There is also the potential for thrombocytopenia due to decreased production of platelets or splenic sequestration of platelets. Prior to dentoalveolar procedures, appropriate coagulation studies must be obtained to verify appropriate levels of coagulation factors and platelets. A partial prothrombin time (PTT) or prothrombin time (PT), along with a platelet count, may be useful in the evaluation of the patient. Routine liver function tests may also be indicated. In addition to bleeding risk, many drugs are metabolized by the liver, with the potential for longer elimination half-lives. Dosing needs to be adjusted accordingly.

Endocrine system

The most common endocrine disorder the dentist is likely to see is diabetes mellitus. Diabetes is classified into insulin-dependent (Type 1) and non-insulin-dependent (Type 2). An insulin-dependent diabetic will usually have a history of diabetes from childhood or early adulthood and is a result of auto-immune destruction of insulin producing cells. Type 2 diabetes results from insulin resistance associated with excessive adipose tissue.

Prior to considering dentoalveolar surgery, the dentist must be familiar with the diabetic patient's medication regimen and glucose levels. If there are concerns that the patient is not well controlled, a hemoglobin A1C can be ordered to assess blood glucose levels over the previous 2–3 months. There are currently short-, intermediate-, and long-acting insulin preparations available. The dentist must be knowledgeable of the type of insulin used by the patient as well as the onset, peak effect, and duration of the insulin preparation. If the patient's diet will be significantly altered due to the surgery, adjustments must be made in medication dosing to avoid hypoglycemia. This is best done in consultation with the treating physician. In all diabetic patients, blood glucose levels should be checked prior to surgery. Short term periods of moderate hyperglycemia in the post-op period are more desirable than risking hypoglycemia.

Diseases of the adrenal cortex may cause adrenal insufficiency. Symptoms of primary adrenal insufficiency include weakness, weight loss, fatigue, and hyperpigmentation of skin and mucous membranes. However, the most common cause of adrenal insufficiency is chronic therapeutic corticosteroid administration (secondary adrenal insufficiency). The stigmata of chronic long-term steroid use include moon facies, buffalo hump, and thin, translucent skin. Theoretically, the patient's inability to increase endogenous corticosteroid levels in response to physiologic stress may cause them to become hypotensive and complain of abdominal pain during prolonged surgery. From a practical standpoint, this Addisonian crisis is rare. A short-term increase of the steroid dose is usually sufficient to prevent this occurrence, while side effects from this steroid bump are minimal.

A thyroid condition of primary significance in oral surgery is thyrotoxicosis, because an acute crisis can occur in patients with the condition. Thyrotoxicosis is the result of an excess of circulating triiodothyronine (T_3) and thyronine (T_4). This is most frequent in patients with Graves' disease, a multinodular goiter, or a thyroid adenoma. Patients with excessive thyroid hormone production can exhibit fine, brittle hair, hyperpigmentation of skin, excessive sweating, tachycardia, palpitations, weight loss, and emotional lability. Exophthalmos, a bulging of the globes caused by increases of fat in the orbits, is a common symptom of patients with Graves' disease. Elevated circulating thyroid hormones, detected using direct or indirect laboratory techniques, leads to a definite diagnosis.

Thyrotoxic patients can be treated with therapeutic agents that block thyroid hormone synthesis and release, surgically with a thyroidectomy, or radioactive iodine ablation. A thyrotoxic crisis can occur in patients left untreated or improperly treated, caused by the sudden release of large quantities of preformed thyroid hormones. Early symptoms of a thyrotoxic crisis include restlessness, nausea, and abdominal cramps. Later-onset symptoms are high fever, diaphoresis, tachycardia, and, eventually, cardiac decompensation. The patient becomes lethargic and hypotensive, with possible death if no intervention occurs.

The dentist may be able to diagnose previously unrecognized hyperthyroidism by taking a complete medical history and performing a careful examination of the patient, including thyroid inspection and palpation. If severe hyperthyroidism is suspected from the history, the gland should not be palpated because that manipulation alone can trigger a crisis. Patients suspected of being hyperthyroid should be referred for medical evaluation before dentoalveolar surgery.

Patients with treated thyroid disease can safely undergo dental procedures. However, if a patient is found to have an oral infection, the primary care physician should be notified, particularly if the patient shows signs of hyperthyroidism. Atropine and excessive amounts of epinephrine-containing solutions should be avoided if a patient is thought to have incompletely treated hyperthyroidism.[5]

The dentist can play a role in the initial recognition of hypothyroidism. Early symptoms of hypothyroidism include fatigue, constipation, weight gain, hoarseness, headaches, arthralgia, menstrual disturbances, edema, dry skin, and brittle hair and fingernails. If the symptoms of hypothyroidism are mild, no modification of dental therapy is required.[1]

Pregnancy

The concern for the pregnant female is not only her welfare but that of the fetus. Potential teratogenic damage from drugs and radiation are serious concerns. It is always best to defer surgery for the pregnant patient, if possible, until after delivery. The patient who requires surgery and/or medication during pregnancy is in a high-risk situation and should be treated as such. Drugs are rated by the FDA as to their possible effect on the fetus. These classifications are A, B, C, D, and X. Drugs classified as A are the safest, whereas D and X are the least safe. The most likely medication to have a teratogenic effect are the D and X drugs, but doses of C and even B drugs should be used with extreme caution (Table 1.4).[6]

Typical drugs used in a dental setting which are considered the safest are acetaminophen, penicillin, codeine, erythromycin, and cephalosporin. Aspirin and ibuprofen are contraindicated because of the possibility of postpartum bleeding and premature closure of the ductus arteriosus.[7] Avoid keeping the near-term patient in a supine position, as that position can compress the vena cava and limit blood flow. In general, elective treatment should be performed in the second trimester. Physician consult is frequently indicated.[8]

Table 1.4 Pregnancy drug categories

Categories	Definitions	Examples
A	Human studies have failed to demonstrate a risk to fetus in first trimester	
B	Animal studies show no risk and there are no human studies —OR—Animal studies have shown adverse effect, but human studies fail to present risk in any trimester	Amoxicillin, augmentin, keflex, oxycodone, lidocaine, ondansetron
C	Animal studies show adverse effect, there are no human studies, BUT potential benefits could outweigh the risk	Hydrocodone, epinephrine, fentanyl, articaine
D	There is positive evidence of risk in fetus in human studies, BUT potential benefits could outweigh risk	ASA, ibuprofen, midazolam, lorezapam, diazepam
X	Studies show fetal abnormalities and/or positive evidence of risk in studies, and risks outweigh the benefits	

Table 1.5 Vital signs for an adult patient

	Normal	High	Low
Pulse rate	60–100 bpm	100 bpm or higher	60 bpm or lower
Respiratory rate	12–18 bpm	25 bpm or higher	12 bpm or lower
Temperature	37°C (98.6°F ± 1°F)	38.3°C (101°F) or higher	36°C (96.8°F) or lower
O_2 saturation (SpO_2)	97–100%		<94%

Table 1.6 Body mass index (BMI)* classification, as defined by World Health Organization (WHO)

Classification	BMI	Risk of comorbidities
Underweight	<18.5	Low
Normal range	18.5–24.9	Average
Overweight	≥25	
Pre-obese	25.0–29.9	Increased
Obese class I	30.0–34.9	Moderate
Obese class II	35.0–39.9	Severe
Obese class III	≥40.0	Very severe

*BMI, defined as {weight (kg)/height (m)^2}, is the accepted measure of obesity in populations and in clinical practice.

Physical examination

The clinician should begin the exam with measuring vital signs (BP, pulse, respiratory rate, temperature, pulse oximetry) (Table 1.5). This both serves as a screening device for unsuspected medical problems and provides a baseline for future evaluations. In addition to blood pressure, a pulse rate should be taken and recorded. The most common method is to palpate the radial artery at the patient's wrist. If there is a weakened pulse or irregular rhythm, elective treatment should not be performed unless the operator has received clearance by the patient's physician. Respirations, performed by counting the numbers of breaths taken by the patient in a minute, can also provide information regarding the patient's respiratory function. When examining respirations, it should be noted whether the patient's breaths

are unlabored or labored, if there is any sound associated with the breaths, such as wheezing, and if the breaths are regular or irregular.

In addition to the vital signs mentioned above, there is other information that should be gathered prior to performing a surgical procedure. The height and weight (in kilograms) of the patient should be recorded. The weight of the patient is used frequently in determining dosages of many medications. The body mass index (BMI) is a useful tool in quantifying obesity (Table 1.6). Obese patients are at a higher risk for having many comorbidities such as CAD, diabetes, and obstructive sleep apnea. The patient's temporomandibular joint (TMJ) function should be documented prior to surgery, by assessing the maximum interincisal opening, lateral excursions, and any pre-auricular tenderness. Patients with limited opening will make dentoalveolar surgery more difficult. Also, if the patient has pre-existing TMJ pain, it must be documented as the surgery could exacerbate the condition. Finally, if the patient is presenting for surgery due to a painful oral condition, it is useful to quantify the level of pain that the patient is experiencing. This is usually done on a 0–10 scale, with 0 being no pain, and a 10 signifying the worst pain the patient has ever experienced.

Most patients can safely undergo dentoalveolar surgery without obtaining preoperative laboratory work. However, patients with a history of current or recent chemotherapy are the exception. Chemotherapeutic agents not only affect malignancy, but can have a significant effect on the hematopoietic system. Thus, the potential for decreased platelet counts as well as decreased white blood cells counts exists. Subsequently, there is the potential for excessive bleeding due to the thrombocytopenia and the potential of infection due to leukopenia. In this subset of patients, preoperative laboratory values must be obtained that assess the adequacy of platelets and white blood cells. If the values are insufficient, the surgery should be delayed or modifications to the treatment considered, e.g. platelet transfusion.

Head and neck examination

The physical evaluation of a dental patient will focus on the oral cavity and surrounding head and neck region, but the clinician should also carefully evaluate entire patient for pertinent physical findings. The physical exam is usually accomplished by: inspection, palpation, percussion, and auscultation. The dentist should also examine skin texture and look for possible skin lesions on the head, neck, and any other exposed parts of the body. Cervical lymph nodes should be palpated. Include examination of the hair, facial symmetry, eye movements and conjunctiva color, and cranial nerves. Inspect the oral cavity thoroughly, including the oropharynx, tongue, floor of the mouth, and oral mucosa for any abnormal appearing tissue, expansion, or induration.

Any abnormalities should be described and noted in the patient's chart. Suspicious lesions must be biopsied or referred for biopsy. Red and/or white lesions are particularly suspicious and must be further investigated (Figures 1.2, 1.3, 1.4, 1.5).

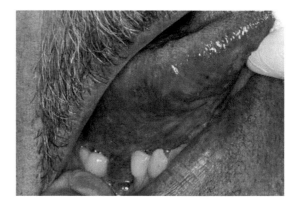

Figure 1.2 Carcinoma *in situ* on the ventral surface of the tongue.

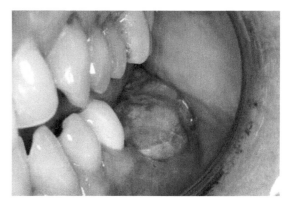

Figure 1.3 Central giant cell granuloma of left mandible.

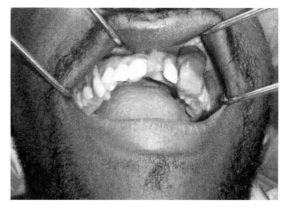

Figure 1.4 Pyogenic granuloma of left anterior maxilla.

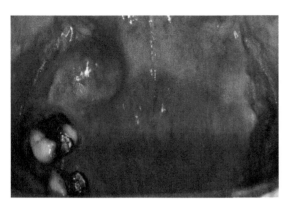

Figure 1.5 Polymorphous low grade adenocarcinoma of the posterior palate.

Conclusion

A responsible and vigilant dentist must recognize the presence or history of medical conditions that may affect the safe delivery of care, as well as any conditions specifically affecting the patient's oral health.

References

1. Becker, DE. Preoperative Medical Evaluation: Part 1: General principles and cardiovascular considerations. *Anesthesia Progress* 2009; 56(3): 92–103.

2. Pickering, TG, Hall, JE, Appel, LJ, et al. Recommendations for blood pressure measurement in humans and experimental animals. *Hypertension.* 2005; 45: 142–161.

3. Simmons BB, Hartmann B, Dejoseph D. Evaluation of suspected dementia. *American Family Physician.* 2011; 84(8): 895–902.Peterson L, Ellis E, Hupp J, Tucker M.

4. Becker, DE. Preoperative Medical Evaluation: Part 2: Pulmonary, endocrine, renal and miscellaneous considerations. *Anesthesia Progress.* 2009; 56(4): 135–145.*Contemporary Oral and Maxillofacial Surgery,* 4th edition. Mosby, St. Louis, 2003.

5. Ainsworth BE, Haskell WL, Whitt MC, Irwin ML, Swartz AM, Strath SJ, O'Brien WL, Bassett DR Jr, Schmitz KH, Emplaincourt PO, Jacobs DR Jr, Leon AS. Compendium of physical activities. *Medicine and Science in Sports and Exercise.* 2000; 32: S498.

6. Pregnancy categories for prescription drugs. FDA Drug Bulletin. FDA, Washington DC, 2008.

7. Little J, Falave D, Miller C, Rhodus N. *Dental Management of the Medically Compromised Patient,* 6th edition. Mosby, St. Louis, 2002.

8. Malamed SF, Orr DL. Medical emergencies in the dental office. 6th ed. St. Louis: Mosby Elsevier; 2007.

CHAPTER 2

Management of the Patient with Medical Comorbidities

David W. Lui[1] and David C. Stanton[2]

[1] Department of Oral and Maxillofacial Surgery, Medical College of Virginia School of Dentistry, Richmond, VA, USA
[2] Department of Oral and Maxillofacial Surgery and Pharmacology, University of Pennsylvania School of Dental Medicine, Philadelphia, PA, USA

Introduction

Once a surgical diagnosis is made after obtaining a focused history and physical examination, clinicians should direct their attention to any pre-existing medical conditions. Significant medical conditions might warrant both risk stratification and further preoperative medical workup or consultation to design a modification scheme that can result in safe treatment for medically compromised patients. The purpose of this chapter is to assist practicing clinicians in their everyday management of outpatient oral surgical patients with concomitant medical comorbidities.

Cardiovascular disease

Coronary artery disease

Coronary artery disease (CAD) is the presence of hardened and narrowed coronary arteries. This architectural change is often the result of atherosclerosis, which describes the buildup of plaque and cholesterol over years. Myocardial oxygen extraction is near-maximal at rest; an increase in oxygen demand must be met primarily by an increase in blood flow at constant hemoglobin levels. CAD may result in an impaired ability to meet an increase in oxygen demand and manifest as stable angina or one of the acute coronary syndromes (ACSs). Stable angina often classically presents with precordial pain lasting 5 to 15 minutes, radiating to the left arm, neck and mandible upon exertion, which is relieved by rest or sublingual nitroglycerin. ACSs describe a continuum of myocardial ischemia, including unstable angina, non-ST elevated myocardial infarction (NSTEMI), and ST-elevated myocardial infarction (STEMI). Symptoms of unstable angina are similar to that of stable angina with increased frequency and intensity. Pain lasts longer than 15 minutes and is typically precipitated without exertion and is not relieved by rest or nitroglycerin. Patients with unstable angina have a poorer prognosis and often experience an acute MI within a short time. NSTEMI is due to partial blockage of coronary blood flow. STEMI is due to complete blockage of coronary blood flow and more profound ischemia involving a relatively large area of myocardium.

The American College of Cardiology/American Heart Association (ACC/AHA) 2007 guidelines on perioperative cardiovascular evaluation and care of non-cardiac surgery may serve as a framework to risk stratify and develop a protocol for ambulatory office-based minor oral surgical procedures.[1] This strategy is essential to determine whether a patient can safely tolerate a planned *elective* procedure. All emergent life-threatening procedures should, therefore, be referred for specialty care in a hospital setting. Risk assessment for the management of patients with ischemic heart disease involves three determinants:

1. Severity of cardiac disease

    (a) Active cardiac conditions are major clinical risk factors for which the patient should undergo cardiac evaluation and treatment. Elective minor oral surgery should be postponed.

    (i) Unstable coronary syndromes: acute (within 7 days) or recent (after 7 days but within 1 month) MI, unstable or severe angina

Manual of Minor Oral Surgery for the General Dentist, Second Edition. Edited by Pushkar Mehra and Richard D'Innocenzo.
© 2016 John Wiley & Sons, Inc. Published 2016 by John Wiley & Sons, Inc.

(ii) Decompensated heart failure: worsening or new-onset heart failure

(iii) Significant arrhythmias: high-grade atrioventricular block, symptomatic arrhythmia or uncontrolled supraventricular arrhythmia

(iv) Severe valvular disease: severe aortic stenosis or symptomatic mitral stenosis

2. Type and magnitude of the oral surgical procedure

   (a) Extensive oral and maxillofacial surgical procedures would fall into the intermediate cardiac risk category under "head and neck procedures," with a 1% to 5% risk

   (b) Minor oral surgery and periodontal surgery, would fall within the low-risk, "superficial surgery" or "ambulatory surgery" category, with less than 1% risk

3. Stability and cardiopulmonary reserve of the patient

   (a) A patient who cannot perform at a minimum of a 4 metabolic equivalent (MET) level without symptoms is at an increased risk for a cardiovascular event. One MET is the oxygen consumption of a 70 kg 40-year-old man at rest. Function capacity is classified as excellent (>10 METs), good (7–10 METs), moderate (4–7 METs), poor (<4 METs).

   (b) Patient with poor functional capacity (<4 METs), in addition to one or more of the following intermediate clinical risk factors may benefit from perioperative heart rate control with beta blockade or preoperative non-invasive cardiac testing, in consultation with a cardiologist.

   (i) History of cardiac disease

   (ii) History of compensated or prior heart failure

   (iii) History of cerebrovascular disease

   (iv) Diabetes mellitus

   (v) Renal insufficiency

Preoperative cardiac testing may include EKG, transthoracic echocardiogram, stress test, perfusion nuclear imaging or cardiac angiography.

The use of vasoconstrictors in local anesthetics may precipitate tachycardia or arrhythmia and may increase blood pressure in patients with history of ischemic heart disease. Local anesthetics without vasoconstrictors may be used as needed. If a vasoconstrictor is necessary, patients with intermediate clinical risk factors and those taking nonselective beta blockers can safely be given up to 0.036 mg epinephrine (two cartridges of 2% lidocaine containing 1:100 000 epinephrine) at a 30–45 minutes window; intravascular injections should be avoided. Stress reduction using preoperative benzodiazepine oral sedation and intraoperative nitrous oxide inhalational sedation may also be considered.

Patients with prior percutaneous coronary intervention with or without stent placement should continue dual-antiplatelet therapy (typically a combination of clopidogrel and aspirin) perioperatively to avoid restenosis; therefore, local hemostatic measures should be employed.

In the event that a patient experiences an acute MI, a patient should be hospitalized and receive emergency treatment as soon as possible with implementation of the MONA protocol:

1. Activate emergency medical service (EMS) system
2. Obtain vital signs and 12-lead EKG if available
3. **M**orphine intravenously for pain reduction and sympathetic output decrease
4. **O**xygen via facemask
5. **N**itroglycerin (0.4 mg sublingually; two additional doses may be repeated at 5-minute intervals if not contraindicated)
6. **A**spirin (325 mg chewable)
7. Additional treatment such as early thrombolytic administration or revascularization may be prescribed after hospitalization

Congestive heart failure

Congestive heart failure (CHF) can result from ventricular or valvular function abnormalities, as well as neurohormonal dysregulation, leading to inadequate cardiac output. CHF may occur as a result of:

1. Impaired myocardial contractility (systolic dysfunction, commonly characterized as reduced left ventricular ejection fraction [LVEF])
2. Increased ventricular stiffness or impaired myocardial relaxation (diastolic dysfunction, commonly associated with a relatively normal LVEF)
3. Other cardiac abnormalities, including obstructive or regurgitant valvular disease, intracardiac shunting, or arrhythmia
4. The inability of the heart to compensate for increased peripheral blood flow or increased metabolic requirements

Left ventricular failure produces pulmonary vascular congestion with resulting pulmonary edema, exertional dyspnea, orthopnea, paroxysmal nocturnal dyspnea, and cardiomegaly. Right ventricular failure results in systemic venous congestion, peripheral pitting edema, and distended jugular veins.

The ACC/AHA stratifies CHF patients into four stages to determine medical management:[2]

1. Stage A: Patients at high risk for CHF, but without structural heart disease or symptoms of CHF
2. Stage B: Patients with structural heart disease, but without signs of symptoms of CHF
3. Stage C: Patients with structural heart disease with previous or current symptoms of CHF
4. Stage D: Patients with refractory CHF requiring specialized intervention

The New York Heart Association (NYHA) also stratifies patients into four classes based on clinical symptoms with physical activities:[3]

1. Class I: No limitation of physical activity by symptoms
2. Class II: Slight limitation of physical activity by dyspnea
3. Class III: Marked limitation of activity by dyspnea
4. Class IV: Symptoms are present at rest; physical exertion will exacerbate symptoms

As mentioned before, compensated CHF (NYHA class I) is an intermediate risk factor whereas decompensated CHF (NYHA class II-IV) is a major risk factor.

Elective minor oral surgery should be postponed in patients with acutely decompensated CHF since they have a high risk for perioperative morbidity (acute MI, unstable angina) and mortality. The primary goal of care for patients with CHF is maintaining cardiac output by optimizing both preload and afterload, preventing myocardial ischemia, and avoiding arrhythmias throughout the perioperative period. Transthoracic echocardiogram is best at providing information such as LVEF, LV structure/function, and valvular pathology. Recommendations for the use of vasoconstrictors and stress reduction protocols are similar to that for patients with ischemic heart disease.

Valvular heart disease

Valvular diseases lead to chronic volume or pressure stress on the atria and ventricles, leading to characteristic responses and remodeling.

Aortic stenosis (AS) is the most common valvular abnormality in elderly patients, due to progressive calcification and narrowing of anatomically normal aortic valve. A bicuspid aortic valve, a result from two of the leaflets fusing during development, is the most common leading cause of congenital AS. Symptoms typically seen in patients with severe AS (an aortic valve area of less than 1 cm^2) include angina, syncope and CHF.

Aortic regurgitation (AR) can be a result of aortic root dilatation due to connective tissue disorders such as Marfan syndrome or infective endocarditis. Symptoms occur after significant left ventricular hypertrophy and CHF due to myocardial dysfunction: dyspnea, paroxysmal nocturnal dyspnea, orthopnea, and angina.

Mitral stenosis (MS) is primarily a sequela of rheumatic heart disease. Signs and symptoms may include left atrial enlargement, pulmonary hypertension, atrial fibrillation, cor pulmonale, dyspnea, and fatigue.

Mitral regurgitation (MR) can be of either acute or chronic in origin. Acute MR can be a result of infective endocarditis or ruptured chordae tendineae/papillary muscle due to acute MI. Chronic MR can be a result of rheumatic heart disease, mitral valve prolapse, Marfan syndrome or Ehlers–Danlos syndrome. Patients may present with pulmonary edema, hypotension, and dyspnea on exertion.

A transthoracic echocardiogram is essential in diagnosis and classification of valvular disease severity and ventricular function. Patients with symptomatic valvular disease on exertion are not good candidates for ambulatory minor oral surgery. The perioperative management of a patient with valvular disease should be formulated in consultation with the cardiologist. Typically, management of a patient with a regurgitant valvular lesion requires maintenance of modest tachycardia, adequate preload and contractility as well as reduced afterload. Management of patient with a stenotic valvular lesion requires maintenance of normal sinus rhythm or a slight bradycardia, as well as increased preload, contractility and afterload.[4]

Prosthetic heart valves can be alloplastic or biologic. Mechanical valves require anticoagulation (such as Coumadin) for life; however, biologic valves (bovine or porcine) may not require anticoagulation after 3 months. The perioperative management of anticoagulation therapy, such as warfarin, is based on a patient's risk for thromboembolism and CVA as well as the type of procedure planned. This will be discussed later in this chapter.

Cardiac conditions associated with the highest risk of an adverse outcome from infective endocarditis for which antibiotic prophylaxis is recommended as per AHA include (Table 2.1):[5]

1. Prosthetic cardiac valve
2. History of infective endocarditis
3. Congenital heart disease (CHD)

Table 2.1 Prophylaxis as per the 2007 AHA Guidelines

Situation	Agent	Regimen: Single Dose 30–60 minutes before procedure	
		Adults	Children
Oral	Amoxicillin	2 g PO	50 mg/kg PO
Unable to take oral medication	Ampicillin	2 g IM or IV	50 mg/kg IM or IV
	Cefazolin or ceftriaxone	1 g IM or IV	50 mg/kg IM or IV
Allergic to penicillins	Cephalexin	2 g PO	50 mg/kg PO
	Clindamycin	600 mg PO	20 mg/kg PO
	Azithromycin or clarithromycin	500 mg PO	15 mg/kg PO
Allergic to penicillins and unable to take oral medication	Cefazolin or ceftriaxone	1 g IM or IV	50 mg/kg IM or IV
	Clindamycin phosphate	600 mg IM or IV	20 mg/kg IM or IV

IM, intramuscular; IV, intravenous; PO, per oram.
Adapted from Fleisher 2007[1].

(a) Unrepaired cyanotic CHD, including those with palliative shunts and conduits

(b) Completely repaired CHD with prosthetic material or device by surgery or catheter intervention during the first 6 months after the procedure

(c) Repaired CHD with residual defects at the site or adjacent to the site of a prosthetic patch or prosthetic device, which inhibits endothelialization

4. Cardiac transplant recipients who develop cardiac valvulopathy

Cephalosporins should not be used in patients who have had an anaphylactic response to penicillin antibiotics.

Arrhythmias

Arrhythmias are usually divided into three categories: bradyarrhythmias, supraventricular tachyarrhythmias, and ventricular arrhythmias. The diagnosis of an arrhythmia requires a 12-lead ECG. Consequently, patients with a history of an arrhythmia might benefit from continuous ECG monitoring during minor oral surgical procedures. Clinicians should assure that patients continue preoperative antiarrhythmic medications. Should an arrhythmia occur during surgery, a certified clinician should follow the advance cardiac life support

(ACLS) protocol to provide appropriate treatment, and EMS activated as indicated.

Hypertension

A hypertensive state is classified according to blood pressure readings:[6]

1. Normal: SBP <120 and DBP <80
2. Prehypertension: SBP 120–139 or DBP 80–89
3. Stage 1 hypertension: SBP 140–159 or DBP 90–99
4. Stage 2 hypertension: SBP 160–178 or DBP 100–109
5. Hypertension urgency: SBP ≥180 or DBP ≥110
6. Hypertension emergency: hypertension associated with end-organ damage (encephalopathy, heart failure, pulmonary edema, renal failure)

In general, patients with blood pressures less than 180/110 mmHg can undergo any necessary minor oral surgery with very little risk of an adverse outcome. For patients with asymptomatic blood pressure of 180/110 mmHg or greater (hypertension urgency), elective procedures should be deferred, and a physician referral for evaluation and treatment within 1 week is indicated. Patients with symptomatic hypertension urgency and hypertension emergency should be referred to an emergency room for immediate evaluation. In patients with uncontrolled hypertension, certain problems such as pain, infection, or bleeding may necessitate urgent treatment. In such instances, the patient should be managed in consultation with the physician, and measures such as intraoperative blood pressure monitoring, ECG monitoring, establishment of an intravenous line, and sedation may be used. A decision must always be made as to whether the benefit of the proposed treatment outweighs the potential risks.

Pulmonary disease

Asthma

Asthma describes bronchial hyper-reactivity with reversible airflow obstruction in response to various stimuli. Despite its reversible nature, chronic airway inflammation is a hallmark of the condition. A reactive airway, or bronchial hyper-responsiveness, is also seen in chronic bronchitis, emphysema, allergic rhinitis, and respiratory infections. Signs and symptoms include shortness of breath, chest tightness, cough, expiratory wheezing, accessory muscle use, tachypnea, and diminished or inaudible breath sounds. Pulmonary function tests can aid with diagnosis and objectively assess severity and response to treatment (forced expiratory volume in 1 s (FEV_1), FEV_1/forced vital capacity (FVC)). A decrease in peak expiratory flow rate to less than 80% of normal value suggests exacerbation. This should be reversible with bronchodilator inhalation in the case of asthma. Management of an asthmatic patient should include the maintenance of all preoperative asthma medications. "Baseline controllers" (such as inhaled steroids, theophylline, leukotriene modifiers, and cromolyn) modify the airway environment. "Rescue medications" (such as beta agonists and anticholinergics) have quick onset for reversal of acute bronchospasm. A typical progressive algorithm for choice of asthmatic medication by most physicians in an outpatient setting includes:

1. Short acting beta agonist (e.g. albuterol as needed)
2. Corticosteroid (e.g. fluticasone)
3. Long acting beta agonist (e.g. salmeterol)
4. Leukotriene receptor antagonist (e.g. montelukast).

Chronic obstructive pulmonary disease

Chronic bronchitis and emphysema are two major categories of chronic obstructive pulmonary disease (COPD). Chronic bronchitis, commonly caused by smoking or from sequelae of respiratory tract infections, is characterized by irreversible airway obstruction, chronic airway irritation, hypersecretion of mucus, and bronchial inflammation. Emphysema is characterized by alveolar destruction and decreased elastic recoil, resulting in increased alveolar size. It is most commonly caused by smoking but can also result from alpha-1 antitrypsin deficiency. The hallmark of COPD is carbon dioxide retention and chronic hypoxemia. Advanced COPD can lead to complications outside of the pulmonary system, such as cachexia, pulmonary hypertension and cor pulmonale. The severity of COPD is determined by spirometry according to Global Initiative for COPD criteria. The diagnosis of COPD requires an FEV_1/FRC ratio < 0.7. Severity is gauged by the postbronchodilator FEV_1:[7]

1. Mild: FEV_1 ≥80% predicted
2. Moderate: FEV_1 50–79% predicted
3. Severe: FEV_1 30–49% predicted
4. Very Severe: FEV_1 <30% predicted

Management of a COPD patient should include the maintenance of all preoperative COPD medications. The perioperative concerns are typically anesthesia-related: avoid nitrous oxide due to its potential accumulation within the multiple bullae, which can rupture and lead to pneumothorax. The potential concern of administering oxygen to COPD patients who rely on a hypoxic respiratory drive is more theoretical than once thought, since ambulatory supplemental oxygen is actually indicated when baseline oxygen saturation is ≤88% or <90% in the setting of pulmonary hypertension or cor pulmonale. In the past, it was believed that COPD patients with high carbon dioxide retention rely on hypoxic respiratory drive; however, recent studies have proven that when COPD patients are in respiratory failure and are supplemented with high concentrations of oxygen, the carbon dioxide level in their blood increases.[8] Therefore, supplemental oxygen via nasal cannula or face mask without suppressing hypercarbic drive in these patients can be beneficial.

Endocrine

Diabetes mellitus

Diabetes mellitus (DM) is categorized into Type 1 and Type 2. Type 1 diabetes is caused by the absence of insulin secretion, resulting in the inability of cells to take in glucose, and resultant hyperglycemia, lipolysis, proteolysis and ketogenesis. Type 2 diabetes is caused by insulin insufficiency or resistance. Type 2 diabetics are usually ketosis-resistant, since their serum insulin concentration is sufficient to prevent ketogenesis. Polyuria, polydipsia and polyphagia may suggest new-onset diabetes. Microvascular and macrovascular disease can result in end-organ damage (cardiovascular disease, cerebrovascular disease, nephropathy, neuropathy, and retinopathy). Therefore, perioperative evaluation of diabetics should assess the involvement and severity of end-organ damage. To assess glycemic control, it is important to inquire about a patient's daily glucose level/range, hemoglobin A_1C level, as well as episodes of hypoglycemia or ketoacidosis, and diabetic medication dosage and frequency. Patients with poorly controlled diabetes are predisposed to impaired wound healing and postoperative infection. During surgery and anesthesia, counter-regulatory hormones are released and cause hyperglycemia and increased catabolism, which may result in complications (sepsis, hypotension, hypovolemia, and acidosis) in uncontrolled diabetics, depending on the nature of surgery. Patients with Type 1 DM are predisposed to diabetic ketoacidosis (DKA), whereas patients with Type 2 DM are susceptible to hyperglycemic hyperosmolar non-ketotic syndrome (HHNK) that may be seen with or without concomitant DKA.

As a general rule, serum glucose should be checked on the day of surgery. If glucose is less than 70 mg/dl, supplemental glucose should be provided preoperatively. If glucose is greater than 200 mg/dl, it may indicate poor glycemic control. For a level greater than 350 mg/dl, the clinician should consider canceling any elective minor oral surgery to stabilize the blood glucose levels and refer to an endocrinologist.

Patients anticipating minor oral surgery performed under local anesthesia should not fast and should not make any adjustment in their medications if the patient will be able to tolerate a normal diet postoperatively. Diabetic patients receiving intravenous sedation, however, would need the following modifications, as oral intake will be prohibited after midnight before surgery:[9]

1. Hold all oral hypoglycemic medications on the day of surgery

   Generally, oral hypoglycemics are discontinued before surgery. The specific class of medication determines how long it should be withheld before surgery.

   (a) The first-generation sulfonylureas should be discontinued approximately 3 days before surgery. These long-acting oral hypoglycemics include tolazamide and chlorpropamide.

   (b) Second-generation sulfonylureas such as glyburide, glipizide, and glimepiride can continue until the morning of the surgery. Thiazolidinediones and metformin should be stopped 48 hours before surgery because of the risk for drug-induced lactic acidosis.

2. For patients on insulin therapy

   (a) These patients should be scheduled as the first case early in the morning.

   (b) Basal insulin (such as glargine) should be administered as usual perioperatively.

   (c) For patients with fair glycemic control, hold all short-acting insulin (such as regular insulin) and administer 50% of the dose of any intermediate-acting insulin (such as NPH) on the morning of surgery.

   (d) For patients with poor glycemic control, intravenous insulin infusion regimen (such as glucose-insulin-potassium infusion) with tight serum glucose monitoring might be required perioperatively, since subcutaneous sliding-scale insulin regimen is usually inadequate to achieve predictable perioperative glycemic control. Therefore, these patients should be treated in an in-patient setting.

3. Use normal saline intravenous solution without glucose for infusion

4. Serum glucose should be checked every 2–3 hours intraoperatively

5. Serum glucose might need to be optimized intraoperatively with sliding-scale insulin

6. Restart preoperative diabetic regimen postoperatively once patient is able to tolerate diet.

Thyroid disease

Hyperthyroidism is categorized into primary or secondary hyperfunctioning. It can be caused by Grave's disease, toxic multinodular goiter, pituitary adenoma, and overdosage of thyroid hormone. Signs and symptoms include tachycardia, atrial fibrillation, weight loss, restlessness, tremor, exophthalmos, and sweating. Treatment usually includes agents that inhibit synthesis of thyroid hormone (such as propylthiouracil or methimazole), radioactive iodine, or surgery. Patients with inadequate treatment of hyperthyroidism may develop thyrotoxic crisis. Early signs and symptoms of extreme restlessness, nausea, vomiting, and abdominal pain have been reported; fever, profuse sweating, marked tachycardia, cardiac arrhythmias, pulmonary edema, and congestive heart failure soon develop. The patient appears to be in a stupor, and coma may follow. Severe hypotension develops, and death may occur. These reactions appear to be associated, at least in part, with adrenal cortical insufficiency. Immediate emergent treatment for the patient in thyrotoxic crisis (thyroid storm) includes propylthiouracil or methimazole, potassium iodide, propranolol, hydrocortisone, and ice packs. In untreated or poorly controlled patients, clinicians should defer elective minor oral surgical procedures and limit use of epinephrine in local anesthesia when providing urgent care.

Hypothyroidism results from decreased circulating levels of the thyroid hormones (thyroxine and triiodothyronine) or from peripheral hormone resistance. It is categorized into primary atrophic, secondary, transient, and generalized resistance to thyroid hormone. Etiologies include Hashimoto's thyroiditis, history of treatment with radioactive iodine or antithyroid medication, thyroidectomy, iodine deficiency, drug-induced, and subacute thyroiditis. Signs and symptoms include lethargy, diminished food intake, constipation, periorbital edema, cold intolerance, bradycardia, and mental slowing. In severe hypothyroidism or myxedema, patients will exhibit impaired mentation, coma, an enlarged tongue, decreased upper airway tissue tone, hypoventilation, CHF, hypothermia and hyponatremia secondary to syndrome of inappropriate antidiuertic hormone secretion (SIADH). Treatment of myxedema requires immediate intravenous thyroid hormone replacement and stress-dose steroids, along with intensive monitoring in a hospital setting. A clinician should determine the severity and tailor an anesthetic plan to the concomitant organ dysfunction. Mild or well-controlled hypothyroidism likely poses no increased surgical risk. Patients with hypothyroidism are sensitive to sedative medications.

Adrenal disease

Disorders of the adrenal glands can result in overproduction or underproduction of adrenal products. Hyperadrenalism results from excessive secretion of adrenal cortisol, mineralocorticoids, androgens, or estrogen, in isolation or combination. The most common type of overproduction is due to glucocorticoid excess. When pathophysiologic processes cause this overproduction the condition is known as Cushing's disease. Adrenal insufficiency is divided into two categories: primary and secondary. Primary adrenocortical insufficiency, also known as Addison's disease, is characterized by destruction of the adrenal cortex with resulting deficiency of all of the adrenocortical hormones. The more common form, secondary adrenocortical insufficiency, may be the consequence of hypothalamic or pituitary disease, critical illness, or the administration of exogenous corticosteroids, with a deficiency of primarily cortisol. However, both of these types of insufficiency downregulate adrenal production of cortisol. One of the most commonly faced clinical scenarios is that of a patient in need of a minor oral surgical procedure with a history of corticosteroid intake. Acute adrenal crisis, characterized by severe hypotension, electrolyte abnormalities and altered mental status, can result if steroid supplementation is not instituted perioperatively. Traditionally, supplemental steroid should be given if a patient has a history of taking greater the 20 mg of prednisone (or equivalent) daily for more than 2 weeks within the past 2 years.[10] The new recommendations, based on evidence-based reviews, suggest that only patients with primary adrenal insufficiency receive supplemental doses of steroid, whereas those with secondary adrenal insufficiency, who take daily corticosteroids, regardless of the type of surgery, should receive only their usual daily dose of corticosteroid before the surgery. The rationale for these new recommendations is that the vast majority of patients who take daily equivalent or lower doses of steroid (5 to 10 mg prednisone daily) on a long-term basis for conditions such as renal transplantation or rheumatoid arthritis maintain adrenal function and do not experience adverse outcomes after minor or even major surgical procedures. In addition, patients who took 5 to 50 mg prednisone daily for several years who had their glucocorticoid medications discontinued within a week before surgery have withstood general surgical procedures without the development of adrenal crisis. Clinicians should recognize that major surgery generally is performed in the hospital setting, in which close monitoring of blood pressure and fluid balance helps to ensure minimal adverse events postoperatively. Although it might be necessary to discuss with the patient's endocrinologist, as a rule of thumb, for minor oral surgical procedures, supplemental hydrocortisone 25 mg IV or equivalent should be administered preoperatively to:[11–13]

1. Patients with a Cushingoid appearance or those taking high-dose steroids (greater than 20 mg/day prednisone or equivalent daily) for greater than 3–4 weeks within the past 6–12 months
2. Patient with primary adrenal insufficiency

Pheochromocytoma, tumors originating from chromaffin tissue of adrenal medulla, commonly presents with signs and symptoms of catecholamine excess. Elective surgery should be delayed to avoid intraoperative hypertensive crisis.

Hematological disorders

Anemia

Anemia is defined as a hemoglobin concentration of <12 g/dl in females and <13 g/dl in males. The etiology of anemia includes decreased hemoglobin production, hemolysis, bleeding, sequestration, and dilution. Among different causes of anemia, sickle cell anemia is perhaps the one that should be discussed here. Sickle cell disease is an inherited hemoglobinopathy characterized by chronic hemolysis, acute painful vaso-occlusive crises, and end-organ damage. Since the reversal of the sickling process is difficult, the focus is on prevention. Therefore, goals for perioperative management include avoidance of acidosis, hypoxemia, dehydration, venous stasis, and hypothermia. Supplemental oxygen, adequate pain control and hydration as well as aggressive treatment of infection are recommended in this group of patients.

Coagulopathy

Abnormalities of platelet function or quantity, of the intrinsic coagulation pathway or extrinsic coagulation pathway may potentially increase the risk of postoperative bleeding.

Spontaneous bleeding occurs with platelet counts <20,000/µl. Minor oral surgery can be safely performed with a platelet count of ≥50,000/µl only if platelet function is normal and no other coagulation abnormalities exist.

Hemophilia is an inherited disorder of hemostasis characterized by a deficiency in clotting factors, resulting in a prolonged PTT. Hemophilia A, B and C have deficiencies of factors VIII, IX, and XI, respectively. The severity of hemophilia A is classified according to the level of activity of factor VIII present. The perioperative management of hemophilia A depends on the severity of disease:[14]

1. Mild hemophilia (factor VIII level 5–30%): use of local hemostatic agents such as Collaplug, Gelfoam, Surgicel®, or thrombin, in addition to transaxemic acid or oral administration of Amicar.
2. Moderate hemophilia (factor VIII level 1–5%): DDAVP IV, SC or intranasally stimulates release of von Willebrand factor from storage sites in endothelium which increases factor VIII levels two to three times.
3. Severe hemophilia (factor VIII level <1%): clotting factor concentrates of recombinant products (Recombinate, Bioclate, and Helixate®) or plasma-derived products (Hemophil-M, Hyate:C®, and Koate® DVI), in conjunction with cryoprecipitate, DDAVP, or Amicar.

Replacement therapy for mild hemophilia B consists of fresh frozen plasma or prothrombin complex concentrates (factors II, VII, IX, X). Factor IX replacement therapy is indicated for severe cases. Local hemostatic measures mentioned above are indicated, but Amicar is contraindicated with concurrent administration of prothrombin complex concentrates.

Von Willebrand factor (vWF) binds and stabilizes factor VIII and mediates platelet adhesion. Often administration of DDAVP before a procedure causes the release of vWF and plasminogen activator from endothelium to prevent bleeding. When patients who have von Willebrand disease are given a single injection of vWF (0.4 mg/kg), there is a considerable increase in platelet reactivity. A hematologist, through dosing and measurements of factor levels, determines the correct dosage of DDAVP necessary for each patient. As with hemophilia, use of adjunctive local agents for hemostasis might be useful.

Most von Willebrand disease can be categorized into three types:[14]

1. Type 1: partial quantitative decrease of qualitatively normal vWF and factor VIII.
2. Type 2: qualitative defects of vWF
3. Type 3: marked deficiencies of vWF and factor VIIIc in plasma, the absence of vWF from platelets and endothelium, and a lack of the secondary transfusion response and the response to DDAVP.

Patients on Coumadin anticoagulation therapy may have a history of atrial fibrillation, a prosthetic heart valve replacement, stroke, myocardial infarction, peripheral vascular disease, deep vein thrombosis, or pulmonary embolism. Perioperative management of this group of patients depends on the underlying indication for anticoagulation therapy, the invasiveness of the planned procedure and preoperative international normalized ratio (INR) value. Generally speaking, for minor surgery such as simple extraction of a few teeth, Coumadin does not need to be discontinued with an INR less than 3.0 if local hemostatic measures (e.g. Gelfoam and meticulous closure) are employed. Infiltration of epinephrine-containing local anesthetics may mask potential post-operative bleeding which could have been controlled if observed intraoperatively. In the case of minor surgical procedures requiring extensive osseous and soft tissue manipulation (such as implant placement or surgical extraction of impacted teeth), Coumadin should be discontinued for 3 days preoperatively in order to achieve a normal INR valve. This should be done in consultation of the patient's physician. If Coumadin cannot be discontinued due to a high risk of thromboembolism, bridging anticoagulation to either Lovenox or heparin may be indicated.

Immunodeficiency

The perioperative considerations of patients undergoing chemotherapy are related primarily to the multiple side effects presented by the various drugs. Bone marrow suppression is a major side effect of nearly all widely used agents. It manifests as pancytopenia. This myelosuppression is reversible and should return to normal 6 to 8 weeks after drug use is stopped. A clinician should therefore allow 6 to 8 weeks after chemotherapy for the bone marrow to recover, and obtain a preoperative complete blood count (CBC) with differential, prior to surgical intervention. As mentioned before, thrombocytopenia with a platelet count of less than 50,000/μl is at high risk of bleeding with even simple tooth extraction. If a patient's absolute neutrophil count (ANC) is 1500/mm³ or less, the patient is considered to be neutropenic with the following classification:[15]

1. Mild neutropenia (ANC 1000–1500): prophylactic antibiotics not required for minor oral surgery without additional risk factors
2. Moderate neutropenia (ANC 500–999): prophylactic antibiotics indicated for invasive procedures
3. Severe neutropenia (ANC < 500): prophylactic antibiotics indicated for minor oral surgery.

Patient with central venous catheters for chemotherapy infusion should receive prophylactic antibiotics prior to surgery, per AHA recommendation.

Hepatitis and cirrhosis

Hepatitis viruses cause most cases of hepatitis worldwide, but hepatitis can also be caused by toxins (notably alcohol, certain medications, and some industrial organic solvents and plants), other infections and autoimmune diseases. End-stage liver disease is usually manifested as cirrhosis of liver, resulting in impaired metabolic and synthetic (clotting factors) function, cholestasis and portal hypertension. Depending on the severity of the disease, signs and symptoms of liver disease include fatigue, nausea, right upper quadrant abdominal pain, jaundice, easy bruising, icterus, hepatosplenomegaly, altered mental status, and asterixis. Elective surgery should be delayed in patients with the acute phase of hepatitis. Preoperative liver function tests, a platelet count and coagulation profiles (PT/INR, PTT) should be obtained. Medications metabolized by liver should be dosed appropriately and best avoided, if possible.

Renal disease

Renal disease can be classified as acute or chronic. Acute renal failure (ARF) is rapid loss of kidney function over the course of days to weeks. While ARF can be further subdivided into prerenal, intrarenal, or postrenal, the two main causative factors of perioperative renal insults leading to ARF are hypoperfusion and nephrotoxic agents. The discussion of ARF is outside the scope of this chapter. Patients with chronic renal failure (CRF) have permanent renal insufficiency that develops over months or years caused by the structural and intrinsic damage of the glomerulus or tubulointerstitial system. The progression of CRF leads to end-stage renal disease (ESRD), which causes death if renal replacement therapy such as dialysis or renal transplant is not provided. The following perioperative management for patients with CRF should be considered:

1. Patients who have ESRD may be susceptible to more intraoperative and postoperative bleeding for multiple reasons.
   (a) Uremia can cause platelet dysfunction.
   (b) Hemodialysis tends to aggravate bleeding tendencies through physical destruction of platelets and the associated use of heparin; therefore, avoid elective procedures on the day of hemodialysis (especially within first 6 hours afterward). Elective procedures should be performed on the day after hemodialysis.
2. On the basis of an apparently low risk, the American Heart Association 2003 guidelines do not include a recommendation for prophylactic antibiotics before invasive dental procedures are performed on patients with intravascular access devices to prevent endarteritis or infective endocarditis, except if an abscess is being incised and drained.[16,17]
3. Anemia develops as renal function declines because of the decreased production of erythropoietin.
4. The dosage and frequency of renally excreted drugs need to be adjusted. Avoid NSAIDs and aminoglycosides.
5. Avoid blood pressure cuff application and intravenous medications in the arm with the arteriovenous shunt or graft.
6. No specific treatment modifications are needed for patients who have indwelling peritoneal dialysis catheters when undergoing minor procedures. However, the presence of a large volume of intraperitoneal dialysis fluid may need to be taken into consideration when positioning a patient for a procedure.

Pregnancy

The care of a pregnant patient undergoing a minor oral surgical procedure requires an understanding of altered physiology of the patient. The following are general recommendations for providing treatment to the gravid patient:

1. Avoid elective procedures in first or third trimester
2. Avoid supine hypotensive syndrome which results from compression of the vena cava by the gravid uterus (usually in the third trimester). The pregnant patient should be placed in the left lateral decubitus position during treatment
3. No intravenous sedation
4. Medications should be prescribed with consideration of fetal risk according to the FDA drug classification:[18]

    (a) Category A: No known risk in the first trimester or later in pregnancy

    (b) Category B: Animal reproduction studies have not shown fetal risk; no controlled studies in pregnant women or animal reproduction studies have shown an adverse effect; human studies have not confirmed adverse effect

    (c) Category C: Adverse effects are shown in animal studies but no controlled human studies are available.

    (d) Category D: Evidence exists of human fetal risk but some use may be acceptable to preserve the health of the mother despite the risk to the fetus

    (e) Category X: Evidence exists of human fetal risk and the risk clearly outweighs any benefit in the pregnant mother.

Neurological disorders

Seizure

Seizure is a spontaneous uncontrolled excessive discharge of cerebral neurons that depolarize in a synchronized fashion and may result in an abrupt suspension of motor, sensory, behavioral or body function. Clinicians should inquire about the nature of a patient's seizures and medications. Patients with uncontrolled seizures or a recent seizure requiring initiation or adjustment of medication may alert clinicians preoperatively of high risk. If seizure activity occurs perioperatively, management is to ensure the patency of the airway and safety of the patient. Repeated seizures over a short period of time without a recovery period are termed status epilepticus, which is a medical emergency. It is most frequently caused by abrupt withdrawal of anticonvulsant medication or an abused substance but may be triggered by infection, neoplasm or trauma. Patients may become seriously hypoxic and acidotic during this event and suffer permanent brain damage. EMS should be activated with concomitant airway management and IV benzodiazepine/barbiturate administration by a trained clinician.

Cerebrovascular accident

Transient ischemic attack (TIA), "mini-stroke", is a brief period of focal neurologic deficit that is of rapid onset, resulting in temporary ischemia and resolution without permanent neurologic damage. Cerebrovascular accident (CVA) or stroke is a serious and potentially fatal neurologic event caused by a sudden interruption of oxygenated blood to the brain due to cerebral vessel blockage or rupture, resulting in ischemia or infarction of the territory of brain deprived of oxygen and nutrients. Patients with a history of cerebrovascular event may take an anticoagulant (Coumadin) or antiplatelet medications (aspirin, Plavix). This may require perioperative management mentioned in the hematologic disorder section. Generally speaking, only emergency treatment should be provided within six months of TIA or CVA.

Head and neck radiation and bisphosphonate therapy

Ideally, all necessary dental extractions should be performed prior to head and neck radiation, which may start after complete mucosalization of intraoral wound. In patients with a history of head and neck radiation for cancer treatment, clinicians may consider the use of perioperative hyperbaric oxygen therapy (HBO) for procedures in which bone is to be exposed. Irradiated tissue is hypovascular, hypoxic and hypocellular. The purpose of HBO is to create a tissue oxygen gradient to promote angiogenesis in the irradiated tissue. HBO therapy should be considered for patients who have received over 5000 cGy of radiation to the operative field. It involves 20 dives preoperatively and 10 dives postoperatively, in an effort to prevent potential osteoradionecrosis of jaw.[19] However, some clinicians do not believe that HBO is necessary for irradiated patients, if an atraumatic surgical technique is employed.

Patients with a history of oral or intravenous bisphosphonate exposure are at risk of medication-related osteonecrosis of jaw (MRONJ). Again, ideally, all necessary dental extractions should be performed prior to the initiation of bisphosphonate administration. Elective minor oral surgical procedures should be avoided in patients with history of intravenous bisphosphonate use. In patients with a history of oral bisphosphonate intake, the following guidelines may be considered:[20]

1. For individuals who have taken an oral bisphosphonate for less than four years and have no clinical risk factors, no alteration or delay in the planned surgery is necessary.

2. For those patients who have taken an oral bisphosphonate *for more than 4 years* OR *for less than 4 years and have also taken corticosteroids concomitantly*, the prescribing provider should be contacted to consider discontinuation of the oral bisphosphonate (drug holiday) for at least 2 months prior to oral surgery, if systemic conditions permit. The bisphosphonate should not be restarted until osseous healing has occurred.

Conclusion

Understanding the pre-existing medical comorbidities of patients allows clinicians to prevent perioperative medically related complications, to optimize patients for surgery and to provide safe treatment. This chapter should provide clinicians a general blueprint in the medical assessment and management of patients who are planned for minor oral surgery procedures.

References

1. Fleisher LA, Beckman JA, Brown KA, *et al*. ACC/AHA 2007 Guidelines on perioperative cardiovascular evaluation and care for noncardiac surgery. *Journal of the American College of Cardiology*. 2007; 50(17): 1701–32.
2. Jessup M, Abraham WT, Casey DE, *et al*. ACCF/AHA Guidelines for the diagnosis and management of heart failure in adults. *Journal of the American College of Cardiology*. 2009; 53(15): 1343–82.
3. Heart Failure Society of America. Executive summary: HFSA 2010 Comprehensive heart failure practice guideline. *Journal of Cardiac Failure*. 2010; 16(6): 475–539.
4. Frogel J. Anesthesia considerations for patients with advanced valvular heart disease undergoing noncardiac surgery. *Anesthesiology Clinics of North America*. 2010; 28(1): 67–85.
5. Nishimura RA, Carabello BA, Faxon DP, *et al*. ACC/AHA 2008 Guideline update on valvular heart disease: focused update on infective endocarditis. *Journal of the American College of Cardiology*. 2008; 52(8): 676–85.
6. Mensah GA. Treatment and control of high blood pressure in adults. *Cardiology Clinics of North America*. 2010; 28(4): 609–22.
7. Huijsmans RJ, Haan A, Hacken NNHT, *et al*. The clinical utility of the GOLD classification of COPD disease severity in pulmonary rehabilitation. *Respiratory Medicine*. 2008; 102(1): 162–71.
8. Cazzola M, Donner CF, Hanania NA. One hundred years of chronic obstructive pulmonary disease (COPD). *Respiratory Medicine*. 2007; 101(6): 1049–65.
9. Yoo HK, Serafin B. Perioperative management of the diabetic patient. *Oral and Maxillofacial Surgery Clinics of North America*. 2006; 18(2): 255–60.
10. Hupp J. Preoperative health status evaluation. In: *Contemporary Oral and Maxillofacial Surgery*. St. Louis, 4th ed, Mosby, St Louis, 2003, pp. 16–17.
11. Fleager K, Yao J. Perioperative steroid dosing in patients receiving chronic oral steroids, undergoing outpatient hand surgery. *Journal of Hand Surgery*. 2010; 35(2): 316–8.
12. George R, Hormis A. Perioperative management of diabetes mellitus and corticosteroid insufficiency. *Surgery (Oxford)*. 2011; 29(9): 465–8.
13. Kohl B, Schwartz S. how to manage perioperative endocrine insufficiency. *Anesthesiology Clinics of North America*. 2010; 28(1): 139–55.
14. Chacon GE. Perioperative management of the patient with hematologic disorders. *Oral and Maxillofacial Surgery Clinics of North America*. 2006; 18(2): 161–71.
15. Ogle OE. Perioperative considerations of the patient on cancer chemotherapy. *Oral and Maxillofacial Surgery Clinics of North America*. 2006; 18(2): 185–93.
16. Baddour LM, Bettermann MA, Bolder AF, *et al*. Nonvalvular cardiovascular device-related infections. *Circulation*. 2003; 108: 2015–31.
17. Hong, CHL, Allred R, Napenas J, *et al*. Antibiotic prophylaxis for dental procedures to prevent indwelling venous catheter-related infections. *American Journal of Medicine*. 2010; 123(12): 1128–33.
18. Ueeck BA. Perioperative management of the female and gravid patient. *Oral and Maxillofacial Surgery Clinics of North America*. 2006; 18(2): 195–202.
19. Marx, RE. A new concept in the treatment of osteoradionecrosis. *Journal of Oral and Maxillofacial Surgery*. 1983; 41(6): 351–7.
20. Ruggiero SL, Dodson TB, Fantasia J, *et al*. American Association of Oral and Maxillofacial Surgeons position paper on medication-related osteonecrosis of the jaw – 2014 Update. *Journal of Oral and Maxillofacial Surgery*. 2014; 72(10): 1938–56.

CHAPTER 3

Minimal Sedation for Oral Surgery and Other Dental Procedures

Kyle Kramer and Jeffrey Bennett

Department of Oral Surgery and Hospital Dentistry, Indiana University School of Dentistry, Indianapolis, IN, USA

Need for sedation and anesthesia in dentistry

At some point in their lives, practically everyone has heard an anecdote or joke that portrays dentistry or dental treatment in a negative light. Often these anecdotes continually served to reinforce the public misconception that dental care is usually accompanied with pain and help to incite fear of the dentist. Clinicians are acutely aware of the generalized fear and anxiety that patients have regarding dental visits and procedures. Fortunately, a large majority of patients are managed satisfactorily using non-pharmacological modalities, such as iatrosedation, behavioral modification and developing excellent communication and rapport with patients. There remains, however, a significant portion of the population that is unable to effectively or comfortably tolerate dental treatment using these commonly deployed methodologies simply because of significant dental anxiety.[1] It is this population who benefits tremendously from the addition of pharmacological interventions.

It is also worth discussing that there are several other groups of dental patients who can benefit from the use of pharmacological interventions besides those with dental anxiety, fear or phobias. These groups would include those with patient management issues, physically, psychologically or medically compromised patients and patients undergoing invasive, extensive or lengthy procedures all of which could impede them from tolerating dental treatment in the traditional office or other clinical environments.[2–4] An example of a patient group with management concerns would include pre-cooperative children. These pediatric dental patients have immature cognitive skills, a highly restricted range of coping abilities, brief or negligible attention spans, and virtually no experience coping with stress, which severely impacts their ability to cooperate perioperatively.[5–7] It may appear counterintuitive initially that medically, mentally, or physically compromised patients can be excellent candidates for sedation or anxiolysis. However, the use of sedation can significantly reduce the patient's physiological and psychological stress levels perioperatively, which is often desired for these patients who may not tolerate such insults without additional complications. Finally, with the explosion of new and innovative dental treatments such as dental implants, and advanced periodontic, endodontic, and restorative therapies, patients are not only retaining their native dentition for far longer, but also often have increased desire and drive to pursue alternative treatment modalities. The prolonged treatment time and invasiveness that often accompanies these alternative treatment options are such that the use of sedation or general anesthesia becomes mutually beneficial for patients and dental care providers. Patients can benefit from reduced anxiety and increased comfort, while dental providers can benefit from a more controlled clinical environment (i.e., less patient movement).

Levels of sedation

In 2004, the American Society of Anesthesiologists (ASA) published *Continuum of Depth of Sedation: Definition of General Anesthesia and Levels of Sedation/Analgesia*,

---

Manual of Minor Oral Surgery for the General Dentist, Second Edition. Edited by Pushkar Mehra and Richard D'Innocenzo.
© 2016 John Wiley & Sons, Inc. Published 2016 by John Wiley & Sons, Inc.

which was reviewed, approved, and amended in 2009.[8] The American Dental Association further utilized these definitions in 2007 when it adopted the Guidelines for the Use of Sedation and General Anesthesia by Dentists.[4,9,10] Defined within these guidelines are the four levels of sedation or anesthesia: minimal sedation, moderate sedation, deep sedation and general anesthesia. The criteria that are used to define each level are stated in Table 3.1. It is critical for dental providers utilizing sedation and anesthesia to have intimate knowledge and complete understanding of the various definitions of sedation. Not only does this permit the practitioner to be able to identify the patient's sedation level and respond accordingly, but it also minimizes the chance of the practitioner unknowingly providing a level of sedation beyond that legally permitted by that practitioner. From a legal perspective, it is imperative that practitioners only provide sedation to the depth that their dental license permits. It must be stated that dental anesthesia providers are expected to identify and appropriately manage patients who have unexpectedly become oversedated. Practitioners must not only be capable of returning the patients to the appropriate level of sedation, but also capable of identifying and appropriately managing any complications that may arise due to the extension beyond the target level of sedation.

Routes of administration

The major routes of drug administration can be categorized as either enteral or parenteral. Topical cutaneous, inhalation and rectal routes of absorption are examples of parenteral routes that bypass the stomach, whereas sublingual and oral/nasal/buccal submucosal routes are a combination of enteral and parenteral routes since a portion of the drug is absorbed directly into the blood while another portion enters after being swallowed. Drugs administered via the enteral route are absorbed through the gastrointestinal tract and are thereby subject to the effects of first-pass hepatic metabolism after they are absorbed into the blood and travel to the liver for metabolism before they can be further distributed to the brain. Drugs administered via the parenteral route bypass the gastrointestinal tract and are not subject to the effects of first-pass hepatic metabolism.[1,11–14] Examples of some of the commonly utilized routes of drug delivery in dentistry are shown in Table 3.2.

Table 3.1 Levels of anesthesia

Level of sedation/anesthesia	Criteria
Minimal sedation	Drug-induced, minimally depressed level of consciousness Patients: • Can independently and continuously maintain their airway • Respond normally to tactile stimulation and verbal command* Cognitive function and coordination may be modestly impaired Ventilatory and cardiovascular functions are unaffected
Moderate sedation	Drug-induced depression of consciousness Patients: • Can maintain their airway without intervention • Respond purposefully to verbal commands, either alone or with light tactile stimulation* Spontaneous ventilation is adequate Cardiovascular function is usually maintained
Deep sedation	Drug-induced depression of consciousness Patients: • May require assistance in maintaining a patent airway • Cannot be easily aroused • Respond purposefully following repeated or painful stimulation Spontaneous ventilation may be inadequate Cardiovascular function is usually maintained
General anesthesia	Drug-induced loss of consciousness Patients: • Often cannot independently maintain ventilatory function • Often require assistance in maintaining a patent airway • May require positive pressure ventilation due to depressed spontaneous ventilation or drug-induced depression of neuromuscular function • Are not arousable, even by painful stimulation Cardiovascular function may be impaired

*Patients whose only response is reflex withdrawal from repeated painful stimuli would not be considered to be in a state of minimal or moderate sedation.

Table 3.2 Routes of drug administration

Route type	Examples
Enteral	Oral (PO)
	Rectal (PR)
Parenteral	Intravenous (IV)
	Intramuscular (IM)
	Subcutaneous (SQ)
	Intranasal (IN)
	Sublingual (SL)
	Inhalational (IH)

Scope of sedation and anesthesia educational training

The ADA has published guidelines that discuss the necessary didactic and clinical curricular components recommended for practitioners desiring to utilize sedation and anesthesia. These guidelines were adopted in 2007 by the ADA and many state dental boards utilize these curricular standards as the licensure criteria for sedation and general anesthesia.[10] Below are listed the various levels of training broken down by level and/or route of sedation, similar to the ADA guidelines.[9,10] Those interested in additional details should refer to the published ADA *Guidelines on Teaching Pain Control and Sedation to Dentists and Dental Students.*[10]

Minimal sedation

The ADA *Guidelines* discuss at length the curricular recommendations for teaching minimal sedation, which includes inhalational (nitrous oxide/oxygen), enteral sedation and combined inhalational/enteral sedation. Most dental school predoctoral curricula contain didactic components and many also provide the clinical components that pertain to teaching inhalational (nitrous oxide/oxygen) minimal sedation. The ADA *Guidelines* recommend at least 14 hours of instruction along with a clinical competency in inhalational sedation. Enteral and combined inhalational/enteral minimal sedation curricular recommendations include at least 16 hours of instruction along with clinical experiences or cases that includes a competency assessment. The ADA Guidelines also recommend clinical experiences involving the management of the compromised airway, similar to the recommendations for parenteral moderate sedation.[10] This is a crucial component as

utilizing multiple drug/route combinations increases the risk of accidental overextension beyond minimal sedation. Practitioners must be aware that they are ultimately responsible for appropriately managing sequelae that may arise. The more serious complications are typically respiratory in nature (airway embarrassment, apnea or hypopnea).[15–18] Depending on the individual state dental laws, practitioners may or may not be required to provide proof of additional training prior to being granted a permit to administer inhalational, enteral or combined inhalational/enteral minimal sedation.[19]

Parenteral moderate sedation

Practitioners who wish to become competent in providing sedation up to and including parenteral moderate sedation can receive appropriate training competency courses that may be available at the predoctoral, postgraduate/residency levels and also as continuing education classes. The ADA guidelines recommend 60 hours of instruction along with 20 patient management cases incorporating the intravenous route of administration. Ideally, a competency case should be included as a capstone experience to demonstrate to the faculty that the student is competent. The guidelines also specifically mention the need for clinical experience in the management of the compromised airway in addition to the demonstration of competency in managing the airway. This is a critical curricular component as the vast majority of perioperative emergencies involving sedation or anesthesia for dentistry involve the airway. Finally, training of this nature is intended for healthy adults, ages 13 and above. The guidelines specifically discuss that additional training is recommended for pediatric or medically compromised patients.[9,10]

Practitioners who are trained and licensed to provide moderate parenteral sedation should also utilize pharmacologic agents with a wide therapeutic index. Common examples of such agents would include benzodiazepines (midazolam and diazepam) and opioid agonists (fentanyl and meperidine).[3] An additional benefit of utilizing these two drug classes only for parenteral moderate sedation is the ability to reverse the drug effects if necessary.

General anesthesia and deep sedation

Currently, there exist two avenues for practitioners to obtain the educational training necessary to become licensed to provide deep sedation and general anesthesia as dentists, complete an advanced education course or residency program in either oral maxillofacial surgery or dental anesthesiology. These programs are regularly evaluated and accredited by the Commission on Dental Accreditation (CODA) to ensure compliance with established didactic and clinical educational standards.

Minimal sedation: anxiolysis

Key Point: The remaining aspects of this chapter will mainly focus on discussions pertaining to minimal sedation as providing this degree of sedation is within the scope of a general dentist who lacks additional anesthesia or sedation training.

As discussed previously, many patients who are planning on undergoing dental or oral surgical procedures would derive significant benefits from the perioperative use of minimal sedation. Historically, this degree of sedation has been known by a variety of descriptors, such as "anxiolysis, stress reduction or twilight sleep" and has even been compared to the sensations that accompany drinking a glass or two of wine.[20,21] While this level of sedation can technically be achieved using a multitude of pharmacological agents and routes, dental providers who have not completed training in deep sedation and general anesthesia should restrict their approach to options with agents or techniques that retain a wide margin of safety such that the unintended loss of consciousness can be avoided.[9,10] Practically speaking, this would include the use of nitrous oxide/oxygen for inhalational minimal sedation, benzodiazepines (diazepam, midazolam, triazolam) administered via the enteral route or possibly a combination of both aforementioned options. An additional benefit of administering an enteral benzodiazepine for minimal sedation is that in an emergency, its effect can be pharmacologically reversed with an antagonist drug if an overdose is suspected to have produced a deeper level of sedation then intended. If a sufficient dose of flumazenil is given parenterally, it can, depending on the total dose of benzodiazepine that was given, temporarily act as a competitive antagonist at benzodiazepine receptor sites and lighten the level of sedation. Likewise, if an enteral opioid were given alone or in combination with the benzodiazepine, it too can be pharmacologically antagonized with a sufficient parenteral dose of naloxone. Finally, so long as the patient is breathing, nitrous oxide can be quickly eliminated in case its combination with an enteral agent produces a level of sedation that is deeper than intended.

Goals and benefits of minimal sedation

The primary concern for any practitioner must be to ensure the safety of the patient. Subsequent goals of sedation utilized for procedures for dentistry and oral surgery ideally are:[1,22]

1. Minimizing pain associated with the procedure
2. Minimizing anxiety associated with the procedure
3. Maintaining normal physiological homeostasis
4. Minimizing intraoperative patient movement
5. Maximizing the chance of success of the procedure
6. Ensuring as short a recovery period as possible

Depending on the pharmacological agents chosen by the practitioner, the benefits to the patient may include:

1. Reduction of the patient's physiological and psychological stress levels
2. Varying degrees of anterograde amnesia
3. Absence of clinically relevant active metabolites
4. Minimal physiologic alterations
5. Mild analgesic effects

There is currently no "magic bullet" or single pharmacological agent capable of fulfilling all of the desired goals and benefits, while avoiding all of the potential unwanted side effects or risks. To overcome this deficiency, practitioners can utilize multiple approaches, such as combining inhalational sedation with local anesthesia. This approach can further minimize risks and side effects as smaller dosages are often sufficient compared to those often necessary if only one agent is utilized. It must be stated that profound anesthesia must be obtained in order for any sedation technique to have the best chance at success. Insufficient blockade of the afferent surgical stimulation with local anesthetic can lead to an increase in sympathetic tone, patient movement, anxiety and pain.

Minimal sedation: pharmacologic agents
Inhalational sedation—nitrous oxide and oxygen

Dentistry has continued to utilize nitrous oxide as an inhalational anesthetic agent, despite the poor response that initially accompanied the "failed" demonstration of the beneficial anesthetic effects of nitrous oxide by Horace Wells early in 1845.[1,23–25] The popularity of using nitrous oxide and oxygen administered concurrently for sedation in dentistry has been somewhat cyclical throughout recent history. In 2007, a survey by the ADA reported that 38.2% of responding dentists used sedation in their practices, of which a resounding 70.3% consisted of inhalational sedation.[26] Nitrous oxide and oxygen continues to be commonly utilized by pediatric dentists as well. A survey in 2011 sent to members of the International Association of Pediatric Dentistry (IAPD) and the European Academy of Pediatric Dentistry (EAPD) demonstrated that inhalational sedation using nitrous oxide and oxygen was the second most frequent type of pharmacologic behavior interventions (46%), behind general anesthesia (52%).[27]

Modern nitrous oxide machines contain several safety devices that help prevent inadvertent administration of hypoxic gas mixtures to patients. As a result, fresh gas delivery is typically limited to a maximum of 70% nitrous oxide and 30% oxygen.[1,24,25] Room air has a concentration of ~21% oxygen, so even at the highest concentration patients receive approximately an additional 9% increase in oxygen. The pharmacodynamic properties of nitrous oxide also contribute to the wide margin of safety that accompanies its use in modern dentistry. Practitioners are usually instructed to administer nitrous oxide by starting at a rather low concentration and titrate upwards until the desired effect or sedative level is achieved. As with all drugs, the response of the patient will fall within a bell-shaped curve, with extremes being hyper- and hypo-responders (Figure 3.1). Nitrous oxide has a minimum alveolar concentration (MAC) of 104%, which reflects its nature of being the least potent inhalational anesthetic.[14,25,28,29] When discussing inhalational anesthetics the concept of a MAC equates to the concentration where 50% of the

patients are unresponsive to a surgical stimulus such as a skin incision.[30] Becker and Rosenberg equated it to the ED-50 (effective dose for 50% of patients) commonly expressed in milligrams for non-inhalationally administered drugs.[25] Clearly, achieving a concentration in excess of 100% is not only incompatible with life, but also not possible under normal clinical conditions. The blood:gas coefficient of nitrous oxide is 0.47 and the fat:blood coefficient is 2.3, which reflects its extreme insolubility and aversion to accumulation within adipose tissue and blood.[28,29,31] This permits nitrous oxide to have an extremely rapid onset in addition to an equally impressive reversal, emergence and recovery; nitrous oxide is an ideal example of titratability of a drug. Care must be taken to protect and ensure that the patient's ventilatory capacity and airway patency remain intact; when nitrous oxide is combined with other sedatives, since otherwise it will become impossible to alter the depth of anesthesia accordingly. Practically speaking, the nitrous oxide won't go away unless the patient breathes it out.

Effects of nitrous oxide

Nitrous oxide administration is known to produce sedation, anesthesia, anxiolysis, and mild analgesia. The main mechanism of action responsible for the anesthetic effects of inhalational agents including nitrous oxide is still under investigation. Existing theories suggest several possibilities including: non-specific expansion of the phospholipid

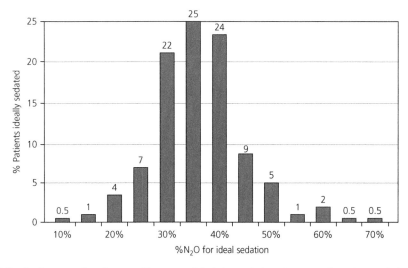

Figure 3.1 Normal distribution curve for nitrous oxide-oxygen inhalation sedation. Source: Malamed SF1, Clark MS. Nitrous oxide-oxygen: a new look at a very old technique. *J Calif Dent Assoc.* 2003 May;31(5):397–403. Reproduced with permission of the *Journal of the California Dental Association.*

bilayer resulting in disruption of various neuronal ion channels; alteration of the fluidity of the neuronal membrane and alteration of the normal function of various ion channels, specifically ligand-gated ion channels such as γ-aminobutyric acid A (GABA$_A$) and glutamate receptors.[28,31,32] Nitrous oxide administration has been proven to cause sedative effects similar to benzodiazepines and analgesic effects similar to opioid agonists. Animal studies have shown administration of benzodiazepine receptor antagonists, flumazenil, leads to reversal of the sedative effects of nitrous oxide, which suggests GABA$_A$ activity involving the benzodiazepine receptor in some fashion. Similarly, multiple studies have shown that administration of opioid receptor antagonists (naloxone) leads to inhibition of the analgesic effects. This suggests that nitrous oxide administration may trigger the release of endogenous opioids or have some agonistic effects within the various opioid receptor subtypes.[32]

Compared to the other inhalational anesthetics used today, nitrous oxide has relatively few deleterious systemic effects. From a respiratory viewpoint, it causes an increase in respiratory rate and a decrease in tidal volume.[29] When administered alone for minimal sedation, nitrous oxide does not significantly depress the respiratory drive. As a gas, nitrous oxide is non-noxious, slightly sweet smelling, unlikely to cause a bronchospasm, and is not a malignant hyperthermia trigger.[33] Nitrous oxide leads to minimal changes from a cardiovascular standpoint, with any mild myocardial contractility depression being offset by a slight increase in sympathetic tone. This could potentially be problematic for those patients who have impaired or insufficient sympathetic reserve. Administered in the acute setting, nitrous oxide does not possess any concerns regarding active metabolites or acute toxicity as it does not undergo any significant metabolism.[29] Prolonged nitrous oxide drug abuse can produce significant neurological problems. Additionally, nitrous oxide, like any gas that is inhaled from whipping cream containers or bulk tanks without supplemental oxygen, can cause hypoxic cellular damage and death.

Absolute contraindications

The use of nitrous oxide and oxygen to achieve minimal or, when combined with other sedative drugs, moderate sedation for dental and oral surgery procedures has few absolute contraindications. The ease and speed at which nitrous oxide can equilibrate within the body and any

associated air spaces are much faster compared to that of nitrogen, which at a concentration of 78% is the main gas present in room air. Essentially, the nitrous oxide molecules are able to enter the air contained within closed spaces in the body faster than the nitrogen molecules can exit. This leads to gas accumulation and generation of potentially significant pressure within these spaces. As such, nitrous oxide is absolutely contraindicated in patients who have entrapped air spaces within their body, such as a pneumothorax, small bowel obstruction, otitis media with Eustachian tube blockage, or following pneumatic retinopexy.[29] Since chronic nitrous oxide exposure has been possibly linked to spontaneous miscarriage and reduced fecundity, nitrous oxide expired waste gas must be scavenged from the dental office atmosphere.[34] Nitrous oxide is classified as a pregnancy C drug, which means that animal reproduction studies have shown an adverse effect on the fetus and there are no adequate and well controlled studies in humans, but potential benefits may warrant use of the drug in pregnant women despite potential risks. Nitrous oxide and oxygen minimal sedation can be utilized for necessary dental procedures during pregnancy assuming the practitioner has discussed the risks and benefits at length with the patient and the risk:benefit ratio strongly favors its use. However, during pregnancy, it is wise to limit exposure of the pregnant patient to only medications that are clearly needed and to postpone clearly elective dental procedures to the postpartum period.[3]

Relative contraindications

There are a few relative contraindications that must be discussed as well. Historically, practitioners have been advised to avoid the use of nitrous oxide in patients with chronic obstructive pulmonary disease (COPD). The main concern of utilizing nitrous oxide and oxygen in patients with COPD is related to the thought that the main factor influencing their respiratory drive is the degree of arterial oxygen tension instead of carbon dioxide. It is thought that patients are at increased risk of hypopnea or apnea due to the administration of supplemental oxygen in addition to the mild blunting of the body's normal response to hypoxemia that can accompany nitrous oxide. Practically speaking, the titratability of nitrous oxide negates this worry as practitioners following the recommended guidelines for nitrous oxide administration. In fact, many of these patients with the most extensive pulmonary disease are prescribed supplemental oxygen for home use. Severe emphysema patients may be at risk of inadvertent air trapping, pressure generation and subsequent rupture of emphysematous blebs or bullae. For this reason, clinicians treating these particular patients with nitrous oxide should proceed cautiously if needed or avoid nitrous oxide altogether.[3,29] Patients who are properly sedated to a depth of minimal or moderate sedation should remain responsive to verbal commands and could simply be told to take a breath if necessary. Exposure to nitrous oxide has been shown to inactivate vitamin B_{12}, which further disrupts the activity of folate synthesis. While this is typically more concerning for drug abusing individuals chronically exposed to high concentrations of nitrous oxide, acute exposure can become problematic for those with predisposing risk factors, such as a pernicious anemia or folate deficiency. Additional relative contraindications are listed in Table 3.3.

Benzodiazepines

Benzodiazepines have a long history of successful use as anxiolytic and sedative agents in medicine and dentistry. Chlordiazepoxide was the first benzodiazepine discovered in 1957 by Sternbach.[35] Within the next decade diazepam was discovered and exploded onto the market. In fact, diazepam was the most frequently prescribed drug in the United States in the 1970s. While

Table 3.3 Nitrous oxide contraindications

Absolute contraindications
Inability to use a nasal hood/mask
• Anatomical or pathological nasopharyngeal obstruction
• Psychological or cognitive inability to tolerate nasal hood/mask
Non-rapidly equilibrating air-containing cavity (closed air spaces)
• Air embolism
• Pneumothorax
• Bowel obstruction
• Intraocular air bubbles
• Otitis media with blockage of Eustachian tube
Pregnancy
• First trimester
Relative contraindications
Chronic obstructive pulmonary disease (COPD)
Pregnancy
• Second and third trimesters
Personality and psychiatric disorders
Borderline or deficient vitamin B_{12}

thousands of benzodiazepine compounds have been discovered and more than a hundred tested clinically, there are several dozen readily available on the market today.[36] Benzodiazepines produce dose-dependent depression of the central nervous system, producing a continuum of clinical effects ranging from anxiolysis to deep sedation and even general anesthesia.[14,28] When used alone in recommended dosages, the likelihood of producing unintended unconsciousness for reasonably healthy patients is very low, as unlike most other central nervous system (CNS) depressants (barbiturates, propofol, volatile anesthetics), benzodiazepines have a relatively wide therapeutic index. Additionally, benzodiazepines have a known reversal agent available, giving clinicians the ability to reverse an unintended overdose if enough is administered and absorbed into the circulation in a timely fashion.[1,3] Benzodiazepines have become very popular with dental clinicians as a result.

Benzodiazepines and GABA$_A$ receptors

GABA is one of the main inhibitory neurotransmitters. GABA binds to vacant GABA$_A$ receptors present on chloride ion channels residing within the neuronal membrane causing a conformational shift of the ion channel. This conformational shift effectively "opens" the channel thus permitting the influx of negatively charged chloride ions. This ultimately leads to further polarization or hyperpolarization of the resting potential of the neuron.[37]

Benzodiazepines specifically bind to the benzodiazepine receptor, located on the gamma subunit of the GABA$_A$ receptors, increasing the ease at which GABA is able to bind to the unoccupied GABA$_A$ receptor.[14,28] This mechanism of action nets an overall increase in GABA agonistic activity.[36] It is crucial for practitioners to understand that benzodiazepines bind exclusively at sites that are specific only to benzodiazepines and that other agents, such as propofol or barbiturates, have alternative binding sites. This fact explains why flumazenil is only useful for reversing the activity of benzodiazepines, as it is a competitive antagonist that is selective only for the benzodiazepine binding site.[28,36]

Enterally administered benzodiazepines: triazolam

The use of enteral sedation using benzodiazepines has become increasing popular in dentistry. This is chiefly due to the wide therapeutic index and relatively large margin of safety that accompanies the use of benzodiazepines as solo sedative or anesthetic agents. There are several popular benzodiazepines available currently for enteral administration, including diazepam, lorazepam and midazolam.[33,37] However, triazolam (Halcion) has become an exceedingly popular agent for use in adults as its pharmacological footprint matches well with most dental and oral surgical procedures, especially with regards to duration of action and rapid recovery.[38–40] Triazolam is absorbed fairly rapidly when administered enterally. It can also be administered sublingually or buccally; however, in addition to an enteral effect from a portion of the drug that is swallowed, those routes are technically also parenteral routes of administration which can lead to increased drug effects beyond those anticipated by untrained or unsuspecting practitioners and will not be discussed within this text.[39] Triazolam is metabolized in the liver by the cytochrome p450 microsomal enzyme system, specifically the 3A4 substrate. As such, patients who are concurrently taking medications or other substances that utilize the same enzyme system can have significant alterations with the clinical effects produced depending on whether those substances serve as inducers or inhibitors of 3A4 activity. Hepatic metabolism of triazolam does produce an active metabolite, α-hydroxytriazolam; however, it does not have significant clinical relevance for the vast majority of patients as it is a relatively short-lived product. The elimination half-life ($\beta 1/2$) of triazolam varies between 1.5–5 hours, which when combined with the variability in absorption following oral administration, can produce variability among patients with regards to the duration of sedation.[33,36,41] One benefit of utilizing triazolam is the lack of a "hangover effect" common with diazepam, produced by continued sedation stemming from the resorption of multiple active metabolites with relatively prolonged and often significant clinical activity.

Triazolam dosing

Triazolam is supplied as either a 0.125 or 0.25 mg tablet. When Halcion was first introduced, it was widely prescribed in a dose of 0.5 mg. At this, and higher doses, Halcion was associated with bizarre behavior, violence, and amnesia. Since then, the 0.5 mg formulation has been taken off the market, and physicians have become more cautious, prescribing Halcion at lower doses.

The dosing ranges for an adult from 0.25–0.5 mg;[36,38–40] 0.125 mg is recommended for small or medically complex adults. Administration of multiple subsequent, incremental or "stacked" doses is not advised. The ADA *Guidelines* state that when the intent is minimal sedation for adults, the appropriate initial dosing of a single enteral drug should be no more than the maximum recommended dose (MRD) stated in the FDA-approved labeling of a drug that can be prescribed for unmonitored home use. However, according to the ADA *Guidelines* for minimal enteral sedation, a single supplemental dose of no more than half of the initial dose of the initial drug may be necessary for prolonged procedures. However, the supplemental dose should not be administered until the dentist has determined the clinical half-life or peak effect of the initial dosing has passed. The total aggregate dose must not exceed 1.5× the MRD on the day of treatment.[9] Being able to reliably assess the peak effect can be difficult especially considering the time to reach peak plasma concentration for triazolam ranges between one to two hours and also factoring in other variables such as delayed gastric emptying times.[36] Clearly, the concern is in the administration of a subsequent dose to a patient, which could inadvertently overextend the sedation beyond the intended level. Some states have mandated that practitioners without additional training are limited to a single dose of triazolam per appointment day. This approach provides a way for practitioners who desire to not proceed until adequate sedation is attained to reappoint patients for whom the initial dose is not sufficient for a subsequent treatment date with a higher dose, which maintains the importance of patient safety as the primary goal of all involved.

Combined nitrous oxide, oxygen and benzodiazepines

The use of multiple CNS depressant pharmacologic agents administered concurrently requires the practitioner to be proficient in the safe use of such agents and intimately knowledgeable regarding the appropriate management of sedated patients. The clinical effects (CNS depression) that can occur when agents are given concurrently can often far exceed those expected when one agent is used alone.[3] As such, dental sedation providers must be ready and willing to intervene should signs of overextension beyond the desired level of sedation be observed.

When combining nitrous oxide, oxygen, and triazolam in order to provide either minimal or moderate inhalational–enteral sedation, it is crucial that the practitioner understands the increased potential for perioperative complications. Ideally, the patient should be given the enteral benzodiazepine with sufficient time such that the practitioner can reliably assess the level of baseline sedation provided by the initial dose. The risk of overextension of the sedation beyond minimal or moderate sedation warrants increased vigilance. Furthermore, it is advisable to have the patient follow the current preoperative NPO guidelines in order to minimize the risk of perioperative vomiting and aspiration risks should the patient become unconscious.[42] With this in mind, patients should be encouraged to utilize the least amount of clear fluid (preferably water) necessary to swallow the orally administered tablet. When administering triazolam, a peak onset time of approximately 45–60 minutes is often recommended unless the patient is at risk for delayed gastric emptying, e.g. a diabetic patient.[1,3] At this point, at a minimum, the patient should be placed on appropriate monitors, under the direct supervision of a dental assistant. It should be understood by all members of the dental care team that sedated patients are never left alone, without direct supervision. Once the baseline level of sedation is established by the practitioner and the monitors are in place, the inhalational sedation can be initiated. The concentration of nitrous oxide should slowly be titrated upwards until the patient reaches the desired level of sedation. The practitioner should continue to monitor the patient throughout the surgical procedure for any signs or symptoms suggestive of oversedation, such as inability to keep their mouth open or respond appropriately to verbal commands. After successful administration of the local anesthetic the level of sedation can often be reduced as the degree of afferent surgical stimulation should be ablated or diminished significantly. Using the combined inhalational-enteral technique, the practitioner can simply decrease the inspired concentration of nitrous oxide. After the termination of the surgical procedure, the nitrous oxide should be stopped with sufficient time (~5 minutes) and 100% oxygen administered in order to minimize the negative sequelae that potentially could arise following abrupt cessation of nitrous oxide. While the patient is still resting quietly and comfortably in the dental chair, the nasal hood should be removed to ensure the patient is able to maintain adequate oxygen saturation while breathing room air. At this point, direct supervision of the patient can safely be transferred back to an auxiliary dental staff member for supervision prior to having the dentist evaluate the patient for discharge. The dentist remains responsible for the patient's care and safety, however, until such time as the patient is discharged from the office.

Monitoring

Rules and regulations for the specific monitors required for the various levels of sedation can differ depending on the state where the dentist practices. Practitioners are responsible for verifying compliance with their state's regulations. Additionally, virtually all national or international dental societies whose members utilize sedation have established guidelines that discuss the care of the sedated patient including the necessary monitors required. These guidelines are updated regularly, which places the responsibility on the individual practitioner to ensure compliance with patient care standards.[4,9,10,43] The ADA sedation guidelines are recommended for dental and oral surgical procedures.

Recommended monitors

First and foremost, it must be stated that the dental sedation provider is responsible for continually providing direct monitoring during the perioperative period. This can easily and often reliably be accomplished by using the practitioner's own perceptive abilities to assess the patient's status and vital functions. For example, is the patient actively breathing, is their upper airway obstructed, are they responsive to commands or are they exhibiting any suspicious or alarming behavior or signs? Significant responses to these types of inquiries often necessitate immediate intervention, accompanied by further assessment and verification with other technological monitors. Of course, to be of sufficient use, the clinician using the monitor must be proficient in understanding the nature of the information provided by the individual monitor. Otherwise, the information provided is useless.

Cardiovascular monitors

Patients undergoing minimal and moderate combined inhalational/enteral sedation should be monitored to ensure adequacy of their cardiovascular function, typically the patient's pulse rate and blood pressure. Although not required for enteral or nitrous oxide minimal sedations, utilizing an electrocardiogram (ECG) permits the practitioner to monitor the patient's heart rate, rhythm as well as any potentially dangerous arrhythmias. The use of a non-invasive blood pressure cuff will permit the clinician to monitor the systolic, diastolic, and mean arterial pressures and pulse rate. This information is used to ensure adequate cardiovascular perfusion and help prevent complications that can accompany hypo- or hypertension.[14]

Respiratory/ventilatory monitors

As mentioned previously, a large majority of the significant complications that arise during the perioperative period for sedated patients are related to disruptions in normal respiratory or ventilatory function. This necessitates that the clinician take appropriate measures to ensure the adequacy of the patient's respiratory capabilities.[4,9] With the advent of pulse oximetry and the spread of other economically viable office monitors, clinicians have the capacity to easily monitor the patient perioperatively for interruptions in respiratory and ventilatory function. Other commonly utilized means to assess ventilation in a sedated or anesthetized patient can include: use of a pretracheal or precordial stethoscope, impedance plethysmography derived from a multi-lead ECG, direct monitoring of the patient's skin/mucous membrane color, movement of the sedation machine's reservoir bag and chest wall.[1,44] These alternative means are best used in conjunction with continuous pulse oximetry and capnography.

Pulse oximetry

Pulse oximetry indirectly and non-invasively provides the clinician with information regarding not only how well oxygenated the patient is but also the patient's pulse rate. Pulse oximeters measure the amount of oxygen carried by hemoglobin molecules in arterial blood, which is displayed as a percentage.[1,14] Practitioners must be proficient in the significance of the values provided by pulse oximetry in order to understand when there is an issue regarding oxygenation of the patient. Not only is a decreased pulse oximetry reading from normal very concerning to the seditionist, but also the rate at which it is declining is also an equally important indication of a respiratory problem.

Capnography

In addition to the use of pulse oximetry, there has recently been tremendous momentum regarding the recommended regular use of capnography for patients undergoing sedation and general anesthesia. Capnography, or non-invasive carbon dioxide monitoring, utilizes infrared gas analysis technology to assess the concentration carbon dioxide in inspired and expired air.[14] Compared to pulse oximetry, which has an inherent delay or lag of 30–60 seconds following changes in oxygenation, capnography is capable of identifying changes in ventilation almost instantaneously.[1] The values provided by capnography are of most use when dilution by ambient air is minimized, such as a patient with a secured airway (endotracheal tube). Despite the obvious limitations that occur with a non-secured airway, capnography has become recommended for use during deep sedations and even some moderate sedations. Capnography provides another non-invasive means of assessing ventilation.[1,9] Most importantly, the loss of the CO_2 waveform immediately signals the possibility of apnea and gives the seditionist more time to diagnose and treat the patient than if later alerted by a decline in pulse oximetry.

Discharge

Patients who undergo dental or oral surgery procedures with concurrent administration of sedation or anesthesia in the ambulatory or office setting do not have the luxury of an extended monitored recovery period commonplace in a post-anesthesia care unit (PACU) in hospital settings. In order to maintain a semblance of efficiency, practitioners who provide dental sedation services must utilize a sedation plan that permits a rapid, smooth emergence and recovery period without delaying patient discharge unnecessarily or compromising safety. Prudent practitioners must realize that patient safety remains the primary goal, which becomes increasingly difficult to ensure once the patient is discharged from the office or ambulatory setting. With this in mind, practitioners must be proficient in assessing the patient's emergence and recovery from sedation and determining whether the patient is fit for discharge.[45] In order to do so, it is crucial for the dental sedation provider to know when the time to the peak effect of any administered drugs has occurred. It is prudent that the patient remain in the office for observation if there is any question of the adequacy of their recovery. Generally speaking, there are several key criteria and additional guidelines that have been established to assist the clinician in determining the patient's fitness for discharge listed below in Table 3.4.[9,46]

Table 3.4 Guidelines for determining patient's fitness for discharge

General discharge criteria
Stability of vital signs:
• Pulse and BP within 20% of preoperative, baseline values
• SpO₂ >95%
Controlled postoperative pain
Minimal/no:
• Postoperative nausea and vomiting
• Surgical hemorrhage
Patient must be:
• Returned to baseline level of consciousness
• Awake and oriented
• Able to ambulate with minimal assistance
Additional guidelines
• Prior to discharge, the patient must be assessed for recovery from the surgical procedure and the anesthetic/sedative plan and deemed safe for discharge home
• Discharge instructions must be reviewed orally with the patient and the patient's escort and given as written instructions as well
• The patient must be given the means to contact the person responsible for postoperative care (the practitioner) should any postoperative concerns arise
• The patient should be instructed to avoid driving, operating heavy machinery, and making important decisions for 24 hours

Rescue

Prevention is best practice

As mentioned previously, practitioners must be proficient in recognizing the signs associated with the various levels of sedation and anesthesia. Practitioners must also understand that they are responsible for ensuring the safety of their patients and must be proficient at managing the possible sequelae that accompany sedation and anesthesia. With this in mind, it is recommended that dentists utilizing sedation remember the following: additional drug can always be given, but once it is given, it can't be taken away. This simple point underlies the importance of slowly titrating drugs to their desired effects. Practitioners who follow the guidelines in regards to patient selection, dosing and clinical protocols are far less likely to accidentally overshoot the desired level of sedation and therefore far less likely to need to rescue their patient from an unintended overdose.

Nitrous oxide rescue

In the unlikely event that a patient who is breathing nitrous oxide and oxygen only for minimal sedation becomes oversedated or possibly unconscious, the appropriate response is simple: immediately decrease the concentration of inspired nitrous oxide. This can be accomplished by either turning down or turning off the inflow of the nitrous oxide gas, increasing the concentration of fresh oxygen, and flushing the system with fresh oxygen, or if an equipment malfunction is suspected, removing the nasal hood and allowing the patient to breathe room air.[1] As discussed above, the key point when discussing the elimination or exhalation of nitrous oxide is that the patient must be breathing adequately. The practitioner must be capable of recognizing signs suggestive of impaired ventilation and be able to intervene appropriately and quickly.

Benzodiazepine rescue

The use of benzodiazepines to produce minimal or moderate sedation carries with it the additional benefit of an effective and rapid reversal agent: flumazenil. Flumazenil is a competitive GABA$_A$ antagonist that specifically functions only at the benzodiazepine receptor.[3,28,36] Because of this selective antagonistic activity, it is only useful for reversing the activity of benzodiazepines and benzodiazepine like agonists. It does not reverse the activity of non-benzodiazepine sedatives (propofol, barbiturates, alcohol, etc.). Flumazenil is intended to be administered intravenously and may not be effective or may not be effective in time to save a patient if administered via slower onset alternative routes, such as sublingually or intramuscularly, despite what may be erroneously taught elsewhere. Additionally, the effective dose of flumazenil depends on the dose of the agonist drug it needs to reverse. A relatively small dose of flumazenil cannot reverse a large dose of a benzodiazepine, even if given intravenously. Practitioners must be aware that the onset and peak effect of flumazenil given intravenously is not instantaneous and may take upwards of 1–3 and 6–10 minutes respectively. As a competitive antagonist, the dosage administered can significantly affect the speed of onset and peak effect. For adult patients who are breathing and stable but otherwise oversedated with benzodiazepines, the recommended dose is 0.1–0.2 mg administered slowly via IV every 3–5 minutes, titrated to effect. For patients who are unstable, a more aggressive approach is recommended. The recommended dose for adult patients is 0.2–0.5 mg administered intravenously every 30–60 seconds. With either scenario, the maximum dose for an adult is 3 mg/hour. The main drawback preventing the use of flumazenil to routinely reverse benzodiazepine sedation is its short alpha half-life of 4–11 minutes, which typically provides clinical reversal of benzodiazepines for approximately 30–45 minutes.[28] Depending on the type and dose of benzodiazepines utilized, it is likely that the patient may become resedated after the flumazenil effects begin to wane. In order to prevent any harm to the patient, it is common practice to monitor any patient who received flumazenil for an extended period of time (i.e. 2–3 hours).

Limitations

It must be remembered that all patients will not benefit equally with the same treatment. There are a multitude of patients who simply will not tolerate minimal or moderate sedation for a large variety of reasons. Practitioners must understand that the use of minimal or moderate sedation still requires a large degree of patient compliance for satisfactory outcomes. Patients who are unable or unwilling to comply with the dentist's perioperative instructions are at risk for failing treatment with minimal or moderate sedation.[1] Examples of these individuals can include pre-cooperative children, patients with a history of substance use and abuse, severe dental phobic patients or those with psychological or physical disorders that preclude them from receiving dental care in the traditional setting.[6] Rather than proceed with treatment in these individuals under less than ideal conditions or risk overdosing them in a vain attempt to make the sedation successful, often the patients can be referred for appropriate care with practitioners who utilize deep sedation or general anesthesia. Nevertheless, minimal and moderate sedation remains a vital treatment adjunct for a large portion of the population undergoing dental or oral surgical treatment and should be increasingly offered as an option to those patients who are deemed suitable candidates.

References

1. Malamed SF. *Sedation : A Guide to Patient Management*, 4th edn. Mosby, St. Louis, 2003.
2. Nathan JE. Managing behavior of precooperative children. *Dental Clinics of North America*. 1995; 39: 789–816.
3. Haas DA. Management of fear and anxiety. In: Yagiela JA, Dowd FJ, Neidle EA, eds. *Pharmacology and Therapeutics for Dentistry*, 5th edn. Elsevier Mosby, St. Louis, 2004, pp. 770–81.
4. American Dental Association A. Policy Statement: The Use of Sedation and General Anesthesia by Dentists, 2007:3.
5. Nathan JE. Effective and safe pediatric oral conscious sedation: philosophy and practical considerations. *Alpha Omegan*. 2006; 99: 78–82.
6. Hicks CG, Jones JE, Saxen MA, *et al.* Demand in pediatric dentistry for sedation and general anesthesia by dentist anesthesiologists: a survey of directors of dentist anesthesiologist and pediatric dentistry residencies. *Anesthesia Progress.* 2012; 59: 3–11.
7. Olabi NF, Jones JE, Saxen MA, *et al.* The use of office-based sedation and general anesthesia by board certified pediatric dentists practicing in the United States. *Anesthesia Progress.* 2012; 59: 12–7.
8. American Society of Anesthesiologists CoQMaDA. Continuum of Depth of Sedation: Definition of General Anesthesia and Levels of Sedation/Analgesia, 2009:2.
9. American Dental Association A. Guidelines for the Use of Sedation and General Anesthesia by Dentists, Chicago, 2007:13.
10. American Dental Association A. Guidelines for Teaching Pain Control and Sedation to Dentists and Dental Students, 2007:17.
11. Yagiela JA. Pharmacokinetics: the absorption, distribution, and fate of drugs. In: Yagiela JA, Dowd FJ, Neidle EA, eds. *Pharmacology and Therapeutics for Dentistry*, 5th edn. Elsevier Mosby, St. Louis, 2004, pp. 18–47.
12. LaMattina JC, Golan DE. Pharmacokinetics. In: Golan DE, Tashjian AH, Armstrong EJ, *et al.*, eds. *Principles of Pharmacology: The Pathophysiologic Basis of Drug Therapy*. Lippincott Williams & Wilkins, Baltimore, 2005, pp. 27–43.
13. Page CP. *Integrated Pharmacology*, 2nd edn. Mosby, Edinburgh, New York, 2002.
14. Stoelting RK, Miller RD. *Basics of Anesthesia*, 4th edn. Churchill Livingstone, New York, 2000.
15. Leelataweedwud P, Vann WF, Jr. Adverse events and outcomes of conscious sedation for pediatric patients: study of an oral sedation regimen. *Journal of the American Dental Association.* 2001; 132: 1531–9; quiz 96.
16. Melloni C. Anesthesia and sedation outside the operating room: how to prevent risk and maintain good quality. *Current Opinion in Anaesthesiology.* 2007; 20: 513–9.
17. Cravero JP, Beach ML, Blike GT, Gallagher SM, Hertzog JH, Pediatric Sedation Research Consortium. The incidence and nature of adverse events during pediatric sedation/anesthesia with propofol for procedures outside the operating room: a report from the Pediatric Sedation Research Consortium. *Anesthesia and Analgesia.* 2009; 108: 795–804.
18. Pino RM. The nature of anesthesia and procedural sedation outside of the operating room. *Current Opinion in Anaesthesiology*. 2007; 20: 347–51.

19. Boynes SG. *Dental Anesthesiology: A Guide to the Rules and Regulations of the United States of America*, 5th edn. No-No Orchard Publishing, 2013.

20. Eckardt MJ, File SE, Gessa GL, *et al*. Effects of moderate alcohol consumption on the central nervous system. *Alcoholism: Clinical and Experimental Research.* 1998; 22: 998–1040.

21. Fairbairn JS. A British Medical Association Lecture on Sedatives In Labour, Particularly "Twilight Sleep." *British Medical Journal.* 1929; 1: 753–5.

22. Sheta SA. Procedural sedation analgesia. *Saudi Journal of Anaesthesia.* 2010; 4: 11–6.

23. Jacobsohn PH. Horace Wells: discoverer of anesthesia. *Anesthesia Progress.* 1995; 42: 73–5.

24. Donaldson M, Donaldson D, Quarnstrom FC. Nitrous oxide-oxygen administration: when safety features no longer are safe. *Journal of the American Dental Association.* 2012; 143: 134–43.

25. Becker DE, Rosenberg M. Nitrous oxide and the inhalation anesthetics. *Anesthesia Progress.* 2008; 55: 124–30; quiz 31–2.

26. American Dental Association A. 2007 Survey of Current Issues in Dentistry: Surgical Dental Implants, Amalgam Restoration, and Sedation, 2008:29.

27. Wilson S, Alcaino EA. Survey on sedation in paediatric dentistry: a global perspective. *International Journal of Paediatric Dentistry.* 2011; 21: 321–32.

28. Morgan GE, Mikhail MS, Murray MJ, Larson CP. *Clinical Anesthesiology*, 3rd edn. Lange Medical Books/McGraw-Hill, New York, 2002.

29. Caswell RE. Nitrous oxide. In: Faust RJ, Cucchiara RF, Rose SH, Spackman TN, Wedel DJ, Wass CT, eds. *Anesthesiology Review*, 3rd edn. Churchill Livingstone, New York, 2002, pp. 107–9.

30. Belmont R, Hall BA. Minimum alveolar concentration. In: Faust RJ, Cucchiara RF, Rose SH, Spackman TN, Wedel DJ, Wass CT, eds. *Anesthesiology Review*, 3rd edn. Churchill Livingstone, New York, 2002, pp. 112–4.

31. Yagiela JA, Haas DA. Principles of general anesthesia. In: Yagiela JA, Dowd FJ, Neidle EA, eds. *Pharmacology and Therapeutics for Dentistry*, 5th edn. Elsevier Mosby, St. Louis, 2004, pp. 271–86.

32. Emmanouil DE, Quock RM. Advances in understanding the actions of nitrous oxide. *Anesthesia Progress.* 2007; 54: 9–18.

33. Haas DA, Yagiela JA. Agents used in general anesthesia, deep sedation, and conscious sedation. In: Yagiela JA, Dowd FJ, Neidle EA, eds. *Pharmacology and Therapeutics for Dentistry*, 5th edn. Elsevier Mosby, St. Louis, 2004, pp. 287–306.

34. Rowland AS, Baird DD, Weinberg CR, Shore DL, Shy CM, Wilcox AJ. Reduced fertility among women employed as dental assistants exposed to high levels of nitrous oxide. *New England Journal of Medicine.* 1992; 327: 993–7.

35. Lopez-Munoz F, Alamo C, Garcia-Garcia P. The discovery of chlordiazepoxide and the clinical introduction of benzodiazepines: half a century of anxiolytic drugs. *Journal of Anxiety Disorders.* 2011; 25: 554–62.

36. Moore PA. Sedative-hypnotics, antianxiety drugs, and centrally acting muscle relaxants. In: Yagiela JA, Dowd FJ, Neidle EA, eds. *Pharmacology and Therapeutics for Dentistry*, 5th edn. Elsevier Mosby, St. Louis, 2004, pp. 193–218.

37. Jedd MB. Benzodiazepines. In: Faust RJ, Cucchiara RF, Rose SH, Spackman TN, Wedel DJ, Wass CT, eds. *Anesthesiology Review*, 3rd edn. Churchill Livingstone, New York, 2002, pp. 165–6.

38. Berthold CW, Schneider A, Dionne RA. Using triazolam to reduce dental anxiety. *Journal of the American Dental Association.* 1993; 124: 58–64.

39. Berthold CW, Dionne RA, Corey SE. Comparison of sublingually and orally administered triazolam for premedication before oral surgery. *Oral Surgery, Oral Medicine, Oral Pathology, Oral Radiology and Endodontics.* 1997; 84: 119–24.

40. Ehrich DG, Lundgren JP, Dionne RA, Nicoll BK, Hutter JW. Comparison of triazolam, diazepam, and placebo as outpatient oral premedication for endodontic patients. *Journal of Endodontics* 1997; 23: 181–4.

41. Flanagan D. Oral triazolam sedation in implant dentistry. *Journal of Oral Implantology.* 2004; 30: 93–7.

42. American Society of Anesthesiologists CoSaPP. Practice Guidelines for Preoperative Fasting and the Use of Pharmacologic Agents to Reduce the Risk of Pulmonary Aspiration: Application to Healthy Patients Undergoing Elective Procedures. *Anesthesiology.* 2011; 114: 495–511.

43. American Academy of Pediatric Dentistry CoSaA. Guideline on the Elective Use of Minimal, Moderate, and Deep Sedation and General Anesthesia for Pediatric Dental Patients. *Pediatric Dentistry.* 2005; 27: 110–8.

44. Moody GB, Mark RG, Zoccola A, Mantero S. Derivation of respiratory signals from multi-lead ECGs. *Computers in Cardiology.* 1985; 12: 113–6.

45. McGlinch BP. Issues in ambulatory anesthesia. In: Faust RJ, Cucchiara RF, Rose SH, Spackman TN, Wedel DJ, Wass CT, eds. *Anesthesiology Review*, 3rd edn. Churchill Livingstone, New York, 2002, pp. 477–9.

46. Marshall SI, Chung F. Discharge criteria and complications after ambulatory surgery. *Anesthesia and Analgesia.* 1999; 88: 508–17.

CHAPTER 4

Surgical Extractions

Daniel Oreadi

Department of Oral and Maxillofacial Surgery, Tufts University School of Dental Medicine, Boston, MA, USA

Introduction

This chapter will provide the reader with general surgical principles and techniques that can be used clinical practice. Surgical removal of teeth is defined in this chapter as extractions that require the elevation of a soft tissue flap, removal of bone, and/or sectioning of the tooth. Surgical extractions are not solely indicated for removal of impacted teeth. In some instances, forcep (simple) extractions turn into surgical extractions requiring a more invasive surgical procedure.

In most situations, a proper preoperative assessment will allow the dentist to predict the degree of difficulty of the extraction.

When used appropriately, surgical techniques applied to surgical extractions may actually be more conservative and cause less morbidity than forceps (simple) extractions.

In some cases, excessive force may be required to luxate and extract a tooth resulting in fracture of surrounding bone, roots or both. For such reason, surgical extraction techniques should be considered in order to allow for controlled removal of bone or the planned sectioning of the tooth and roots, leading to a more predictable outcome.

General principles

A clear understanding and knowledge of the anatomy is important for anyone performing surgical extractions. Several principles should be followed which include proper preoperative evaluation, the patient informed about the risks and complications associated with the procedure, proper development of a soft tissue flap so that adequate access for visualization is obtained, use of controlled force to decrease the risks of root or bone fracture, and proper re-approximation of the soft tissue flap. Adherence to sound surgical techniques will ensure success.

Preoperative evaluation

The extraction of teeth is one of the most commonly performed surgical procedures in oral surgery. Table 4.1 presents the main indications for tooth removal.

A thorough review of the patient's medical history, medications, allergies and social history is mandatory prior to any surgical procedure. The dentist should also perform comprehensive clinical and radiographic evaluations. Panoramic X-rays are recommended, in addition to individual periapical radiographs, as they allow for proper evaluation of the tooth or teeth to be extracted.

Such careful evaluation will allow the dentist to predict the difficulty of the extraction thus minimizing the incidence of complications.

Clinical exam

When clinical evaluation of the tooth to be extracted is performed, many factors need to be taken into consideration. Some of them would raise concern and can be used as predictors of difficulty (Table 4.2).

Limitations in surgical access

Access to the tooth may be difficult causing the procedure to become challenging. Difficulties can result from limited mouth opening that minimizes access and

Manual of Minor Oral Surgery for the General Dentist, Second Edition. Edited by Pushkar Mehra and Richard D'Innocenzo.
© 2016 John Wiley & Sons, Inc. Published 2016 by John Wiley & Sons, Inc.

Table 4.1 Indications for tooth removal

 1. Caries
 2. Periodontal disease
 3. Orthodontic treatment
 4. Prosthetic reasons
 5. Teeth associated with pathology
 6. Radiation therapy
 7. Chemotherapy
 8. Malpositioned teeth compromising the health of adjacent teeth
 9. Infected teeth
10. Socioeconomic reasons
11. Teeth in the line of fracture
12. Traumatized and unrestorable teeth

Table 4.2 Clinical factors predicting the difficulty of extractions

1. Limitations to surgical access
2. Limited access to the tooth in the dental arch
3. Extensive loss of tooth structure
4. Limitations due to conditions of the supporting bone
5. History of root canal therapy
6. Increased age of the patient

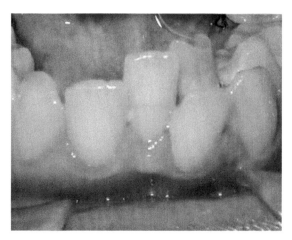

Figure 4.1 Severe crowding in the dental arch can limit access to the application of a forcep.

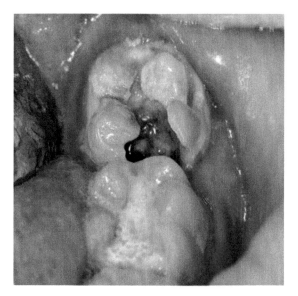

Figure 4.2 Extensive dental caries weakens the coronal tooth structure. These teeth are better approached surgically.

visibility especially in the posterior region. Depending on the degree of access required, a routine forcep extraction might be converted to a surgical extraction because of the inability to obtain an adequate grasp. Some of the causes for restricted mouth opening are odontogenic infections affecting the masticator spaces, radiation-induced fibrosis, temporomandibular joint disorders, trauma, and microstomia.

Difficult access can also result from the location of the tooth in the dental arch. Access to the maxillary third molar may be challenging, even in a patient with no restriction in mouth opening due to the interference created by the coronoid process when the patient fully opens his/her mouth. Access into this area can be improved by having the patient close slightly and move the mandible laterally towards the side of the tooth to be extracted. This will allow the coronoid process to move away from the surgical site thus improving access.

Severe dental crowding is another cause of difficult access which limits availability of the clinical crown of the tooth to be extracted. This type of limited access is most commonly seen in the mandibular anterior and premolar teeth. Damage to adjacent teeth could result

when attempting extractions in severely crowded areas (Figure 4.1).

Loss of tooth structure

The presence of extensive caries or even large restorations (Figure 4.2) weakens the tooth and often results in unwanted fractures or inability to properly adapt the forcep around the remaining tooth structure which will require a surgical intervention. Once tooth surface is lost, a soft tissue flap is required in order to expose

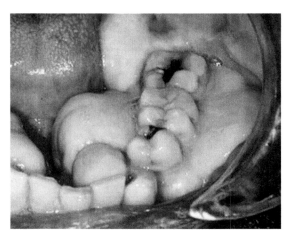

Figure 4.3 Large exostoses can limit the amount of buccal bone expansion. These teeth are better approached surgically.

enough root surface to allow for subluxation and subsequent extraction of the tooth or removal of bone if necessary.

Condition of the supporting bone

Successful tooth removal depends on the expansion of the buccal bone. If the supporting bone is thick or dense, adequate expansion in less likely, increasing the risk of tooth fracture at the time of extraction. As we age the bone tends to become denser as compared to the bone in younger patients. Individuals with parafunctional habits such as dental grinding often have thick and dense alveolar bone. The presence of buccal exostoses also makes bone expansion challenging (Figure 4.3).

Consideration should be given to perform surgical extraction if the presence of thick and dense bone is suspected in order to decrease the risk of both dental and/or buccal plate fracture during extraction and to ensure a predictable outcome.

Radiographic evaluation

Thorough radiographic evaluation is of great importance when planning surgical extractions. Imaging of diagnostic quality provides important information that cannot be obtained from the clinical evaluation alone. Panoramic X-rays are the standard of care in our specialty; however, the use of periapical X-rays is of high benefit when thoroughly evaluating a tooth in particular. Occasionally, an occlusal radiograph can be used to evaluate the buccolingual or buccopalatal location of an impacted tooth.

Table 4.3 Radiographic factors predicting the difficulty of extractions

1. Severely divergent roots
2. Root dilacerations
3. Endodontically treated teeth
4. Increased number of roots
5. Evidence of external or internal tooth resorption
6. Presence of hypercementosis/bulbous roots
7. Long roots
8. Dense bone
9. Root fracture

The radiographic factors predicting the degree of difficulty for dental extractions to be considered while performing a thorough radiographic evaluation are listed in Table 4.3.

Cone Beam computerized tomography (CT) scan may be useful in determining the location of impacted teeth as well as their relationship to vital structures.

Dental anatomy

It is important to evaluate the length and number of roots as well as the presence of dilacerations. The longer, thinner, and more curved roots the more difficult the extraction and the higher the risk of root fracture. Teeth with dilacerated roots can be challenging to extract, and surgical extraction may be indicated.

For multirooted teeth, the degree of root divergence should also be evaluated. The greater the degree of divergence, the greater the difficulty of the extraction. A way to evaluate for such difficulty is to compare the dimension at the point of maximum divergence of the roots to the widest dimension of the tooth crown at its contact points. If the former is greater than the latter, then the extraction most likely will be difficult and sectioning of the tooth will probably be required to create an adequate path of removal (Figure 4.4A and B).

Anatomic structures and their relation with teeth

Careful evaluation of the important anatomic structures in the vicinity of the tooth to be extracted is of paramount importance when planning for a surgical extraction. The inferior alveolar nerve and the maxillary sinus can frequently be seen in close proximity to the roots of teeth to be extracted. Involvement or injury to the aforementioned structures is considered a

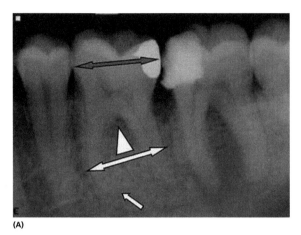

(A)

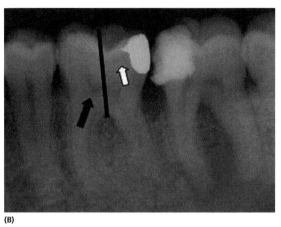

(B)

Figure 4.4 (A) When evaluating this periapical radiograph, a measurement is made at the widest portion of the root (double-headed white arrow) and compared to a measurement at the contact points of the crown (double-headed dark arrow). If the root measurement is greater than at the contact points, this indicates an inadequate path of withdrawal. Also note the curvature on the mesial root (single white arrow). This tooth is best approached by sectioning the tooth between mesial and distal roots. Some bone should be removed from the buccal in the furcation area (white triangle) before tooth sectioning. (B) On the lower first molar, the distal root should be removed first (white arrow), and then the mesial root (black arrow). This sequence will prove easier because of the curvature on the mesial root.

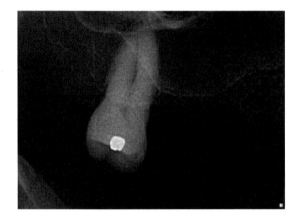

Figure 4.5 An isolated first molar with roots into a pneumatized sinus.

complication and therefore care is always taken to avoid them.

Great variations exist in the relationship of the maxillary posterior teeth to the maxillary sinus. The roots of some bicuspid and molar teeth might extend beyond the floor of the sinus increasing the chance of sinus involvement after their extraction (Figure 4.5).

In general, the degree of maxillary sinus pneumatization increases with advancing age and loss of posterior dentition. Various degrees of maxillary sinus involvement can result from the removal of maxillary posterior

Table 4.4 Teeth at risk of sinus exposure

1. Lone-standing maxillary molar with pneumatized maxillary sinus
2. Roots projecting into a severely pneumatized maxillary sinus with minimal coronal bone visible radiographically
3. Long and divergent roots with a pneumatized sinus into the trifurcation area
4. Teeth with advanced periodontal disease but without mobility

teeth and range from displacement of a root tip into the sinus to the development of an oro-antral communication or fistulous tract.

Those teeth with a greater risk of sinus exposure are best approached by surgical extraction (Table 4.4). Tooth sectioning with or without elevation of a flap and possible bone removal may be of benefit when trying to avoid maxillary sinus involvement.

The approximate incidence of inferior alveolar nerve injury when removing impacted third molars ranges from 0.41 to 7.5%, and such incidence decreases as we move anteriorly in the dental arch towards the midline. For that reason it is important that we carefully evaluate the proximity of the nerve to the roots of those teeth to be extracted. Attention to the appearance of the inferior alveolar nerve canal during panoramic radiograph examination may provide information about

Table 4.5 Radiographic features associated with increased incidence of inferior alveolar nerve injuries

1. Close proximity of the roots to the inferior alveolar nerve canal
2. Loss of cortical integrity of the canal
3. Narrowing of the canal
4. Diversion of the canal
5. Darkening of the roots
6. Nerve canal irregularities
7. Narrowing of the roots

the proximity of the roots therefore indicating the likelihood for injury (Table 4.5).

Tooth integrity and bone appearance

It is important to evaluate for dental structure defects such as internal or external root resorption. If extensive resorption is present, fracture of the root can be expected at the level of the resorption and such extraction should better managed surgically (Figure 4.6). A tooth that has been endodontically treated, unless treatment occurred within a year, tends to be very brittle and fractures easy. Furthermore, an endodontically treated tooth often presents with large restorations or a crown, further complicating the extraction. For this reason, endodontically treated teeth may be better treated by elective surgical extraction. The possibility of ankylosis should be ruled out. The periodontal ligament space around the tooth should be visible, otherwise the tooth might be considered ankylosed and such teeth should be approached as a surgical extraction. The same applies to teeth with hypercemetosis (Figure 4.7), which can be difficult to extract due to an inadequate path of withdrawal. A surgical extraction should be performed in these situations so that the roots are sectioned or an adequate path of withdrawal is created.

The bone surrounding the tooth to be extracted should be carefully evaluated. Assessment of the relative density can be performed using a good quality radiograph. Bone that appears relatively radiolucent is less dense and is more likely to expand making the extraction easier to perform. However, bone that is relatively radio-opaque is denser and less likely to expand which could potentially cause fracture of the roots.

The same rule applies for patients with a long history of bisphosphonate therapy where the bone becomes denser as a result of the decrease of their osteoclastic activity. A difficult extraction could be expected in this patient group.

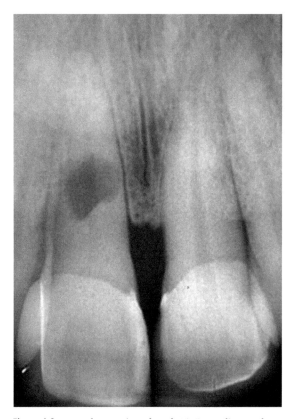

Figure 4.6 Internal resorption of tooth #9. Depending on the extent of the internal resorption, the tooth can fracture at the level of the resorption during extraction, requiring surgical removal of the root tip.

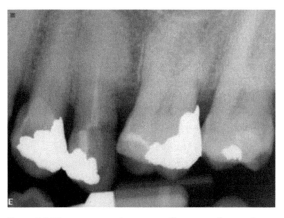

Figure 4.7 Hypercementosis on a maxillary second premolar with a bulbous root.

Ethnic background needs to be also considered. Patients of African-American descent are known to have long-rooted teeth and denser bone.

Surgical extractions: flap design and technique

Flap design

Before beginning any surgical extraction, one should review the overall treatment plan and incision design. A well-designed treatment plan with the necessary equipment available will allow a potentially difficult surgery to be performed efficiently and painlessly for both the patient and the surgeon.

Paramount to any surgical treatment plan is the development of an appropriate flap. Adequate design of the flap plays a vital role in exposure and access for the surgical extraction of teeth. Sound surgical principles and good surgical techniques help minimize tissue trauma and delayed healing.

It is important to consider the position of the chair and the patient as well as the ergonomics of the operator in order to achieve a successful outcome during dental extractions. A correct position will allow the surgeon to keep the arms close to the body providing stability and support. Such support will prevent instrument slippage causing soft tissue injuries to the patient and will also allow the surgeon to maintain the wrists straight enough to deliver the necessary force with the arm and shoulder instead of the hand.

Extractions are generally performed from a standing position. For a maxillary extraction the chair should be inclined backwards so that the maxillary occlusal plane is at an angle of about 60 degrees to the floor. The height of the chair should be enough so the patient's oral cavity is at or slightly below the operator's elbow level. For extraction of the mandibular teeth, the patient should be placed in an upright position so that the occlusal plane is parallel to the floor when maximum opening of the mouth is achieved.

The decision to reflect a flap should be carefully made prior to beginning the extraction procedure in order to avoid unnecessary trauma and discomfort to the patient. The indications to reflect a flap are generally to allow for adequate access and complete visualization of the surgical field, to allow for bone removal and tooth sectioning and to prevent unnecessary trauma to soft tissue and bony structure. Once the decision to raise a flap is made the surgeon must decide what type and design of flap is to be made. In the design process, several factors should be taken into consideration, including vascular supply to the flap, regional anatomy, underlying bony

anatomy, health of the tissues to be incised, and the ability to place an incision in a discrete and cosmetic location that can be repositioned postoperatively in a tension-free fashion.

Generally, most surgical extractions will require the elevation of a full-thickness mucoperiosteal flap. Such flaps include the overlying gingiva, mucosa, submucosa, and underlying periosteum as one entity. In order to properly develop this type of flap, one must create sharp, discrete, full-thickness incisions that extend completely to the underlying bone.

When considering flap design, the surgeon must decide which flap will allow the most effective visualization and execution of the surgical procedure while maintaining minimal invasiveness. A few basic surgical principles must be kept in mind. First, when outlining the flap, the base must be broader than the apex to allow for maintenance of an adequate, independent blood supply (Figure 4.8). If this basic principle is violated, the risk of flap necrosis is increased. Second, the margins of the flap should never be placed over a bony defect (Figure 4.9); this could lead to dehiscence and healing by secondary intention. Third, margins should never be placed over a bony prominence as this may prohibit tension-free repositioning. Additionally the flap must be designed to avoid underlying vital structures such as the mental or lingual neurovascular bundles.

Around the lower third molar region, incisions should be well away from the lingual aspect of the ridge to avoid accidental severance of the lingual nerve,

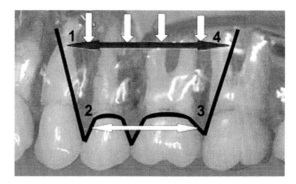

Figure 4.8 This picture shows a trapezoidal or four-cornered flap. The base of the flap (double-ended blue arrow) should be wider than the coronal aspect of the flap (double-ended white arrow) to allow adequate blood supply (single-ended white arrows).

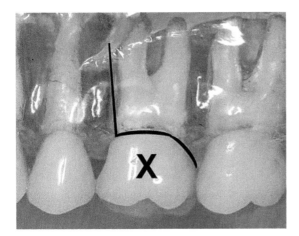

Figure 4.9 Avoid making a releasing incision too close to or directly over the area of the extraction. An incision near a bony defect can result in a dehiscence and delayed healing. In this example, the release is too close to the tooth being extracted.

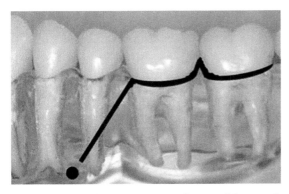

Figure 4.10 Avoid releasing incisions in the area of the mental nerve, as shown here.

which may lie supraperiosteally in that area. Likewise, apical to the mandibular premolars lies the mental nerve. Incisions should be placed well anterior and/or posterior to this structure to avoid iatrogenic damage (Figure 4.10).

An incision placed too high in the maxillary posterior mucobuccal fold could penetrate into the area of the buccal fat pad. This becomes more of a surgical annoyance and usually does not represent a true complication. If this should occur, the pad can be repositioned easily and the mucosa can be closed postoperatively; however, it tends to create a visual obstruction to the surgical field during the procedure.

Table 4.6 Flap design considerations

Avoid	Result if not avoided
1. Incision over bony prominence	Tension, dehiscence and delayed healing
2. Incising through papillae	Dehiscence, periodontal defect
3. Incision over facial aspect midcrown	Dehiscence, periodontal defect
4. Incision not placed over sound bone	Collapse and delayed healing
5. Vertical incision in area over mental foramen	Injury to the mental nerve
6. Lingual releasing incisions in the mandible	Injury to the lingual nerve (posteriorly), dehiscence, delayed healing
7. Vertical releasing incision in the palate	Bleeding, injury to the greater palatine neurovascular bundle

When a palatal incision is necessary, attention must be paid to the greater palatine and incisive neurovascular bundles. The greater palatine artery provides the major blood supply to the palatal tissues, and therefore, releasing incisions should be avoided at all cost. Anteriorly, if tissue must be reflected to access an impacted or supernumerary tooth in the area of the incisors, transection of the incisive neurovascular bundle usually will not lead to significant bleeding, and the nerve tends to redistribute quickly. In addition, the altered sensation subsequent to this nerve's severance usually does not lead to significant morbidity for the patient. A good understanding of the regional anatomy is of utmost importance to avoid inadvertent damage or exposure of vital structures (Table 4.6).

The next decision to be made after identification of the surrounding anatomy is the design of the mucoperiosteal flap to be utilized. Intraorally, there are a number of designs to choose from. These include the simple crestal envelope flap (Figure 4.11); crestal envelope with one releasing incision (three-corner flap) (Figure 4.12); crestal envelope with two releasing incisions (Figure 4.13), or semilunar incision (Figure 4.14).

For surgical extractions, the most common flap is the sulcular envelope (with or without releasing incisions). For this flap, a full-thickness incision is created intrasulcularly around the buccal and lingual aspects of the teeth. The papillae are kept within the body of the flap, which is reflected apically in a full-thickness fashion. This flap provides great access to the coronal part of the

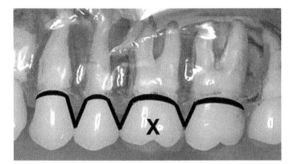

Figure 4.11 Envelope flap. Ideally, this type of flap should be extended one tooth posterior and two teeth anterior to the one being extracted in order to provide adequate reflection with minimal tension on the flap.

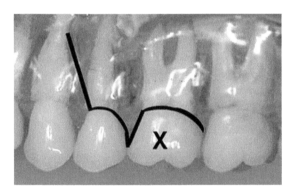

Figure 4.12 The correct design for a three-corner flap. Releasing incisions should be 6–8 mm anterior and/or posterior to the extraction site.

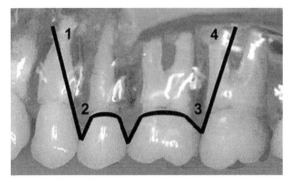

Figure 4.13 The correct design for a four-corner flap.

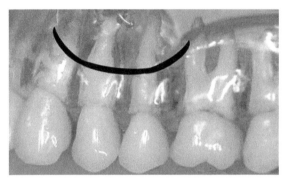

Figure 4.14 Semilunar flap.

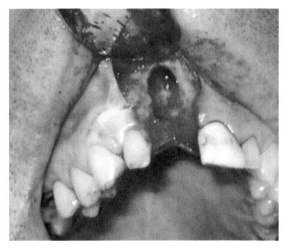

Figure 4.15 Releasing incisions can be created either at the mesial or distal side of the flap.

tooth, allowing for better visualization, instrumentation, bone removal at the crest level, and tooth sectioning when needed. Additionally, it can be easily converted into a three-corner flap if access to the apical area is required.

Generally speaking, most surgical extractions can be performed without a releasing incision; however, occasionally extended reflection is necessary for tension-free visualization and to avoid unwanted soft tissue tears. The release can be created at either the mesial or distal end of an envelope, but in most cases, it is placed anteriorly and the flap reflected posteriorly (Figure 4.15) The releasing incision should be located at a line angle of a tooth and should not directly transect a papilla (Figure 4.16) or cross over a bony prominence like the canine eminence in the maxilla. Papilla transection could lead to necrosis and loss of

the papilla postoperatively, thereby causing cosmetic and periodontal problems. When a procedure begins with a short envelope flap, the use of a release provides greater access, especially to the apical area. This is

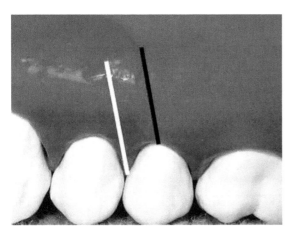

Figure 4.16 Releasing incisions should not transect the papilla (white line). Also, releasing incisions should not be placed in the midbuccal surface of the tooth (black line).

occasionally necessary in the posterior regions of the oral cavity, particularly in the maxilla, where visualization is often challenging.

When a release is necessary, it is very rare that a four-corner flap (two releases) will be required. However, in cases of fractured roots in the posterior maxilla near the sinus, this flap design may be beneficial – especially if there is the potential for an oral–antral communication requiring soft tissue advancement for primary tension-free closure. Semilunar incisions are of limited use in surgical extractions, as they provide limited access to the apical region. They are used more often for periapical surgery and for that reason it will not be included in this chapter.

Once all the previous information is considered, the technique for the development of a surgical flap is relatively straightforward.

Technique

Since the most common flap used for surgical extractions is the sulcular envelope with or without a release, this is the technique that will be described. Most incisions are created using #15 or #12 blades. A bite block should be always used to aid in stabilization regardless of the tooth to be extracted.

The chair should be lowered enough so the surgeon's arm is inclined downward to approximately 120-degree angle at the elbow, which provides a comfortable, stable position.

The incision is created intrasulcularly down to the alveolar bone. It begins at the distobuccal line angle, one tooth posterior to the tooth being extracted and extends anteriorly. If an envelope flap is planned, the incision should be extended at least two teeth anterior to the tooth to be extracted. When a three-corner flap is planned, the incision is then carried one tooth anteriorly and a releasing incision is then made to include or exclude the papilla in the design of the flap.

If a release is used, it is begun at the sulcus and extends in an anteroapical direction towards the vestibule. A Seldin or other broad retractor (not a dental mirror) is used to tense the alveolar mucosa to allow a clean, smooth incision to be made without tearing the tissue. Once the incision is completed, elevation of the flap is achieved by using the sharp end of a periosteal elevator. Reflection is begun at the anterior sulcular extent of the incision. The elevator is positioned underneath the full-thickness flap and run posteriorly along the sulcus, elevating all of the papillae and buccal tissue down to the alveolar bone. The papillae are reflected by simply inserting the elevator and performing a rotation motion while on an outward direction.

The crestal gingiva is always reflected first along the entire extent of the incision prior to reflecting the mucosa apically. If any area of the crestal incision is difficult to reflect or if it appears that the incision is not completely down to the bone, the blade is run over the previously made incision to ensure a smooth full-thickness cut to the bone. Next, the sharp end of a periosteal elevator is run along the release incision against bone, and the tissue is elevated in a posteroapical direction and always against alveolar bone making sure the flap remains as full-thickness. When the anterior portion of the flap is raised, it is often helpful to place the broad end of a retractor under the flap and against the alveolus to assist in visualization while the rest of the flap is fully raised. At this point, the broad end of the periosteal elevator is normally used to complete the reflection into the depth of the vestibule.

Once the tooth or root tip has been exposed, establishing a proper path of removal is one of the main principles in extracting erupted or impacted teeth. Failure to achieve an unimpeded path of removal results in failure to perform a successful surgical extraction. This is commonly achieved either by sectioning the tooth or removing bone with a surgical handpiece next to the root to allow for its delivery. The preferred sequence is to initially section the tooth, which will convert a multi-rooted tooth into single-root components. Elevation of each root separately will allow for removal of the tooth in the majority of the cases. If needed, bone can be carefully removed to achieve a path of withdrawal. This sequence will preserve the most alveolar bone around the extraction socket and such preservation is important especially when future placement of dental implants is planned.

In some instances, reversing this sequence is necessary (bone removal followed by tooth sectioning), especially when the location of the furcation cannot be visualized. Removing bone buccal to the tooth to expose the furcation is then recommended to allow sectioning of the tooth.

Once the previous maneuvers have been performed and the teeth/roots are completely exposed, one must consider a key aspect of tooth extraction, which is the use of controlled force. The surgeon needs to keep in mind that slow, steady movement should be used during extractions at all times. The use of excessive and uncontrolled force can result in fracture of the tooth and possibly the alveolar bone. When the tooth cannot be extracted with reasonable force, it should be surgically removed which involved sectioning the tooth and removing bone as necessary after reflecting a flap.

Technique for surgical extraction of a single-rooted tooth

The surgical extraction of a single-rooted tooth is relatively straightforward. After an adequate flap has been reflected, the need for bone removal is assessed. Often, the improved visualization and access afforded by the flap makes bone removal unnecessary. This is because after a flap has been reflected, elevators can be used effectively and forceps can be seated more apically creating a better mechanical advantage.

If bone removal is indicated, the tooth/root and, if necessary, a small portion of buccal bone may be grasped with the forcep. The tooth is then removed along with that small portion of bone (Figure 4.17).

Other options when bone removal is necessary include removal of buccal bone using a surgical bur and surgical handpiece or chisel. The width of the bone removed should be approximately the same as the mesiodistal dimension of the root, and the most

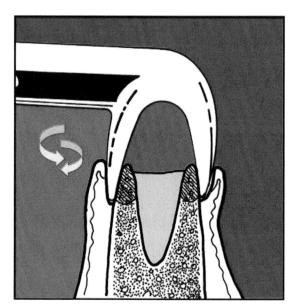

Figure 4.17 A forcep is shown being used to remove the root with a small portion of the alveolus.

common vertical length of the bone removed is approximately one-third to one-half the length of the root. The tooth can then be extracted using a straight elevator and/or forcep (Figure 4.18A). It is important to keep in mind that the amount of bone removed should be just enough to allow for successful extraction of the tooth. Excessive bone removal should be avoided; this is especially critical in patients whose treatment plan includes implant placement.

If extraction of the tooth is still difficult after bone removal, a purchase point can be made. The purchase point should be made as apically as possible on the root in order to create a better mechanical advantage. It should be large enough that the instrument to be used is able to engage. The author's recommendation is to use a Crane pick or Cogswell B. The adjacent bone will be the fulcrum during elevation movement (Figure 4.18B).

The surgical site should be inspected after the tooth has been removed. All bony spicules should be removed and all sharp bony edges smoothed. Sharp bony edges are assessed by replacing the flap and palpating over it with a finger. A rongeur or bone file may be used to smooth all sharp edges.

It is important to always use copious irrigation with a sterile solution to remove all debris. Special attention

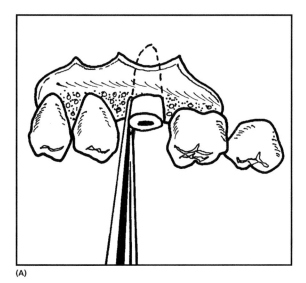

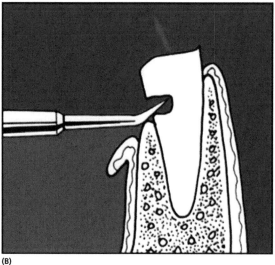

(A)   (B)

Figure 4.18 (A) When adequate bone has been removed with a bur or chisel, the root is luxated and removed with an elevator, or a forcep can be seated onto sound root structure for its removal. (B) The placement of purchase point has three essential requirements: (1) The purchase point should be placed close to the level of the bone. (2) The purchase point should be deep enough to allow for placement of the instrument. (3) Enough tooth structure (3 mm) should be left coronal to the purchase point to prevent tooth fracture during elevation.

should be paid to the area at the base of the flap, as debris tends to collect in this area and could potentially cause infection of the surgical site.

Always remember to use copious amounts of irrigation when using high-speed instruments to remove bone or section a tooth to keep the site cool and avoid overheating of the bone. The use of a pneumatic drill instead of an air-propelled one is of extreme importance when performing tooth or bone resection in order to avoid direct flow of air into an open wound which can cause dissection of soft tissues causing air entrapment and emphysema with increases risk of infection in addition to other complications.

Once the surgery is completed, the surgeon must return the flap into its original anatomical position or, if necessary, arrange it in a new position in order to provide complete coverage to supporting structures.

Technique for surgical extraction of a multi-rooted tooth

The technique for the surgical extraction of a multi-rooted tooth is essentially the same as that for single-rooted ones. The main difference is that a multi-rooted

tooth can be divided with a surgical bur to convert it into multiple single-rooted teeth to facilitate their removal.

After an adequate flap has been reflected and held in proper position, the need for sectioning of the tooth and bone removal is assessed. As in the case for a single-rooted tooth, the improved visualization and access afforded by the flap might make bone removal and tooth sectioning unnecessary. In such cases, the more apical (to the bone level) positioning of the elevators and forceps allows for a more effective extraction avoiding the need for tooth sectioning or bone removal.

If further measures are deemed necessary for removal of a tooth, it is preferable to start by sectioning the tooth before removing any bone. Using this approach will either eliminate the need for bone removal or decrease the amount of bone removed. As in the case for single-rooted tooth, it is important that the amount of bone removed is just enough to allow for the extraction to be completed. Remember that excessive removal of bone should be avoided especially in a patient who desires implant placement to replace the extracted teeth.

Bone removal prior to sectioning of the tooth is usually not necessary when the furcation of the tooth can be visualized after the flap has been reflected. Sectioning of the tooth is accomplished with a fissure surgical bur, the roots are then separated and elevated using a straight elevator and removed separately using a forcep.

After the extraction, the same care taken after extracting a single-rooted tooth is taken with multi-rooted teeth. Thorough irrigation with sterile solution, 0.9% such as normal saline should be performed after adequate removal of any sharp bone spicules and smoothing the bony edges using a combination of a rongeur forcep and/or bone file.

The flap is then repositioned and sutured into place.

Considerations for the removal of root tips

No matter how experienced and careful the surgeon is, roots can fracture during extractions. When that occurs, the surgeon should make the decision as to whether the root tip can be left in place or whether it should be removed. Usually, small root fragments of about 3 mm or less, not infected, from a non-carious tooth can be left in place and monitored over time especially if in close proximity to the inferior alveolar nerve or maxillary sinus (Table 4.7). Another condition in which the risks of removing a fractured root tip outweighs the benefit of removing it is when excessive bone is needed to be removed in order to retrieve the root fragment. The patient should always be informed about the decision to leave the root in place. The most important reason for this is that the possibility exists of a future complication associated with the retained root segment. Proper documentation should detail the entire conversation along with the reasons behind the decision of leaving the root segment in place.

Radiographic documentation of the root tip should be obtained and recorded in the patient's chart. The patient should also be instructed to follow up every six months or every year to make sure no problems arise.

Surgical technique for removal of root tips

As with any other surgical procedure, it is important to work under adequate conditions such as good lighting, access and proper suction.

Careful evaluation of the tooth that has been removed to determine the location and size of the fractured segment is important. This is especially critical in the case of a multi-rooted tooth. If the location and size of the root tip cannot be determined clinically, a radiograph (preferably a periapical X-ray) should be obtained.

For a small root tip (4–5 mm or less), the irrigation–suction technique may be used for retrieval. This technique is useful only if the tooth was well-luxated and mobile before the root fractured. The socket is irrigated vigorously and suctioned with a fine suction tip. This way, the root fragment may occasionally be retrieved with the suction. Good visualization is essential during this technique as small fragments may be suctioned without the surgeon's knowledge.

Another technique is the use of a root tip pick. The fine tip of the instrument is inserted into the periodontal ligament space and the root tip is gently teased out of the socket. A surgical hand-piece with a fine surgical bur can be used to enlarge the space between the bone and the root tip when placement of the root tip pick is difficult.

Care must be taken not to exert excessive force apically which could result in the displacement of the root tip into deeper spaces such as the mandibular canal, maxillary sinus or submandibular region. Excessive lateral forces could also result in bending or fracture of the instrument and, in the worst case scenario, displacement of the broken instrument fragment into other anatomic locations.

An endodontic file might also be used. The file can be inserted into the canal to engage the root tip which is subsequently removed by grasping the file with a hemostat. This technique is useful only if the root has a visible canal and if it does not have a severe dilaceration that prevents adequate access and easy retrieval.

If attempts failed using the preceding techniques, and visualization or access is impaired and a flap has not been reflected, the decision to reflect one should be made.

Table 4.7 Indications for leaving a root tip

1. Small root fragment (4 mm or less)
2. No evidence of periapical pathology or infection associated with the root fragment
3. Inability to visualize the root tip
4. Removal of root tip will cause extensive bone loss
5. Proximity to the inferior alveolar nerve
6. Proximity to the maxillary sinus
7. Uncontrolled hemorrhage

Following the reflection of a flap, the use of a periodontal probe could be helpful in determining the exact location of the root tip from the crest of the bone. The size of the root tip is also measured from the periapical radiograph. A window or fenestration is then created in the bone at the apex of the root tip. The tip can be retrieved using a root tip pick. This technique is especially useful when bone on the buccal aspect is thin and must be preserved for implant placement or orthodontic movement of a tooth into the area (Figure 4.19A–D).

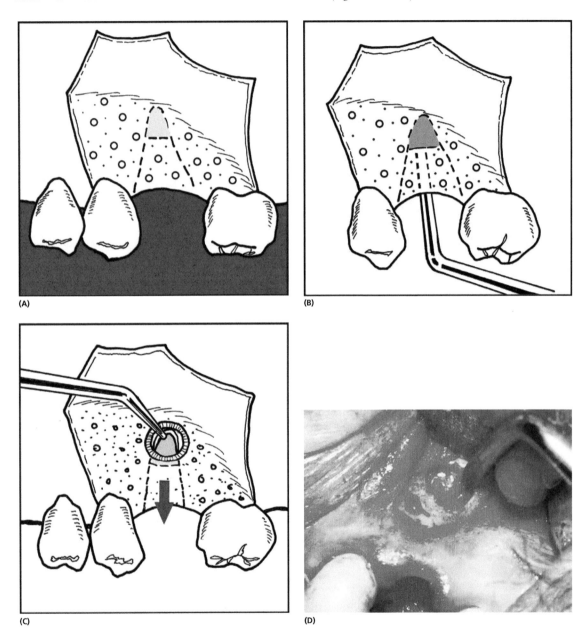

(A)

(B)

(C)

(D)

Figure 4.19 (A) To remove a small, inaccessible, buccal root tip in the maxillary arch, a flap should be reflected with adequate exposure to the tooth's apical portion. (B) The location of the root tip is measured using a periodontal probe. (C) The measurement is transferred to the buccal bone, and a window is created through which a root tip pick or similar instrument can be used to push the fragment coronally. (D) Clinical example of the procedure using a semilunar flap.

Technique for extraction of multiple teeth

It is common for a patient to require extractions of multiple adjacent teeth or all of their remaining teeth. In this situation, certain principles should be followed so that the transition from a dentulous state to an edentulous one is as smooth as possible. The goal is to allow proper functional and esthetic rehabilitation with removable or fixed prostheses after the extractions.

The order in which the teeth should be extracted is important (Table 4.8). Generally, maxillary teeth should be extracted before mandibular teeth for several reasons. Local anesthetics tend to have a more rapid onset and a shorter duration of action in the maxillary arch. This means that surgery in the maxillary arch can begin sooner after the administration of local anesthetics, but it also means that the surgery should not be delayed. In addition, extractions of maxillary teeth first will prevent debris from falling into the mandibular extraction sites if mandibular extractions were performed first.

Adequate hemostasis should be achieved in the maxillary arch before starting the extractions in the mandibular arch to prevent obstruction in visualization. Extractions should also progress from posterior to anterior teeth, this allows for the more effective use of straight elevators in luxating and mobilizing the teeth before using the forceps to extract them. However, since the canine tends to be the most difficult tooth to extract due to its long root, it should be extracted last. Extractions of the teeth on each side of the canine weakens the bony housing, potentially making the canine easier to extract, although it is recommended to luxate the tooth while adjacent teeth are still present in order to achieve a successful extraction.

In cases of multiple tooth extractions, the reflection of a flap improves access and visibility. It also allows for bone removal and sectioning of teeth when necessary.

Selective alveoplasty is usually required following multiple extractions. This is especially true in the area of the canine prominence. The goal of the alveoplasty is to remove all sharp bony edges. Areas of large undercuts should also be removed in patients who are to receive removable prostheses.

Excessive removal of bone should be avoided. Adequate height and width of the alveolar ridge should be maintained as much as possible to allow for proper rehabilitation. The alveoplasty may be performed with a rongeur or a 4 x 8 mm oval surgical bur (commonly known as "Pineapple Bur") (Figure 4.20).

Table 4.8 Multiple extractions sequence

1. Maxillary teeth
2. Achieve hemostasis prior to moving to lower arch
3. Mandibular teeth
4. Posterior to anterior
5. Reflection of a minimal buccal flap if needed to facilitate extractions
6. Alveoplasty
7. Irrigation
8. Suturing
9. Postoperative instructions

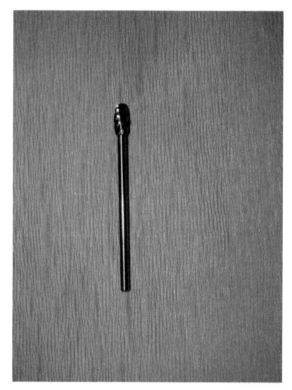

Figure 4.20 Oval surgical bur (4 × 8 mm) used for alveoplasty.

Final smoothing should be performed using a bone file followed by copious amounts of irrigation with sterile saline solution.

The flap can then be replaced and sutured in position. Attempts to achieve primary closure by advancing the flap should be avoided in order to prevent decrease depth of the vestibule which will negatively affect prosthesis stability in those situations when patients receive immediate dentures. In some cases, when treating patients who have been radiated or treated with bisphosphonate or any other antiresorptive medications, primary closure is beneficial.

Principles of flap repositioning and closure

Sutures perform multiple functions; the most important is to approximate wound margins holding the flap in position. They also aid in hemostasis and prevent the development of hematomas. Sutures help maintain bone covered by soft tissue which is extremely important to avoid bone necrosis, delayed healing and the possibility of infection.

A wide array of suture material is available depending on the type of soft tissue and the necessary properties expected from that particular suture. Polyglactin or chromic gut sutures are both commonly used when suturing oral mucosa. If greater tensile strength is required, Nylon sutures are recommended. Sutures are available in various sizes but most incisions in the oral cavity can be closed with a 3-0 or 4-0 size suture. A 3-0 suture is thicker than a 4-0 suture.

Different suturing techniques can be used based on the amount of tissue to be re-approximated. Simple interrupted or a figure of 8 are used in cases when a suture is needed over a single extraction site (Figure 4.21A–E).

Continuous suturing can be used when many contiguous extractions are performed and an envelope flap or the gingival margins are re-approximated (Figure 4.22A–E). Different continuous suturing techniques exist—locking and non-locking (see Figure 4.23 for the non-locking technique).

Horizontal mattress sutures can also be used when single or multiple tooth extractions are performed, however they are used with less frequency (Figure 4.24).

Common mistakes and complications

Careful preoperative planning, a good surgical technique and attention to postoperative instructions will minimize the occurrence of complications following tooth extractions.

Common mistakes that are made during extraction of teeth include attempting a forcep extraction when the preoperative evaluation indicated that a surgical extraction was required. Poor flap design, inadequate reflection of the flap, use of uncontrollable force, inadequate seating and adaptation of the forceps, attempting removal of subgingival root tips without a flap, inadequate irrigation of the surgical site prior to re-approximation of the flap and poor suturing technique are all mistakes that can lead to possible complications.

Under normal circumstances, following a tooth extraction, a socket should stop bleeding in less than 10 minutes. When a patient presents with post-extraction hemorrhage, contributory treatment factors such as anticoagulant medications or systemic conditions should be excluded. The area should then be irrigated copiously with sterile saline solution with the use of good illumination and suction in order to identify the bleeding point. Local pressure usually controls the bleeding although this can be aided by the application of a hemostatic agent such Gelfoam or Oxidized Cellulose (Surgicel). Control of the persistent hemorrhage may require the administration of local anesthesia, placement of sutures, diathermy (cautery) or ligation of vessels.

Alveolar osteitis (dry socket) is an acutely painful condition, which can complicate tooth extractions. It is characterized by the onset of pain 24 to 72 hours postoperatively. Examination usually reveals halithosis, erythema of surrounding soft tissues and an exposed bony socket from which the clot has been lost and which has often become filled with debris. Suturing with primary closure generally minimizes its occurrence.

Osteomyelitis is an infection of the bone which, if not treated effectively, can lead to major complications requiring extensive additional treatment.

Bone necrosis can occur especially in patients at risk (patients with history of radiation therapy to the head and neck region and history of treatment with Bisphosphonate or any other antiresorptive medications). Proper preoperative considerations need to be taken prior to performing any surgical procedures on these patients.

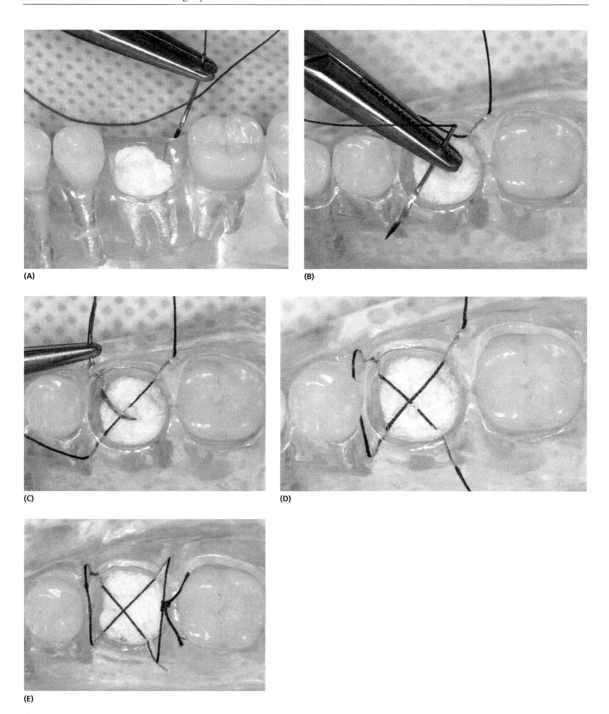

(A)

(B)

(C)

(D)

(E)

Figure 4.21 (A) Figure-eight suture. This is commonly used when the socket is packed with Gelfoam™ or Surgicel™. The needle is passed at the distobuccal papilla. (B) Through the mesiolingual papilla. (C) Through the mesiobuccal papilla. (D) Through the distolingual papilla. (E) The suture is tied.

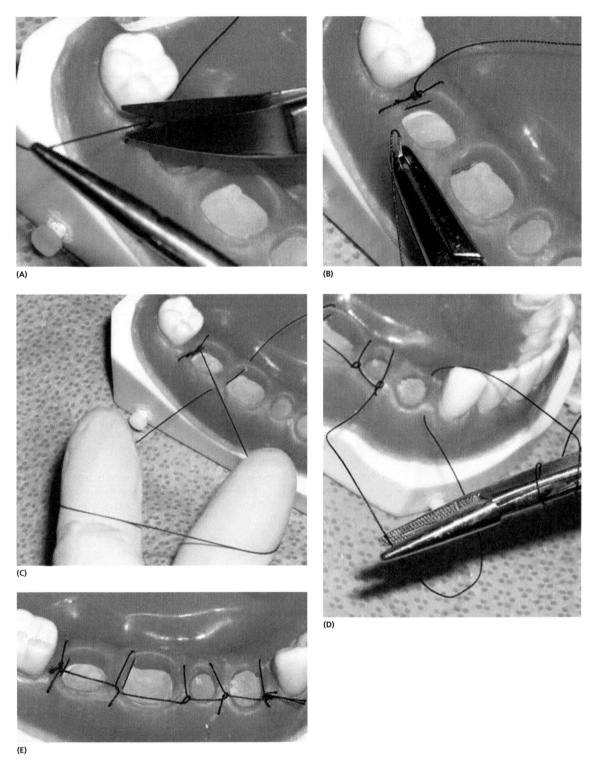

Figure 4.22 (A) Continuous locking suture. Initially a simple suture is tied, only the short end of the suture is cut. (B) Then the needle is passed through the adjacent buccal and lingual papilla. (C) A loop is created. That loop is twisted once and the needle is passed through it, after which the loop is pulled through. (D)The procedure is repeated until the last pass, where a final loop is made – which is used to place the final knot. This last loop functions as the short end of a simple interrupted suture. (E) Final continuous locking suture.

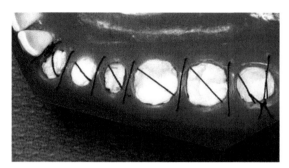

Figure 4.23 Continuous non-locking suturing.

Table 4.9 Complications with extractions

1. Pain
2. Bleeding
3. Infection
4. Swelling
5. Injury to adjacent teeth
6. Maxillary sinus involvement
7. Inferior alveolar and lingual nerves damage
8. Bone spicules necessitating additional surgery
9. Alveolar osteitis
10. Temporomandibular joint problems

Complications can occur when performing surgical extractions (Table 4.9). Detailed preoperative evaluation and proper execution of surgical technique are paramount in prevent complications and ensuring successful outcomes.

Further reading

Anderson L, Kahnberg KE, Pogrel MA. *Oral and Maxillofacial Surgery*, Wiley-Blackwell, New York, 2010.

Dym H, Ogle OE. *Atlas of Minor Oral Surgery*. WB Saunders, New York, 2001.

Fonseca RJ, Turvey TA, Marciani RD. *Oral and Maxillofacial Surgery*, 2nd edn WB Saunders, New York, 2008.

Ghali GE, Larsen PE, Waite PD. *Peterson's Principles of Oral and Maxillofacial Surgery*, 2nd edn. BC Decker, New York, 2004.

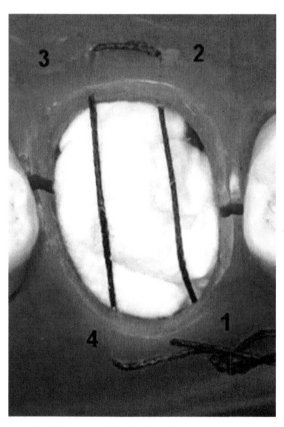

Figure 4.24 Sequence of the horizontal mattress suture.

CHAPTER 5
Third Molar Extractions

George Blakey

Department of Oral and Maxillofacial Surgery, University of North Carolina School of Dentistry, Chapel Hill, NC, USA

Introduction

Third molar extraction is a common procedure performed in dental and oral surgery offices daily. In many cases, the third molars are impacted, requiring more complicated surgery. Impaction refers to the inability for the tooth to have a natural path of egress into the oral cavity. Teeth can be impacted by adjacent teeth, bone, or excessive soft tissue. Third molars are most commonly impacted by adjacent teeth impeding their path of eruption, or by malposition in the bone, as in the case of distoangular impactions and inverted teeth. One of the most common questions of general dentists regarding impacted third molars is whether they should be extracted. Extraction is a generally accepted treatment for symptomatic third molars, or those with associated pathology, but what about asymptomatic third molars? Symptom free does not necessarily mean disease free, and up to 71% of asymptomatic third molars have either periodontal disease or caries. Additionally, only 11% of people with four third molars are both asymptomatic and free of caries or periodontal disease at any third molar site.[1]

Impacted teeth must be evaluated radiographically and clinically, and treatment can vary from observation alone, to surgically assisted eruption, to extraction. When evaluating impacted teeth, it is important to take into account the radiographic appearance of the teeth, clinical presentation, and age of the patient. Impacted third molars are commonly extracted, because both the degree of difficulty of the surgical procedure and recovery time increase with age. Additionally, full bony impacted teeth may result in the formation of various jaw cysts or tumors. It is vitally important that the general dentist or specialist take all of these factors into account when planning for third molar surgery. This chapter discusses the basic principles for management of impacted third molars, from preoperative assessment and planning through surgical execution and postoperative care.

Indications for removal of third molars

Caries

The health of first and second molars is predictive of the health of third molars. Patients with first and second molar caries are more likely to develop caries on third molars.[2] Due to their distal position in the arch and frequent partially impacted position, third molars are often difficult to maintain caries-free (Figure 5.1A, B). Gingival pocketing around the coronal aspect of the third molar can lead to coronal tooth structure that is difficult to clean and susceptible to colonization by oral flora. Additionally, the anaerobic environment provided by the tissue overlying the partially erupted coronal tooth portions leads to the development of particularly pathogenic caries-producing bacteria. Dental caries resulting in pulpal necrosis contribute to the increased number of third molar extractions due to caries with increasing age. Restorative treatment on third molars is contraindicated when they are impacted, and it is difficult to achieve sound restoration on fully erupted third molars; therefore the definitive treatment of caries on third molar teeth is extraction.

Manual of Minor Oral Surgery for the General Dentist, Second Edition. Edited by Pushkar Mehra and Richard D'Innocenzo.

© 2016 John Wiley & Sons, Inc. Published 2016 by John Wiley & Sons, Inc.

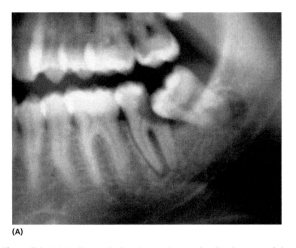
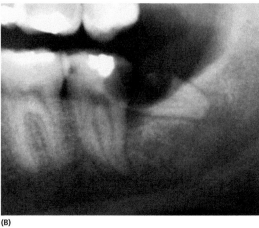

(A) **(B)**

Figure 5.1 (A) Radiograph showing caries on the distal aspect of the second molar secondary to an impacted third molar (B) Radiograph showing caries on both second and third molars.

Pericoronitis

Pericoronitis is an inflammation of the gingival tissue surrounding the crown of a partially impacted tooth (Figure 5.2). The excessive coronal soft tissue overly a partially impacted third molar is problematic because it is difficult to clean these "pseudopockets" and they are often a region ripe for the development of the cariogenic and periodontal pathogenic bacteria found in oral flora. If the balance between host defenses and bacterial growth is disturbed, an infection can result in the area, resulting in pain and inflammation on the pericoronal tissues consistent with pericoronitis. Left untreated, the infection may spread in the typical tissue planes of the head and neck. Traumatic occlusion of the inflamed tissues lead to a vicious cycle of increased inflammation, and creates new sites for bacterial overgrowth and continued infection. Additionally, tissue pseudopocketing around third molars can entrap food debris in the pericoronal tissues, further contributing to pericoronitis secondary to streptococci and anaerobic oral microbes.

Treatment of pericoronitis is mechanical debridement under the operculum or pseudopocket. Antibiotics such as penicillin can specifically target the bacterial load, and chlorhexidine rinses can be used as an adjunct. The patient should be instructed on hygiene methods for these areas with use of a monoject syringe and cleaning under the operculum with normal saline rinses. The patient should be instructed to cleanse the area gently and to avoid forceful use of the syringe, as this may result in hydrodissection and propulsion of the bacteria into deeper pockets.

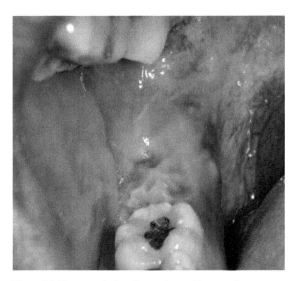

Figure 5.2 Photograph showing pericoronitis around an impacted third molar tooth. Note the erythema of the gingival surrounding the third molar.

Operculectomy is an alternative treatment for pericoronitis, provided that operculectomy will expose sufficient coronal tooth structure to allow for maintenance of oral hygiene in the area and self-cleansing embrasures. Impacted teeth cannot be definitely treated with the above local measures because the environment is not permanently altered, and bacterial colonization under the operculum or in pseudopocketing is favored. Therefore, extraction is the indicated treatment of pericoronitis in patients with bony or soft tissue impaction.

Periodontal disease

The health of the third molars also affects the health of teeth more anterior in the mouth. For example, retention of the third molars in the presence of periodontal disease is associated with significantly increased levels of interleukin-6, intercellular adhesion molecule-1, and C-reactive protein, and leads to increased periodontal pocketing of adjacent second molars and a predisposition to increased periodontal disease in more anterior teeth. Increased periodontal pockets on retained third molars (>4 mm) is associated with worsening of periodontal pocketing on all other teeth at 4-year follow up. Therefore, extraction of third molars with periodontal pockets greater than 4 mm is indicated to prevent spread of periodontal pathogenic bacteria to more anterior sites, which may result in first and second molar mobility and/or necessitate future periodontal surgical intervention. Additionally, mesioangular impaction of lower third molars often results in increased periodontal pocketing of the adjacent distal surface of the second molar. Finally, note that patients presenting with pericoronitis at the third molar site have overall greater levels of periodontal disease throughout the mouth.

Root resorption

Proximity of the third molar to a second molar root can predispose the second molar to root resorption. The most common site for root resorption of the second molar is the middle third of the distal root.[3]

Preprosthetic

Impacted third molar teeth must be evaluated when planning for a removable prosthesis. Downward pressure from the prosthesis, alveolar resorption, and bony remodeling can lead to exposure of a previously impacted tooth into the oral cavity or ulceration of the soft tissue overlying the impacted tooth. The tooth is then at risk for caries or periodontal infection. There is an additional risk of extraction of third molars in this situation because the mandible may be atrophic and susceptible to fracture (Figure 5.3).

Orthodontic, including preparation for orthognathic surgery

Orthodontic treatment planning may require extraction of third molars. The presence of an impacted third molar may interfere with eruption of more anterior teeth. Additionally, vertically and mesially or horizontally impacted third molars may cause continuous mesially directed forces that contribute to relapse after orthodontic treatment. Removal of third molars may facilitate distalization of the teeth by creating space posteriorly in the arch. Consideration should be given to removal of third molars before orthodontic treatment is initiated, and again at completion of orthodontic treatment if the third molars are still present. Age of the patient, dental and skeletal development are all taken into consideration.

When a patient is being evaluated for orthognathic surgery, or if orthognathic surgery is part of their orthodontic and surgical treatment plan, the presence of impacted third molars should be noted. It is the

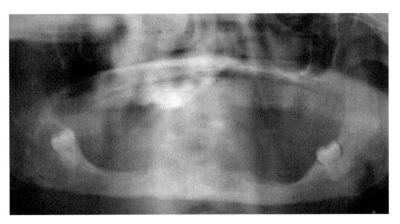

Figure 5.3 Radiograph of a 70-year-old patient with third molars exposed to the oral cavity due to prolonged denture wear. This patient had recurrent episodes of pericoronitis and was treated by removal of the offending teeth. Performing third molar extractions in this kind of patient is complex due to the presence of an atrophic mandible. There is increased risk of jaw fracture and inferior alveolar nerve injury during surgery.

surgeon's preference whether third molars should be extracted intraoperatively or preoperatively. Access to maxillary third molar is often superior intraoperatively during a LeFort osteotomy. If lower third molars are extracted pre-operatively, then they should be removed at least 6–9 months prior to the procedure to allow for adequate bone healing prior to osteotomy.

Pathology

Impacted third molars can be associated with various types of tumors and cysts (Figure 5.4A, B). The most commonly associated cysts are dentigerous cysts, which are derived from the dental follicle. Tumors in the third molar region include keratocystic odontogenic tumors (previously known as

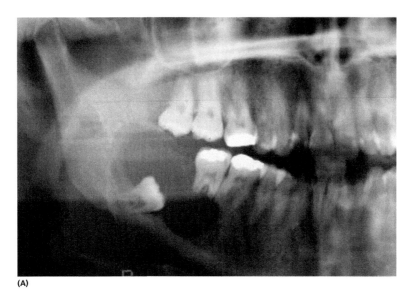

(A)

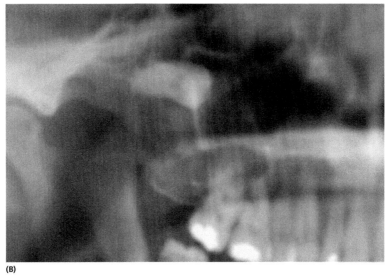

(B)

Figure 5.4 (A) Panoramic radiograph of an impacted third molar in a 17-year-old female with a pericoronal radiolucency causing root resorption of the second molar. Upon histopathological examination, this radiolucency was found to be an ameloblastoma. (B) Panoramic radiograph of an impacted third molar in a 46-year-old male with a large pericoronal radiolucency in the maxillary sinus area. The impacted third molar has been displaced into the sinus and towards the infratemporal fossa. Upon histopathological examination, this radiolucency was found to be a dentigerous cyst.

odontogenic keratocysts), ameloblastomas, or a variety of others. These tumors arise from the dental follicle and require excision with surgical margins. Any cystic structure surrounding an impacted third molar should be sent for histopathological examination with the associated tooth. Note that the frequency of odontogenic cysts and tumors arising from impacted third molars is low at approximately 3%[4] that the removal of asymptomatic third molars with unenlarged follicles to prevent development of cysts or tumors is not supported.

Fracture

While still somewhat controversial in the literature, in general, impacted teeth in the line of fracture should be removed (Figure 5.5). Fractures that extend through

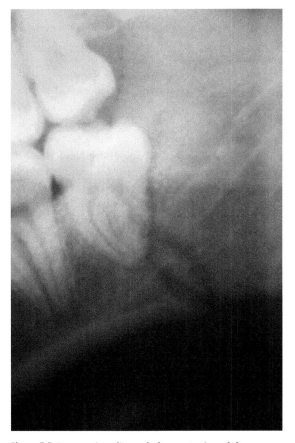

Figure 5.5 Panoramic radiograph demonstrating a left mandibular angle fracture, which runs through the impacted third molar area.

the periodontal ligament space are considered open fractures. The fracture line serves as a conduit for oral bacteria to invade deeply into bone and around the impacted tooth, potentially causing caries in the impacted tooth or acute infection of the fracture. Teeth in the line of fracture are generally removed at the time of fracture repair, unless there are tooth fragments that are grossly mobile and present a risk for aspiration, in which case the mobile tooth portions should be removed on initial exam.

In some cases, an impacted tooth may contribute to the risk of developing a pathologic mandible fracture in an atrophic ridge. Because the tooth is embedded in the mandible, it necessarily lessens the osseous bulk at that site by occupying a space that would otherwise be occupied by bone, thereby contributing to the strength of the mandible. The position of the impacted tooth may permit only minimal continuity of bone, predisposing the patient to a pathologic fracture at that site. Removal of the tooth under controlled circumstances may minimize the overall risk of pathologic fracture. While there is risk of iatrogenic fracture at the time of tooth extraction or in the first six weeks postoperatively, the incidence is low, and removal of the tooth may be a beneficial procedure for the patient.

Management of facial pain

The etiology of facial pain is often multifactorial, and assessment and diagnosis may be complicated by multiple contributing sources of pain. For those patients with facial pain of unknown origin, a referral should be made to a facial pain specialist for evaluation. Additionally, diagnostic local anesthetic blocks can be useful in determining whether pain of odontogenic origin is contributing to facial pain. The proximity of the third molar roots to the inferior alveolar nerve may contribute to facial pain. If the patient has no contraindications for third molar extraction, the removal of these teeth should be considered as—or as an adjunct to—treatment. In these situations the patient should be informed that there is no guarantee that extraction of third molars will ameliorate their condition, and they should also be counseled that there are risks associated with extraction of third molar that may cause increased pain, such as alveolar osteitis and nerve injury resulting in dysesthesia.

Contraindications to removal of impacted third molars

Damage to adjacent structures

Impacted teeth may be located directly adjacent to nerves, the sinuses, and other teeth. Their radiographic position should be evaluated to determine if the risks of damage to these structures during extraction outweighs the benefits of tooth extraction. The most commonly injured adjacent structures to impacted mandibular third molars are nerves. Both the inferior alveolar nerve and the lingual nerve can be in close proximity to an impacted mandibular third molar. The inferior alveolar nerve canal can be identified on panoramic radiograph. When lower third molars are fully impacted in bone, they are often very close to the inferior alveolar canal, and the risks of iatrogenic nerve damage, and intraoperative bleeding must be weighed against comparatively low risk of developing pathology around the third molar if left in place. In Figure 5.6, the fully impacted tooth #32 is in close proximity to the radiographic inferior alveolar nerve canal, the patient was asymptomatic, and therefore the decision was made to observe the tooth, and not extract the it. However, in the case of symptomatic impacted teeth that are in close radiographic proximity to the inferior alveolar nerve, the risks of non-extraction outweigh the risks of iatrogenic injury. In those cases, a 3-dimensional image such as a cone beam computerized tomography (CT)

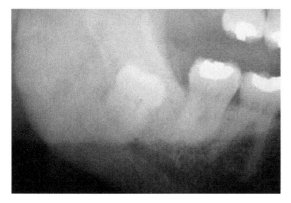

Figure 5.6 Deeply impacted mandibular third molar in very close proximity to the inferior alveolar nerve in a 48-year-old male. Note the dense bone overlying the impacted tooth. In view of the difficulty of the surgery, age of the patient, and asymptomatic nature of the impaction, elective extraction was not recommended.

scan will help to localize the buccolingual position of the nerve canal and assist with surgical planning for extraction.

Maxillary third molar teeth are often closely related to the maxillary sinus antrum. Extraction of impacted maxillary teeth can result in a tearing of the Schneiderian membrane and oroantral communication. Risk factors for persistence of the oroantral fistula include fistula size >2 mm, incomplete primary closure over the fistula site, and smoking. Prior to elective extraction of maxillary third molars, their vertical position in relationship to the maxillary sinus should be assessed along with patient-level risk factors such as smoking. The risks associated with extraction of high vertically impacted third molars may outweigh the benefits.

Adjacent to all teeth, including impacted third molars, is bone. Bony defects caused by troughing with a drill around the impacted molar may result in a permanent bony defect. This is particularly true in elderly or medically compromised patients where bone healing may not be as robust as in the younger population.

Chronologic age, dental, and skeletal maturity

Impacted third molars do not necessarily remain impacted but their eruption may be difficult to predict. In one study, by age 24, 17% of all third molars failed to erupt, despite adequate space in the arch for eruption. According to some studies, third molar teeth that appear impacted at age 18 may have a 50% chance of erupting by age 25.[5] The required extent of bone removal and difficulty of extraction should be considered when determining if a patient is at the appropriate age for third molar extraction. Consider a 13-year-old male with third molars present, but without any significant root formation and in deep vertical impaction. In this case, a large amount of bone removal would be required for extraction and there would be increased morbidity associated with both the risk for nerve damage and the difficulty of recovery. Ideally, third molars are extracted when two-thirds of the root is formed. This allows for ease of extraction and sectioning if required, with minimal risk to the nerve. There are some indications for third molar extraction at a young age, before third molars are significantly developed and still in deep vertical impaction; for example, a patient undergoing intravenous

(IV) sedation for extraction of premolars for ortho-dontic treatment plan. It may be prudent to remove third molars at the same time if there is any concern for the need for space for distalization of the arch in the orthodontic treatment plan, therefore avoiding two separate procedures for extraction.

Medical compromise

Compromised medical status must be taken into account in planning for extraction of third molars. This includes psychiatric health, the ability to tolerate the procedure, and ability to comply with the recommended postoper-ative course. Anesthesia options are affected by the patient's medical status. A thorough patient evaluation is indicated to determine which anesthesia option the patient will require and can tolerate. In the case of severe medical compromise, a risk–benefit analysis should be made to determine the appropriateness of extractions. Asymptomatic third molars should not be removed in a patient population where life expectancy is very short or in cases where the stress of surgery or general anesthesia puts the patient at risk for more serious complications.

Finally, consideration should be given to whether to extract asymptomatic third molars in patients with severe mental retardation, where it would be difficult to determine if the patient is experiencing postoperative pain, and also difficult to follow routine postoperative instructions that include keeping the sites clean, or in some cases taking oral antibiotics.

Presurgical considerations

Informed consent

As for all dental procedures, informed consent is required prior to extractions. Informed consent requires that the dental care provider explain the benefits of the procedure and the most common risks of the opera-tion. Benefits have been generally referred to previ-ously in this chapter but can be summarized by prevention of caries, periodontal disease, and pathology associated with third molars. Risks include bleeding, swelling, infection, pain, nerve damage, damage to sinuses, damage to any adjacent structures, and alve-olar osteitis "dry socket." In the absence of a previously undiscovered coagulopathy, bleeding can generally be well controlled intraoperatively with the use of coagulant agents such as Gelfoam or Surgicel. Postoperative swelling should be expected; it peaks within 72 to 96 hours postoperatively and then slowly diminishes. Intraoperatively, a steroid dose can be given via IV or postoperatively, an oral steroid taper can be used to minimize swelling. Infection is rare and is not anticipated. There is no indication for postoperative antibiotics in the absence of obvious infection at the time of surgery. Postoperative infection usually pres-ents between 5 and 7 days, or can sometimes present weeks to months after surgery, as in the case with subperiosteal abscess. Pain should be expected after removal of impacted third molars and adequate pain medication should be prescribed for the anticipated duration of pain (usually 3–4 day tapering supply of narcotic pain medication such as hydrocodone or oxy-codone is sufficient). The patient should also be advised that they can take over-the-counter pain medication (such as ibuprofen) as long as there is no medical contraindication. In the event of extraction of maxil-lary teeth the possibility of oroantral communication should be clearly explained, as well as the general postoperative instructions should an oroantral com-munication occur (such as no nose blowing). Some people blow their noses so frequently that the sugges-tion that a complication may arise that they would not be able to blow their nose for 2 weeks by itself is enough to avoid the surgery. The patient should also be informed that here is a low, but present, risk of nerve injury and particularly the distribution and function of the nerves involved (which are the inferior alveolar nerve and the lingual nerve). It should also be clear that no infected root tips measuring less than 5 mm may be left in place in order to avoid damage to the sinuses or nerves. The risk of damage to adjacent teeth should be explained and a plan should be in place should damage to adjacent teeth occur. The patient should verbalize understanding of these risks and benefits and have the opportunity to ask ques-tions. Finally, the patient should be advised that the overall costs associated with retaining third molars may exceed those of extraction. Observation and biyearly follow up for 20 years for two impacted man-dibular third molars has an estimated cost of $2300 to the patient, while extraction of two full bony impacted third molars has an estimated cost of $1200.[6] The con-sent should be signed in the presence of a witness who is not directly involved in the surgical procedure.

Radiographic analysis

As in many aspects of dentistry, radiographic analysis of the third molars is imperative prior to extraction. The panoramic radiograph is the standard of care because a large field can be visualized that includes the condyles, sinuses, inferior alveolar nerve canal, and any intrabony or tooth-associated pathology that may exist and need to be addressed with prior to, or during extraction. Proximity of the maxillary third molars to the sinus and mandibular third molars to the inferior alveolar nerve canal can be helpful in predicting the risks associated with extraction. In some cases CT scan is beneficial to better characterize the position of the inferior alveolar nerve (IAN) to the mandibular third molar, because panoramic radiographs cannot give buccolingual position information. Rarely, an occlusal radiograph can be used, but patient intolerance to such a posteriorly positioned film may preclude the use of this modality.

Surgical instrumentation

The appropriate surgical instrumentation is required prior to beginning extraction. Some surgical items may only be necessary in the event that a root tip is fractured, or if the surgeon encounters excessive bleeding. These scenarios may be rare, but the operator should be prepared to address them. The following surgical instrumentation and supplies are recommended in the set-up for all third molar extractions:

#15 Bard–Parker blade
#9 Molt periosteal elevator
#1 Woodson elevator
Minnesota retractor (alternative is Austin retractor)
Seldin retractor
"Sweetheart" lingual retractor
Small, medium, and large straight elevators
Cryer elevators ("east–west" elevators)
Root tip pick
Millers, Potts, or Cogswell elevators
Bone file
Upper universal extraction forceps
Lower universal extraction forceps
Cowhorn forceps
Ronguer
Hemostat
Needle holder
Suture scissors
Suture material (3–0 or 4–0 chromic gut or Vicryl)
Gelfoam or Surgicel

Irrigation syringe
Normal saline
Frasier tip suction
Yankauer suction
Gauze
Surgical drill (such as a Hall drill or other non-air-powered drill. It is important that a standard front-vented dental drill is not used for bone removal as this may result in dangerous air emboli, or air emphysema)
Fissure and round burs
Supplemental oxygen via nasal cannula if necessary.

Mandibular third molar impactions

Mandibular third molar impactions are classified based on their angulation, position relative to the occlusal plane, and position relative to the anterior portion of the mandibular ramus. These can all be important considerations in assessing difficulty of extraction and the planned surgical approach for extraction. Angulation refers to the direction of the long axis of the tooth. Mesioangular direction is the most common, and occurs when the crown of the third molar tooth is positioned mesial to the root apex. A vertical impaction is the second most common type of impaction; in this case, the third molar crown is centered over the root structure vertically, but the tooth has not fully erupted to the occlusal plane. Distoangular impaction occurs when the long axis of the third molar is position such that the crown of the tooth is distal to the root apex. Horizontal impaction occurs when the third molar is so mesially inclined that it is perpendicular to the ideal long-axis of the second molar.

Pell and Gregory devised a system of classification of impaction of third molar teeth based on their position (Figure 5.7). There are two parts to this classification system—the first part categorized at either 1, 2, or 3 is based on the position of the coronal portion of the tooth with respect to the anterior portion of the ascending mandibular ramus. If the coronal portion of the tooth is completely anterior to the anterior portion of the ramus, this is considered Class 1. If 50% of the coronal portion of the tooth is covered by the ramus then the impaction is considered Class 2. If the entire crown of the third molar is positioned posterior to the anterior aspect of the ascending ramus, then is it considered Class 3. Class 3 impactions require more bone removal,

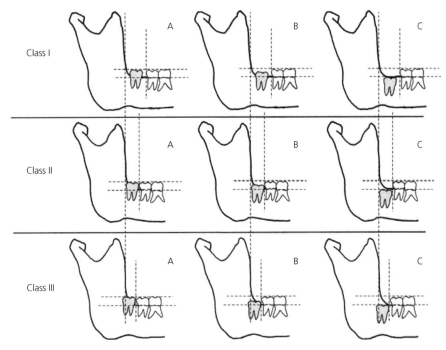

Figure 5.7 Pell and Gregory classification of third molar impactions.

and are therefore considered more challenging and are associated with greater morbidity. The second part of the Pell and Gregory classification system is based on the vertical position of the third molar relative to the occlusal plane and is categorized as class A, B, or C. Class A refers to an erupted third molar where the occlusal plane is at the level of the occlusal plane of the second molar. Class B impaction is a tooth that is partially erupted such that the occlusal plane of the third molar is situated between the occlusal plane of the erupted second molars and the cemento-enamel junction of the second molar. Class C refers to the case in which the occlusal plane of the third molar is completely submerged below the level of the CEJ of the second molar. Since Class C impacted teeth are the most deeply impacted, they require more bony removal and are considered more difficult than Class A.

Facial form

Obese patients and patient with large cheeks can make third molar extraction very difficult. The cheek tissue can be difficult to retract fully, and adequate exposure may challenging. Accessing the maxillary third molar is often the most challenging in these patients, excess cheek tissue and the coronoid process moving inferiorly with mouth opening can obscure the view and access to these teeth, thus requiring tooth extraction while the mouth is essentially closed so the cheek tissue have maximum laity and the coronoid process is in its most retruded position. This should be determined in the preoperative appointment, and be taken into consideration in determining the difficulty of extraction.

Root morphology

Root maturity is one of the most important factors in assessing difficulty and surgical planning. Ideally, third molars are extracted when root formation is between 1/3 and 2/3 completed (Figure 5.8A). This allows for adequate root structure to grasp the tooth, and or section it into mesial and distal segments. A fully developed root may have apices that are close to the inferior alveolar nerve. Incomplete root apices are usually blunted, and less likely to be intimately associated with the nerve. Very immature teeth without significant root structure are difficult to remove because they have no long axis, and therefore roll around and are difficult to section (Figure 5.8B).

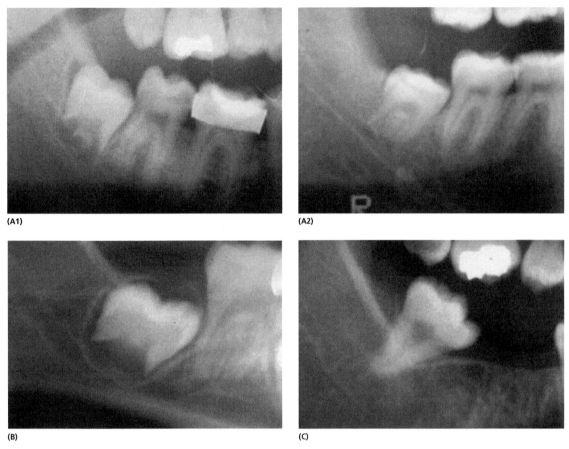

(A1) (A2)

(B) (C)

Figure 5.8 Root morphology affecting complexity of surgery. (A1, A2) Roots are approximately 1/3 to 2/3 developed, therefore, these are easier extractions. (B) Roots have not developed—may be a difficult extraction. (C) Conical roots morphology—easier extractions.

The length of the root should also be considered. Long thin roots are easily fractured during extraction and removal of root tips can be difficult and risky if their position is close the inferior alveolar bundle. Bulbous roots may also pose a challenge for extraction, and may require a large amount of bone removal to gain an unimpeded path of exit (Figure 5.8E). Dilacerated roots may cause a similar problem both with the requirement of large amount of bone removal to create an unimpeded path of egress, and also with the need to remove a fracture root tip that may be in close proximity to the inferior alveolar bundle (Figure 5.8D). A conical root form is generally the most favorable for extraction as there is generally an already unimpeded path for egress (Figure 5.8C). Because panoramic radiographs cannot show the buccolingual orientation, it may at times be difficult to determine what type of root form is present.

A root that appears conical may actually have a buccal or lingual dilacerations and be very difficult to extract. A third molar may also have an additional root that is not clearly evident on radiograph. When extraction of an apparently easy tooth becomes difficult, the operator should think of these other possibilities and tailor his/her surgical technique to accommodate these situations.

Anesthesia

Adequate and profound anesthesia is paramount for extraction of both maxillary and mandibular third molars. When extracting a mandibular third molar, an inferior alveolar nerve block should be performed as well as a long buccal block. Anesthesia is tested by asking the patient if the lower lip on the side of the extraction is numb, and by testing the gingival tissue with a periosteal elevator. The most common anesthetic

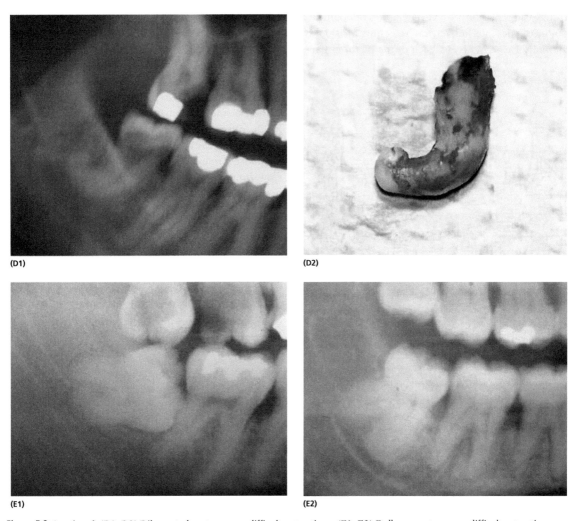

(D1)

(D2)

(E1)

(E2)

Figure 5.8 (*continued*) (D1, D2) Dilacerated roots—more difficult extractions. (E1, E2) Bulbous roots—more difficult extractions.

used is 2% lidocaine with 1:100,000 epinephrine. The epinephrine causes vasoconstriction, and decreases the distribution of the local anesthetic while also minimizing bleeding at the surgical site. Other local anesthetics can also be used, for example bupivacaine (Marcaine) can provide local anesthesia for approximately 6 to 8 hours and be a useful adjunct for pain management in the immediate post-operative period. Mepivacaine (Carbocaine) is often in preparations without epinephrine. This can be appropriately selected for those patients in whom epinephrine is a relative contraindication. Local anesthetics without epinephrine are often useful in cases where profound local anesthesia is difficult to achieve (missed blocks). In this case

the large distribution of the local anesthetic can obviate the need for precisely placed nerve block in a setting where there is an unusual position of the inferior alveolar nerve.

Flap design

The flap used for extraction of teeth is always a full thickness mucoperiosteal flap. This type of flap is created by incising from the epithelium to bone, then dissecting subperiosteally to elevate the flap. Subperiosteal elevation is created with a periosteal elevator with the concave surface of the elevator against the bone and the convex surface against the periosteum. Flaps for mandibular third molar surgery may be envelope (no releasing incision); however, more commonly, a distobuccal or anterior vertical releasing incision is required for ease of access. Each of the pictured flaps

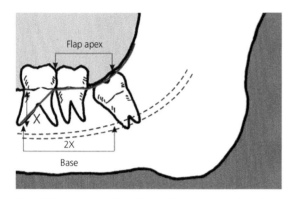

Figure 5.9 Basic principles of flap design: The base of the flap should be wider than the apex of the flap. The releasing incision(s) should be divergent in relation to the site of exposure so as to not undermine the blood supply of the raised flap. The ratio between the height of releasing incision(s) and length of base should not exceed 2:1.

can be modified based on surgeon preference. Basic principles of flap design should always be followed. The base of the flap should be wider than the apex, ensuring that the blood supply to the apical portion of the flap is not compromised. The flap must be fully subperiosteal, and raised in such a way to prevent tearing of the tissue or periosteum. The ratio of the height of the releasing incision and the length of the base should not exceed 2:1 (Figure 5.9). When using a distobuccal releasing incision (Figure 5.10A, B, C, D) care should be taken to ensure that when the tissues are not retracted, the incision site is distobuccal. To accommodate tissue retraction, the incision can be directed straight buccal while the tissues are retracted so that when the tissues are released the incision is oriented distobuccally. If a releasing incision is made in the distobuccal direction while the cheek tissues are retracted, then when the tissues are released the incision may actually be only distal and thus compromise the lingual nerve. Kiesselbach *et al.* found that in approximately 17% of the population the

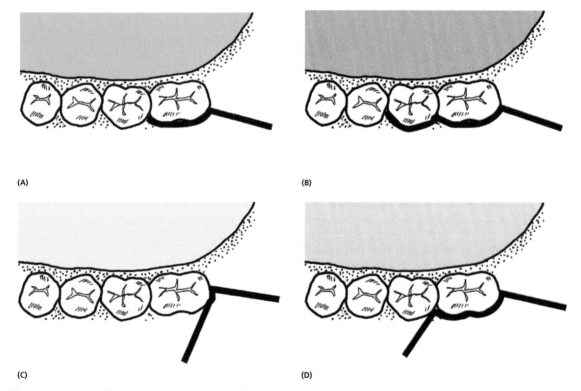

(A)   (B)

(C)   (D)

Figure 5.10 Common flap designs for mandibular third molar surgery. (A) Short envelope flap. (B) Long envelope flap. (C) Short triangular flap. (D) Long triangular flap.

lingual nerve lies at or above the alveolar crest in the tissues distal to the third molar.[7]

Almost all flaps begin with a sulcular incision around the second molar. This can be extended to the first molar for increased visibility. A distobuccal releasing incision is made at the distobuccal line angle of the second molar. To increase access and anterior releasing incision can be made either at the mesiobuccal line angle of the second or first molar.

Triangular flap (three-cornered flap)

More exposure can be obtained with both a distobuccal releasing incision and an anterior releasing incision. In cases where the third molar is deeply impacted, the addition of an anteriorly place releasing incision may greatly improve access and thus decrease the degree of difficulty of the extraction. The anterior aspect of the flap may be placed at the mesiobuccal line angle of the second or first molar. Alternatively, in cases where no sulcular incision is created, the anterior releasing incision may begin at the distobuccal line angle of the second molar and proceed anteriorly and inferiorly (Figure 5.10C).

The design of the flap should optimize exposure and access to the tooth. However, larger flaps result in increased post-operative pain and edema. The skill in flap design is to obtain adequate visualization and access, while minimizing trauma to tissues, flap reflection, and flap size. The level of expertise often dictates flap size; novice surgeons often require increased exposure to perform the procedure, while experienced surgeons are often able to perform the operation with a minimal amount of reflected tissue. Flap design is based on personal preference, clinical and radiographic evaluation of tooth position, and the operator's level of expertise.

Bone removal

After adequate soft tissue reflection, the impacted tooth must be exposed. Exposure of the crown of the tooth from the buccal aspect is the initial step and this is completed with the use of a bur on a handpiece under copious irrigation to prevent burning the surrounding bone. When using the handpiece, is it critically important that the soft tissues of the lip, cheek, and full thickness mucoperiosteal flap are protected with an retractor such as a Minnesota. The goal of bone removal is to create a path of egress to deliver the tooth from the alveolus,

while sparing as much bone as possible. Therefore, bone removal should be carefully planned at the appropriate sites, and not haphazardly remove a large amount of buccal bone for extraction (Figure 5.11A–D).

The first step in bone removal should provide visualization of the coronal portion of the tooth (Figure 5.11A). This is true for full bone impacted teeth and teeth that are incompletely impacted. For full bony impacted teeth a round bur can be used at occlusal and superior buccal aspect of the mandibular alveolus just distal to the second molar. Bone removal is continued with a round bur until the crown is identified and the orientation of the crown is evident (Figure 5.11B). Once the orientation of the crown is evident (as with a partially impacted tooth) a fissure bur can be used to create a buccal trough adjacent to the tooth with the long axis of the fissure bur parallel to the long axis of the tooth (Figure 5.11C). The purpose of the trough is to remove bone immediately adjacent to the tooth while leaving a ledge of bone laterally. This facilitates the use of straight elevators for luxation with the buccal ledge of bone used as a fulcrum. It is therefore important the trough is just wide enough to accommodate the straight elevator, but not so wide that the elevator freely rotates in the trough. The trough can be extended distally around the posterior aspect of the tooth into the mandibular ramus provided that there is adequate tissue retraction and protection of all tissues that may house the lingual nerve. This can be completed with a Minnesota or Austin retractor by placing the edge of the retractor in direct contact with the distal bone. With excellent soft tissue retraction and protection it is safe to remove bone in this area and adequate bony removal to the middistal of the impacted tooth will allow for adequate room for egress of the tooth.

Troughing should never extend to the lingual aspect of the tooth. Soft tissue elevation should not occur on the lingual tissues and perforation of the lingual cortex poses a risk for lingual nerve injury. Violation of the lingual cortex may also provide a communication to the floor of the mouth, into where fragment of tooth or debris can be dislodged. This poses a challenge for retrieval of tooth fragments from the floor of the mouth.

The depth of the trough should be extended to the level of the furcation at the buccal aspect of the tooth. Access to the furcation allows for ease of sectioning the tooth into mesial and distal parts if necessary. Extension should be far enough anteriorly to allow access to the

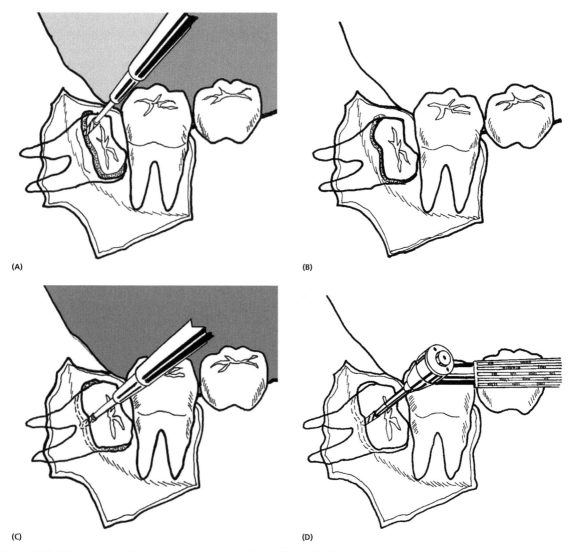

Figure 5.11 (A) Bone removal for a mesioangular impacted mandibular third molar surgery. Bone removal from the occlusal aspect. (B) Bone removal from the buccal aspect. (C) Troughing of bone on the buccal aspect with a straight handpiece. (D) Troughing of bone on the buccal aspect with a surgical high-speed handpiece.

mesial–buccal aspect of the third molar root structure, but should not extend so far mesially to cause a periodontal defect at the distal aspect of the second molar or compromise second molar distal root structure.

Luxation

Once adequate bone removal has been achieved exposing the crown of the tooth, the operator may make an attempt at luxation. In order for luxation to be successful, there must be an unimpeded path of egress. The opening in the bone must be larger than the occlusal surface of the crown of the tooth, and the roots must not be convergent so that the interseptal bone hinders a straight path of egress or divergent so that there is no straight path of egress. If all of these conditions are satisfied, is it reasonable to attempt luxation at the buccal aspect of the tooth in the trough with the goal to deliver the tooth in its entirety. The elevator should be directed along the long axis of the tooth and the apex of the elevator should provide superiorly directed pressure allowing the tooth to emerge from its bony housing. If the tooth does not have an unimpeded path of egress, then it should be sectioned and each section should have its own unimpeded path.

Tooth sectioning

Tooth sectioning refers to splitting the tooth from the buccal aspect using a drill under irrigation. The tooth can be initially sectioned into mesial and distal parts, or the crown can be sectioned from the root surface. In either case, a fissure bur is used to make a groove either vertically along the tooth long axis in the buccal groove of the tooth toward the furcation, or horizontally (perpendicular to the long axis) just coronal to the cementoenamel junction to separate the crown from the root structure. It is very important that the groove does not extend more that ¾ of the way into the tooth. This is an adequate extension so that the tooth can be divided into the desired sections, but not so far that there is risk of penetration of the bur into the lingual cortex and potential trauma to the lingual tissues housing the lingual nerve. Once the groove is extended ¾ of the way through the tooth a small straight elevator is inserted into the tooth and rotated to complete the split. Determining whether the tooth should be split into mesial and distal aspects or coronal and root portions is based on the anatomy of the tooth and the type of impaction.

Mesioangular impactions

Mesioangular impactions are the most common type of mandibular third molar impaction. In these types of impactions, the distal aspect of the crown of the second molar is impeding the egress of the mesial aspect of the crown of the third molar. Sectioning the tooth can be completed in a variety of way that will allow for extraction. The easiest way is to section the tooth into mesial and distal parts through the furcation (Figure 5.12A), the distal aspect of the tooth is removed first. The mesial portion can be removed with elevator luxation anteriorly with and gentle posterior pressure. At times the mesial portion of the crown is still trapped under the crown of the second molar. In this case the remaining coronal portion on the mesial section can be removed, followed by the mesial root. (Figure 5.12B). Alternatively, the same tooth can be approached with a transverse cut parallel to the cementoenamel junction to separate the crown from the root trunk (Figure 5.12C).

The crown is removed with forceps, followed by an attempt at removal of the root structure. Removal of the roots may require more troughing in the area buccal to the roots, or sectioning at the furcation into mesial and distal roots (Figure 5.12D).

An important principle in sectioning teeth is to have adequate exposure to ensure that the groove is oriented in the appropriate direction. The inexperienced surgeon will attempt to section the tooth into mesial and distal parts with the long axis of the bur directed at a shallower angle than the long axis of the tooth. This can result in a segment of the distal portion of the crown separating from the remainder of the tooth, but no progress in separating the crown from the roots. In addition to, or in some cases instead of, sectioning a tooth that already have unimpeded egress but is difficult to luxate, a bur can be used to make a purchase point in the buccal aspect of the tooth. A crane pick, Cryer, or Cogswell B elevator can be inserted into the hole and force directed coronally to push the tooth out of the mandible.

Horizontal impactions

Horizontal impactions can be treated the same way as mesioangular impactions. The trough is created buccally, and a window is made in the crest of the alveolar ridge and at the anterolateral aspect of ramus so that the coronal portion of the tooth can be accessed. It is important that the soft tissues overlying the anterior ramus are protected with a retractor to avoid injury to the lingual nerve. It is also important that bone removal does not extend to the lingual aspect of the ascending ramus. Once the coronal portion of the horizontally impacted tooth is fully visualized, the crown can then be sectioned from the root trunk. The crown is delivered first. If a path of exit exists for the root structure, then both roots can be extracted simultaneously. If no path exists then the roots should be sections and taken out individually (Figure 5.13).

Vertical impaction

The vertical impaction is also a common presentation for impacted mandibular third molars. When a third molar presents this way the operator needs to be cautious of injury to the second molar and also to the nerve. To prevent injury to the second molar, the trough should not be extended so far mesially that bone from the distal aspect of the second molar is removed. Troughing distally is almost always necessary for

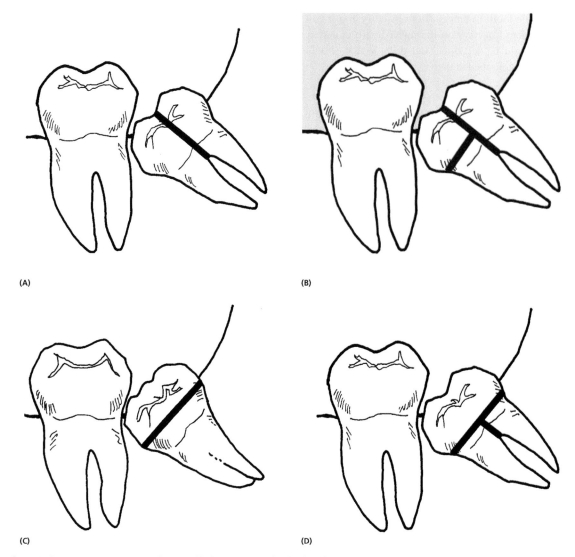

(A)

(B)

(C)

(D)

Figure 5.12 (A) Sectioning options for mandibular mesioangular third molar impactions. This view shows a cut longitudinally through the furcation. (B) Same as (A), but with an additional cutting of the mesial crown, which is wedged under the second molar. (C) Crown and root separation. The crown is removed and then the root is delivered into the original crown space. (D) Crown removal as in option (C), but then the roots are divided longitudinally through the furcation and moved into the crown space for removal.

removal of vertically impacted teeth, again this should be completed with great care to protect the lingual tissues overlying the anterior and lingual aspect of the ramus to avoid injury to the lingual nerve. The path of removal should be occlusally oriented, so the crestal bone overlying the occlusal aspect must be removed. If a substantially large amount of bone removal is required distally to gain and unimpeded path of removal, then the distal

portion of the crown can be removed separately from the remainder of the tooth. Once a trough is completed and the tooth is luxated with straight elevators, it can be removed with forceps. On occasion, it may be easier to make a purchase point with a bur in the buccal aspect of the tooth near the furcation, then use a Cogswell B or Cryer elevator to apply directed force occlusally to deliver the tooth. If the tooth is

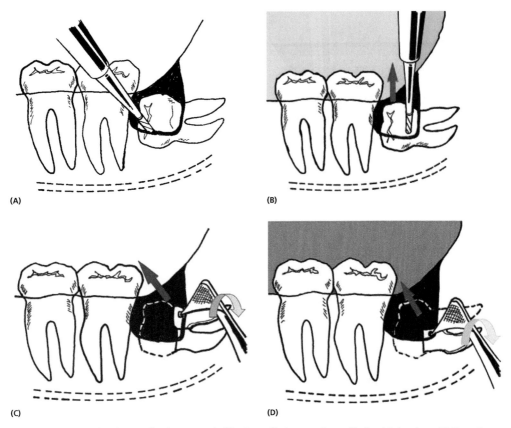

Figure 5.13 Common surgical technique for the removal of horizontally impacted mandibular third molars. (A) Bone is removed from the superior surface of the tooth and from the buccal—and also perhaps from the occlusal aspect of the crown if there is sufficient bone thickness distal to the second molar. (B) Crown is sectioned from root, and then removed. (C) Roots are delivered together. Occasionally, a purchase point can be made to facilitate delivery. (D) Roots have been split and delivered separately.

impacted under the distal aspect of the second molar (similar to a mesioangular impaction), and unimpeded path of removal may require sectioning of the roots, and their removal individually. In this case a purchase point can be placed on the distal root for elevation. The mesial part of the tooth is delivered with a straight elevator using rotary and a lever-type of motion (Figure 5.14).

Distoangular impaction

Distoangular impactions are often considered one of the most difficult scenarios for third molar removal for three reasons. First, visualization can be difficult because a large amount of bone removal may be necessary to visualize the crown of the tooth. Second, access is often troublesome, because a fissure bur

cannot parallel the long access of the tooth. And third, delivery of the tooth is distally directed. The plan for distoangular impacted teeth follows the same basic principles as other types of impactions. First, gain visualization and access by removal of bone. Bone is removed occlusally, creating a path of removal for the tooth, and troughing should be completed on the buccal, mesial, and distal aspects of the tooth, with great care to protect the soft tissues overlying the anterior and lingual aspect of the ramus. Sectioning the crown from the root trunk is a useful technique because the crown can often be easily delivered thought the occlusal access. Extraction of the roots is then completed by first sectioning the roots, and then delivering each one independently, either by creating a purchase point in each root and providing superiorly directed force, or

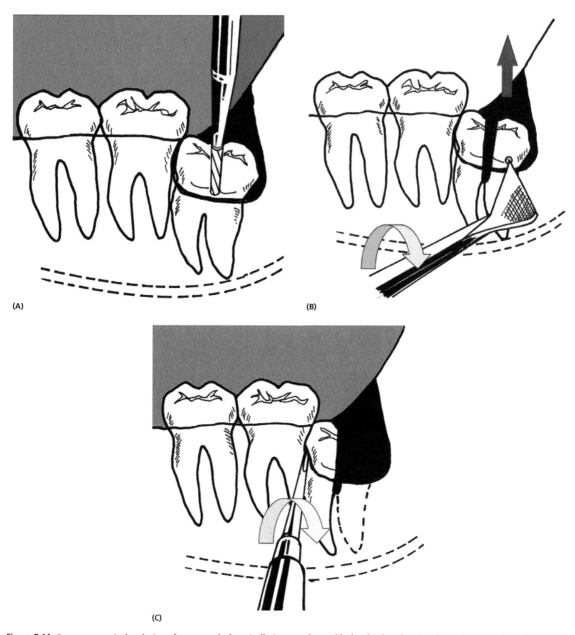

(A)

(B)

(C)

Figure 5.14 Common surgical technique for removal of vertically impacted mandibular third molars. (A) Bone is removed on the occlusal, buccal, and distal aspects. (B) After sectioning lengthwise through the tooth the posterior aspect is delivered first with purchase point and an elevator. (C) The mesial part of the tooth is delivered with a straight elevator using rotary and a lever-type of motion.

elevation with a small straight elevator. In some instances, removal of the crown will provide enough space for removal of the roots without sectioning, this can be facilitated with a mesiobucally placed purchase point and elevation with a Cryer elevator (Figure 5.15).

Closure

Prior to closure the operator should be certain that all portions of the tooth have been removed. This is especially true for tooth enamel, which, if left, will almost certainly result in post-operative infection or wound healing

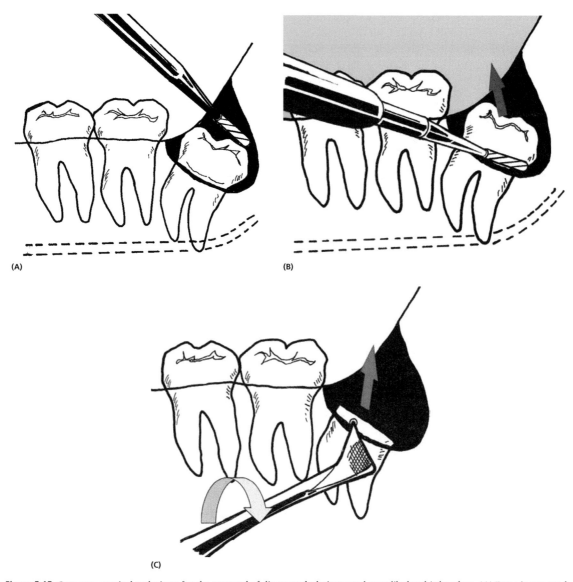

Figure 5.15 Common surgical technique for the removal of distoangularly impacted mandibular third molars. (A) Bone is removed on the occlusal, buccal, and distal aspects. More distal bone removal is usually required in these cases. (B) The crown of the tooth is sectioned from the root and delivered with straight elevators. (C) A purchase point is made and an elevator is used to deliver both roots. Sometimes, roots may need to be split into separate halves and delivered separately.

complication. Fragments of root structure less than 5 mm in length can be left if (1) the tooth is not infected and (2) its removal jeopardizes other adjacent structures such as the IAN nerve or if a large amount of bone removal is required that would greatly increase the patient's risk of jaw fracture. If any root structure is intentionally left, a panoramic radiograph should be completed at the end of the case, and the size and location of the root tip should be documented in the patient's chart along with the indication for leaving it. This should also be clearly explained to the patient prior to their dismissal and at the follow-up appointment. Antibiotics should be prescribed.

The extraction site should also be cleared of any remaining follicle. This can be done with small hemostats to remove any soft tissue inside the extraction site. Once grossly obvious soft tissue is removed, all of the bony margins should be thoroughly curettaged with a dental curette until only hard tissue is felt at all margins. Follicle left in place due to inadequate curettage has the potential to develop into an odontogenic cyst or tumor. The patient's treatment record should note that all follicle was removed from the extraction site and that the site was thoroughly curettage. Any granulation tissue should be removed with the curette or if exuberant granulation tissue exists, careful removal with an end cutting ronguer is appropriate.

Inspection of the extraction site should include a view inferiorly to determine if the inferior alveolar nerve is visualized. Curetting should be performed with great care if the nerve is visualized to avoid damage to the nerve. If the nerve is visualized, a comment should be made in the chart as to its integrity (completely intact, partially intact, or transected). The lingual cortex should also be inspected, and any damage to the lingual bone or perforation in the cortex should be noted in the event that the patient presents with lingual nerve paresthesia at a follow up visit.

Next, bone margins at the trough areas should be smoothed with a bone file until no sharp margins exist. Bone filing is followed by copious irrigation of the extraction site and under the periosteum of the flap. While it is important to thoroughly irrigate these areas, it is also important to avoid too much irrigation under pressure so that bone filing are dislodged further under the flap. The irrigation should be gentle yet thorough to lift all bone dust and debris upward and out from under the flap. If bone or loose fragments are not thoroughly removed from under the periosteum, a subperiosteal abscess may present in weeks to months after the extraction.

It should be noted at this time whether adequate hemostasis has been achieved. If not, the source of bleeding should be identified. Local infiltration of lidocaine with epinephrine may help with hemostasis temporarily, but does not provide long term control. In cases where the patient is on anticoagulant medications, or may be non-compliant with post-operative instructions, a thrombotic agent, such as Gelfoam can be place in the extraction site to assist with hemostasis.

Closure should reapproximate natural landmarks. In cases of fully impacted teeth this is simple, because the corner of the distobuccal releasing incision is easily reapproximated to obtain complete closure over the site. In cases where a portion of the crown had erupted, then reapproximate of the flap corner will still leave a large opening at the extraction site. In this case, advancement of the corner of the flap at the distobuccal releasing incision to the distolingual tissues of the second molar will provide closure over the site. The choice of suture material is at the discretion of the operator, but a resorbable material such as chromic gut is an excellent choice, given its time frame for resorption and non-braided structure.

Maxillary third molar impactions

Classification

Maxillary third molar impactions are classified in the same way as mandibular impactions with the exception that there is no classification based on the anterior ramus. Therefore, the classification is limited to the level of the impacted tooth to the level of the occlusal place at the erupted second molar. Unlike mandibular impactions, the angle of maxillary impaction very rarely changes the surgical approach, unless the angulation is very severe. Visibility can be extremely difficult in the maxilla, especially when attempting to visualize a high vertically impacted tooth. The coronoid process moves anteriorly as the jaws open, obscuring visualization and access to the posterior maxilla. As the jaws close, cheek retraction is easier, and the tooth may become visible, but elevation may be difficult because the jaws are fully closed.

Flap design

Flaps in maxillary surgery are designed in exactly the same way as flaps for mandibular surgery. A sulcular incision is created around the second molar and a distobuccal releasing incision allows for superior elevation of the flap. The flap can be extended in a sulcular fashion around the second molar only, or anteriorly to the first molar. In contrast to the mandible, a simple envelope incision without a releasing incision may not, at times, provide enough access for extraction. Some surgeons routinely use an anteriorly based vertical releasing incision sparing the papilla of the second molar tooth. This vertical release allows for easier visualization and access to the mesial aspect of the tooth (Figure 5.16A–D). As in all extraction surgery, a full thickness mucoperiosteal flap should be developed. This can be accomplished with

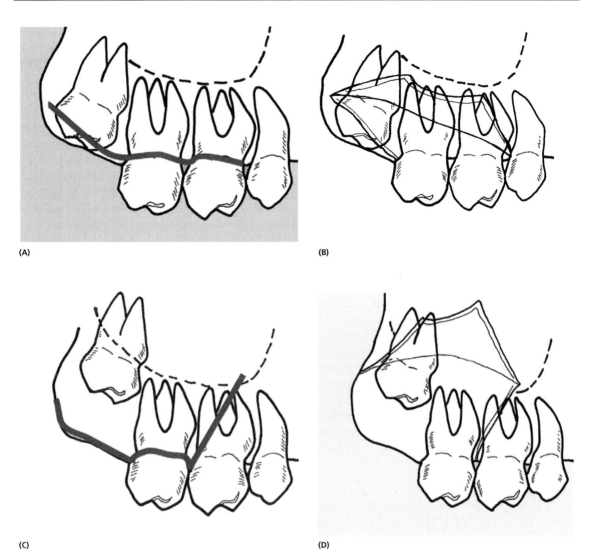

Figure 5.16 (A) Envelope flap showing the extent of the nearly linear incision. (B) When the envelope flap is reflected, this is the access that is achieved. (C) This drawing shows the outline of a typical triangular flap. (D) When the triangular flap is reflected, this is the access that is achieved. It allows greater visibility than the envelope flap.

a #9 Molt periosteal elevator or Woodson elevator. The soft tissues at the palatal aspect of the site should also be gently undermined to prevent tearing of the tissues with delivery of the tooth.

Bone removal

Unlike the mandible, bone removal with a bur is rarely required in the maxilla secondary to the less dense quality of the maxillary bone. Typically, a Woodson #9 Molt elevator can be used to remove

small amounts of buccal bone in order to identify the crown of the impacted third molar. The same instrument can be used to gain access to the mesial aspect of the tooth and create a site for elevator placement. In patients with thicker buccal bone, some practitioners prefer a chisel and mallet to remove bone, but this is relatively uncommon. If rotary instrumentation is necessary, the bur should be placed on the buccal bone and directed posterior to and along the long axis of the second molar in order to expose crown of the impacted third molar and gain access to an elevator to its mesial aspect.

Luxation and delivery

A straight dental elevator can be inserted at the mesiobuccal aspect of the tooth with the point directed towards the patient's opposite ear canal. Alternatively, a Cogswell B, or Bayonet elevator can be used. It is crucially important that forces are not directed superiorly. This can cause dislodgement of the instrument into the sinus. Forces should be directed so that the tooth emerges in a buccal and slightly distal direction (Figure 5.17). This is accomplished with rotation of the straight elevator away from the operator in a counterclockwise direction. If access is difficult with a straight instrument, then a Miller elevator or a dental elevator with an offset handle can be used (such as a California elevator). The Miller elevator is designed to contour around the mesial aspect of the tooth and engage from the palatal aspect to create buccally directed force.

Misdirection of forces can be dangerous during extraction of the maxillary third molar. It is important to prevent displacement of the tooth behind the tuberosity and into the infratemporal fossa. A retractor should be placed just distal to the tuberosity to avoid this complication. Additionally, misdirected forces superiorly may

dislodge the tooth into the sinus, so the operator should maintain direct visualization of the tooth at all times so the vector of forces can be appreciated.

Maxillary third molars typically present with conical shaped root structure. However, various types of root morphology exist. If the tooth has aberrant root morphology that can be discerned preoperatively from the panoramic radiograph, and the tooth is non-carious, the patient should be informed preoperatively that a portion of root may be left in place if the tooth fractures in order to avoid dislodgement into the sinus. Tooth sectioning is generally not necessary for maxillary third molar removal, and can be very difficult secondary to difficult access. If the root morphology is obviously divergent, it may be necessary to section the tooth to accommodate extraction. This can be done by sectioning the tooth into three distinct crowns with root portions, with a centrally located trifurcation on the occlusal surface. Removal of the crown separately from the removal of roots is not advised because access to the roots is limited by difficult visualization.

Distoangular impacted third molars should be identified preoperatively and fracture of the tuberosity should be anticipated. This is because the crown of the impacted tooth undermined the integrity of the tuberosity, and inferiorly directed forces result in fracture. Fracture of

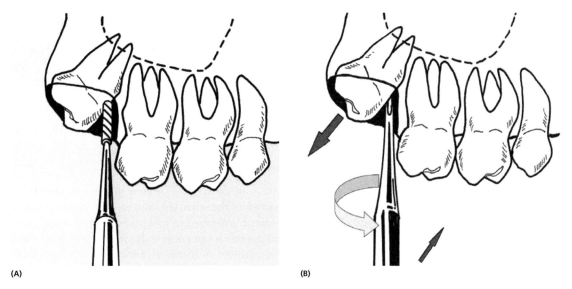

(A)   **(B)**

Figure 5.17 (A) Surgical technique for extraction of maxillary impacted third molars. If the tooth is not visualized once soft tissue has been reflected, bone is removed from the buccal and occlusal aspects. This can be accomplished with hand instruments (such as a periosteal elevator) or with rotary instruments. (B) The tooth is delivered with straight elevators applied on the mesiobuccal with rotational and lever types of motions. The tooth is always delivered in a distobuccal and occlusal direction.

the tuberosity can lead to difficulty with fitting dentures later in life. It can also result in sinus exposure intraoperatively. To prevent fracture, the operator must establish unimpeded pathway for removal. In the case of distoangular impacted tooth, this may include removal of a portion of the tuberosity bone to allow for tooth delivery distobuccally. If a fracture of the tuberosity is noted during luxation, the surgeon should cease luxation, and use a fissure bur to attempt to relieve the tooth from the fractured bone. This will prevent removing a large piece of the tuberosity bone with the tooth. If removing a section of tuberosity is unavoidable, then that segment should be carefully dissected free with a Woodson or periosteal elevator to prevent tearing of the palatal soft tissue upon extraction.

Closure

Closure of maxillary flaps follows the same basic principles as mandibular flaps. The entire contents of the extraction site are curettaged and any follicle is removed. The site is inspected with a dental mirror to ensure that here is no sinus perforation. Any intentionally left root structure should be documented. If any oroantral communication exists, its size should be noted and documented. All sharp bone edges should be bone filed until smooth, and the site and flap should be thoroughly irrigated. The mesial aspect of the flap should be closed first by approximating the papilla. In the case of the partially erupted third molar extraction, there is no need to advance the corner of the distobuccal releasing incision to create complete closure over the site. Gelfoam or any similar local hemostatic agent can be used at the discretion of the operator to provide hemostasis, and a figure-eight suture is usually placed over the Gelfoam for retention. Resorbable, non-braided suture material is an excellent choice.

Postoperative management

Postoperative management begins preoperatively, with a thorough explanation of the typical postoperative course during the consult visit. This explanation should include the anticipated days of pain, anticipated time off from work, and any anticipated limitations, such as a soft diet, and not smoking.

Patients should be advised about postoperative pain. A moderate amount of discomfort is anticipated for 2 to 4 days postoperatively. The level of discomfort increases with increased amount of bone removal and proximity to the inferior alveolar nerve. Ibuprofen is an excellent pain reliever for uncomplicated extractions and also helps in minimizing edema. A narcotic pain medication can be provided if the operator deems it necessary based on the complexity of the extractions. It is important to prescribe the correct amount of narcotic pain medication, if too many days' worth is prescribed, the patient may continue taking the pain medication long after you anticipate that they should no longer need the medication. This can be problematic because symptoms of acute postoperative complications such as infection may be masked by continued use of narcotic pain medication and therefore present at a more advanced stage when the patient runs out of narcotics. Therefore it is prudent to prescribe only the number of days' worth of narcotic pain medication that you anticipate the patient will need; if they require more, then a visit to the office for evaluation is warranted to ensure that there are no complications.

Hemostasis should be achieved prior to closure; however, it is prudent to have the patient bite on gauze upon completion for additional hemostasis postoperatively. The patient can replace this gauze once after 30 minutes, if required. It is important to remind that patient that the gauze will have both saliva and blood on it; this may create the appearance of a large amount of blood-saturated gauze. Remind the patient that as long as the gauze is pink and not saturated with bright red blood, that it is normal. A small amount of blood may be present on the patient's pillow in the morning, and that is also normal.

Instructions should be given to the patient on oral hygiene that include brushing teeth after all meals, and maintaining meticulous oral hygiene in the postoperative period. They should be instructed to avoid brushing directly on the surgical site or on the sutures. On occasion, an irrigation syringe may be provided if the extraction socket is left open. In this case the patient can be instructed on gentle irrigation with warm salt water at the extraction site. The patient should be instructed to avoid smoking, and this should be documented in the chart. The diet should be soft, so that the flap is not damaged by hard pieces of food, and the patient should avoid foods with very small pieces such as sesame seed buns, as these can become trapped in the extracted site and provide a nidus for infection. Spicy food should be avoided in the immediate postoperative period as this can irritate the extraction site tissues. The patient should rinse carefully after all oral intake and avoid any forceful spitting. The use of straws should also be avoided for 48 hours. Spitting can dislodge the blood clot and predispose the patient to alveolar osteitis.

A follow-up appointment should be provided for all patients undergoing surgical extraction of impacted third molars. This can be planned for approximately 1 week postoperatively.

Management of complications

Inevitably complications will occur, and despite excellent surgical technique and planning, many of them are often unavoidable.

Damage to soft tissues

Soft tissue damage may take place at or near the site of extraction, with damage to the surrounding tissues or flap tissues, or further away from the extraction site. Soft tissue damage at the extraction site is usually secondary to trauma caused by over-zealous instrumentation with elevators and forceps. Elevators should be placed in a manner so that luxation does not cause repeated tissue trauma to the papilla or gingival tissues. Additionally, the proper use of a finger rest on the shaft of an elevator will help prevent slipping and tissue puncture. Poor flap design can also result in tissue trauma. The papilla adjacent to the tooth to be extracted should be included in the flap, and retracted away from instrumentation. Forceps should also be placed carefully to avoid their placement on gingival tissue. This is especially true when using cowhorn forceps on mandibular teeth. The lingual aspect may be difficult to visualize and cause trauma to tissues overlying the lingual cortex. Injuries caused by forceps can lead to macerated tissue, or tissue puncture—and both are difficult to repair. In general these types of tissue injuries are best left alone to heal on their own after copious irrigation of the site.

Lacerations to tissue are more straightforward. They can be cause by an aberrant stroke of the #15 blade, or more commonly with poor execution of periosteal elevation around the lingual tissues of the mandibular third molar and the distopalatal tissues around the maxillary third molar. When a firm attachment is not removed between this tissue and the tooth, forceps extraction can tear these tissues resulting in lacerations. In the maxilla, the tissue should be carefully dissected off the tooth, and the laceration should be repaired with non-braided resorbable suture material such as monocryl or chromic gut. In the mandible, tearing of the lingual tissues with forceps extraction can cause injury to the lingual nerve. Any tissue attached to the third molar should be carefully dissected free. Any lacerations should be repaired with 4–0 resorbable suture after copious irrigation.

Injuries to soft tissues can also result from improper retraction. The retractor edge should always contact bone. If flap tissue becomes trapped under the retractor, it can result in maceration or laceration of that portion of the flap. If there is great trauma to the flap, a #15 may be used to remove the traumatized edge to create a new tissue margin for closure. Basic principles of flap creation still apply, and it is important to keep the base of the flap wider than the apex. If after removal of injured tissue, the flap cannot close primarily, a #15 blade can be used gently on the undersurface of the flap to score the periosteum. This allows for increased laxity of the tissues and will often allow enough tissue stretch for primary closure.

Further away from the site of extraction, injuries can occur to the lip and cheeks. Retraction of the lips for a prolonged period of time can cause lip splitting and chapping of the lip commissure. This may be prevented with the use of a petroleum-based balm applied to the commissures preoperatively. If trauma at the lip commissure does occur, it is important to counsel the patient that this injury improves over time, continuous use of petrolatum jelly can provide some relief, and despite the injury appearing worse 2–3 days postoperatively, with increased scabbing at the lip commissures, it generally resolves without scarring. The lips are also a common site for burns. The shank of the handpiece should be shielded from the lip tissue, and care should be taken to ensure that the handpiece does not touch the lip tissue. Burns can be treated with application of Silvedene, and if necessary, referral to a surgeon.

Pain and swelling

Pain should be anticipated after extraction of impacted third molars. The anticipated length of the duration of pain should be predicted by the difficulty of extraction and patient age.[8] An appropriate amount of narcotic pain medication such as hydrocodone-acetaminophen can be provided for approximately 3 days for control of postoperative pain. It is important to avoid giving a prescription for too many tablets that would exceed use for the intended period of time; this is not because there is a likelihood of addiction to narcotics in the postoperative period, but rather because if the patient continues to have pain requiring narcotic pain medication for longer than you anticipate, it is important for them to return to the office for evaluation. Ibuprofen is also an excellent choice for pain medication, and 600 mg orally every 6 hours postoperatively can reduce pain and swelling.

Swelling peaks at approximately 72 hours. In some cases intraoperative steroids are administered to reduce swelling in the early postoperative period. Typical doses rage from 4 to 10 mg IV dexamethasone. If there is severe postoperative swelling, the patient may experience trismus. The application of ice packs postoperatively may be palliative, but does not decrease swelling. Swelling usually resolves within 5–7 days. Severe pain or swelling that last longer than anticipated, or begins to worsen after initial improvement, requires evaluation.

Infection

Infection as a result of extraction of third molars is rare and incidence ranges from 1.7 to 2.7%.[9] Acute postoperative infections present with increased pain and swelling at the extraction site and may be suppurative. Symptoms of increased swelling after 72 hours, severe or increasing pain, trismus, extraoral erythema, fever and dysphagia or odynophagia, require evaluation. Treatment of acute infection is establishment of drainage, which can usually be accomplished by removing sutures to open the flap with minimal subperiosteal dissection, and copious irrigation under the flap. The typical oral pathogens are the cause of the postoperative infections so treatment with a penicillin or clindamycin for 7-day course is acceptable. In contrast to acute postoperative infections that present between 4–8 days postoperatively, subperiosteal infections often present later in the postoperative course (generally 4–12 weeks). These are usually caused by debris left under the mucoperiosteal flap. Treatment is incision, drainage, antibiotics for 7 days and re-evaluation until the infection has cleared.

Alveolar osteitis

Alveolar osteitis, also known as dry socket, is generally considered a phenomenon of early lysis or dislodgement of the clot in the extraction site (although the exact mechanism of this pathology remains unknown). The typical presentation occurs at 3–4 days postoperatively with increased pain radiating to the ipsilateral ear and characteristic mal-odor. Unlike acute infection, there is an absence of fever or increased edema. Alveolar osteitis does not typically occur at maxillary sites. Bacteria are all likely contributor to the onset of alveolar osteitis given that pre-operative systemic antibiotics have been shown to decrease incidence.[10] The incidence of dry socket also seems to be high in patients who are female, smoke, and use oral contraceptives.[11,12] Examination of the extraction site will typically reveal exposed bone or open socket with no clot present, together with tenderness to palpation.

Alveolar osteitis is self-limiting, and the goal of treatment is to alleviate pain. The site should be thoroughly irrigated to remove any debris from the extraction site. This is followed by placement of a sedative obtundant dressing, and if necessary the use of pain medication. The dressing typically contains eugenol, and needs to be changed daily until the symptoms are fully resolved which is usually within 1 week. A number of commercially available obtundant preparations exist. A small strip of gauze conservatively covered with one of these preparations should be placed inside the affected socket. Placement of the dressing may be painful but pain typically resolves within minutes of placing the dressing. Local anesthetic can be used at the operator's discretion.

Bleeding

Mild postoperative bleeding can be expected for up to 48 hours. The patient should be advised that it is normal to have a small amount of diminishing oozing from the site during the first 48 hours, and that even a small amount blood mixed with saliva can have the appearance of a large amount of bleeding. Concern should not arise unless the patient is saturating gauze with dark or bright red blood. Postoperative bleeding beyond 48 hours should be evaluated. It is often the result of direct trauma to the tissues by brushing or mastication. If no obvious source of bleeding is determined, a medical evaluation should be completed for possible underlying coagulopathy. Prolonged bleeding beyond 72 hours postoperatively, even if mild, can be dangerous. Decreasing hemoglobin levels in a patient with coronary artery disease can increase cardiac work load and therefore predispose a patient to myocardial oxygen insufficiency.

Postoperative bleeding is controlled similarly to intra-operative bleeding. The site should be irrigated and explored to examine for an obvious source. Direct pressure is the mainstay of bleeding control, and direct pressure by biting on gauze or finger pressure may provide adequate hemostasis, or enough temporary hemostasis to determine the source of bleeding. Infiltration of local anesthetic with epinephrine will also provide temporary hemostasis. For the patient who calls in with continued bleeding, they can be advised to apply direct pressure with gauze or bite on a black tea bag (the tannin in the tea has some hemostatic properties). In the office, local hemostatic agents such as Gelfoam (absorbable gelatin sponge), Surgicel (regenerated oxidized cellulose), and topical thrombin can be used at the site. Sutures can also be used to control bleeding, and, tight tissue reapproximation, and contact with underlying bone often provides adequate hemostasis.

Patients who have systemic medical conditions that predispose bleeding or are taking medication that prevents adequate hemostasis should be identified preoperatively. If taking warfarin, an international normalized ratio should be checked with in 24 to 48 hours preoperatively. Alternatively, a low-molecular-weight heparin bridge (Lovenox) can be used to maintain adequate anticoagulation in the perioperative period. This author does not endorse discontinuation of Plavix or aspirin therapy preoperatively, but if the operator deems this necessary, a discussion with the patient's prescribing provider is required. Patients on anticoagulant therapy may require more surgical intervention to control post-operative bleeding—such as the use of electrocautery or exploration in the operating room.

Damage to adjacent teeth

The possibility of damage to adjacent teeth should be explained to the patient at the preoperative consult appointment. Damage may occur at the time of surgery, or later in the postoperative course. During the operation adjacent teeth may become luxated and mobile. Highly carious teeth may be fractured, and adjacent restorations may become dislodged. Prevention of these injuries starts with identification of the risks. The operator should not place a straight elevator next to an adjacent periodontally compromised tooth, deeply carious tooth or tooth treated with a crown. In each of these situations, there is high risk for damage to that adjacent

tooth, and a different approach to tooth extraction should be considered, such as forceps extraction, or tooth sectioning to decrease the necessary applied force for extraction. The patient should be notified if there is any obvious damage to the adjacent tooth, or if future damage is anticipated, as in the event of bone removal that may compromise the periodontal health of the adjacent tooth. All of these incidents should be included in the chart, as well as a notation that the complication was explained to the patient.

Nerve dysfunction

Nerve dysfunction of the inferior alveolar nerve or lingual nerve in the form of hypoesthesia, paresthesia, or dysesthesia, occurs in approximately 3% of patients undergoing extraction of impacted third molars.[13] This risk should be carefully explained at the preoperative consult appointment and should include a description of the anatomy affected by these nerves. In the case of inferior alveolar nerve injury, numbness of the ipsilateral lip and chin can be seen. For lingual nerve injuries there can be numbness or dysesthesia of the ipsilateral tongue, as well as dysguesia. Radiographic signs that are highly correlated with increased risk of inferior alveolar nerve injury are diversion of the path of the canal, darkening of the root tip at the radiographic canal, and interruption of the canal.[14]

All patients undergoing surgical removal of impacted third molars should receive a follow-up appointment approximately 1 week postoperatively. At that time, nerve function should be evaluated. If a sensory deficit exists, the area of deficit should be clearly charted and followed on a biweekly or monthly basis. A referral should be made to an oral and maxillofacial surgeon specializing in nerve repair is recommended for all nerve injuries. At 9 months to 1 year postoperatively, any remaining nerve deficit is likely permanent. Treatment and thorough evaluation of nerve injuries is beyond the scope of this text.

Displacement of teeth or roots

Dislodgement of teeth or root fragments is multifactorial and can occur in the maxilla or mandible. In the mandible, teeth can be dislodged into the floor of the mouth or inferior alveolar canal. This is usually the result of lingually directed force pushing the tooth or root through the thin lingual cortical plate. If this occurs, extraoral finger pressure should be used to push upward onto the floor of the mouth along the lingual aspect of the mandible and re-present the tooth into the extraction site. While this maneuver risks injury to the lingual nerve, an attempt should still be made at retrieval. The patient should also be carefully monitored for floor of mouth bleeding or hematoma formation postoperatively.

Maxillary teeth can be dislodged into the maxillary sinus or into the infratemporal space. This is because there is very thin bone surrounding a deeply impacted third molar separating it from the maxillary sinus or infratemporal space posterosuperiorly. To prevent dislodgement into the infratemporal space, a retractor should be placed at the tuberosity and extraction forces should be directed buccally and inferiorly. The same is true for prevention of displacement into the maxillary sinus. Even small forces that are misdirected can lead to this type of dislodgement. If a small root tip remains after extraction of the bulk of a maxillary tooth, consideration should be given to leaving the root tip. If the tooth is non-carious then this may be the prudent choice in order to avoid dislodgement. If the tooth becomes no longer visible during an extraction, and there is suspicion that the tooth was dislodged into the maxillary sinus or infratemporal fossa, the practitioner should gain access and visualization prior to making any further efforts to remove the tooth. If the tooth is dislodged into the infratemporal fossa, an attempt can be made at retrieval by placing inferior finger pressure high at the posterior aspect of the maxillary vestibule near the pterygoid plates. If this is unsuccessful, the tooth should be left in place to re-address after fibrosis has occurred in approximately 4 weeks. Referral to an oral and maxillofacial surgeon is necessary. The tooth will be removed in the operating room under general anesthesia after localization with CT scan.

For a tooth or tooth root displaced into the maxillary sinus, an initial attempt at retrieval can be made with a Fraser tip or yankauer suction. If neither of these is successful, a panoramic radiograph or in-office CT scan can help localize the tooth, and a Caldwell–Luc procedure can performed by a specialist to remove the tooth. The surgical technique for Caldwell–Luc is beyond the scope of this text.

If referral is necessary, the patient should be informed and be placed on sinus precautions. The instructions should be given to the patient verbally and in writing and should include: complete abstinence from smoking, no use of straws, sneezing should occur with the mouth open, the patient should not attempt to blow his nose. An antibiotic that covers typical sinus pathogens, such as amoxicillin or cephalexin, should be prescribed for 7–10 days. Pseudoephedrine or similar oral systemic decongestant should be used as an adjunct to keep the sinus mucosa dry and help prevent infection; typical doses are 30 mg orally two to four times daily.

A tooth or tooth fragment may be dislodged into the patient's posterior oropharynx. In this situation the patient should be placed in the Reverse-Trendelenberg position and encouraged to cough while using yankauer suction at the posterior oropharynx. If this unsuccessful, and the patient continues coughing or experiences difficulty breathing, there should be high suspicion that the tooth has dislodged into the airway, and EMS should be called immediately. If the patient does not experience coughing or breathing difficulty, the tooth may have been swallowed. In this case the patient should be referred to the emergency department for chest and abdominal radiographs.

Oroantral communication

The sinus lining is, in many instances, closely positioned next to the roots of the maxillary teeth. This anatomy can sometimes be visualized preoperatively on the panoramic radiograph. In cases where the sinus is in close contact with the roots of the third molar, the patient should be notified beforehand that there is a risk of oroantral communication that may be unavoidable. If at the time of extraction an oroantral communication is suspected, the operator should seek to determine if one exists first by direct visualization, then very gentle probing with a periodontal probe in the extraction site to feel the bone walls superiorly. If neither of these techniques reveals a communication, then a dental mirror should be placed for view of the extraction site, while the patient's nares are squeezed closed, the patient should be instructed to blow gently through the nose. Bubbles from the extraction site or condensation on the mirror indicates that an oroantral fistula exists. If the fistula is less than 5 mm in greatest diameter, then Gelfoam can be placed into the site to occlude the fistula and a figure of eight suture should be placed for retention. The patient should be placed on standard sinus precautions as noted above in the tooth displacement section. If the size of the fistula is greater than 5 mm, then the patient should be referred to an oral and maxillofacial surgeon for evaluation and definitive closure. The operator should still use Gelfoam in the site and a figure-eight suture. An attempt should be made to primarily close the site by scoring the periosteum of the flap.

Jaw fracture

Jaw fracture is uncommon in third molar surgery but is a known risk that should be reviewed at the preoperative visit as part of the informed consent process. Factors that may predispose to this include findings on a preoperative panoramic radiograph like a deep impaction with very little bulk at the inferior border, an atrophic mandible, or cyst associated with the impacted tooth causing a bony defect. In these cases pre-operative planning is critically important. Sectioning the tooth as well as a judicious amount of bone removal may be required while avoiding excessive extraction forces.

If jaw fracture is suspected intraoperatively, the procedure should be aborted unless the tooth can be easily removed. A panoramic radiograph is required to document the location and displacement of the fracture. The patient needs referral to an oral and maxillofacial surgeon for evaluation and possible repair. The patient should be placed on a full liquid diet and instructed not to chew anything. An antibiotic such as penicillin should be prescribed for 1 week duration, and the patient should be instructed to use chlorhexidine rinses. Narcotic pain medication will likely be necessary for pain control. If possible at the time of fracture the patient should be placed into maxillomandibular fixation with Ivy loops or Erich arch bars.

Delayed mandible fractures often occur 2–4 weeks postoperatively and are more common than intraoperative fractures. This is because bony remodeling includes osteoclastic activity which further weakens bone. Generally, 2–4 weeks after extraction, the patient feels well enough to resume a regular diet, however, the bone is not fully healed, and in a patient where risk factors for fracture have been identified, this is the most risky time. These patient should be instructed postoperatively what to avoid and remain on a pureed diet for 6 weeks. The patient with a postoperative fracture will complain of increased pain and edema, and sometimes will report an incident where they felt a "pop," usually during chewing. Examination will often reveal malocclusion and trismus.

These patients should be given the same instructions and medications as noted above for intraoperative fractures and also be referred to an oral and maxillofacial surgeon for definitive treatment.[15]

Acknowledgment

The author would also like to thank Dr. Pushkar Mehra and Dr. Shant Baran for their work on the previous edition of this chapter, and whose contributions are still contained in the current text.

References

1. White RP, Fisher EL, Phillips C, Tucker M, Moss K, Offenbacher S. Visible third molars as a risk indicator for increased periodontal probing depth. *Journal of Oral and Maxillofacial Surgery*. 2011; 69(1): 92–103.
2. Divaris K, Fisher E, Shugars D, White RP. Risk factors for third molar occlusal caries: a longitudinal clinical investigation. *Journal of Oral and Maxillofacial Surgery*. 2012; 70: 1771–80.
3. Nitzan D, Keren T, Marmary Y. Does an impacted tooth cause root resorption of the adjacent one? *Oral Surgery*. 1981; 51: 221–4.
4. Guven O, Keskin A, Akal UK. The incidence of cysts and tumors around impacted 3rd molars. *International Journal of Oral and Maxillofacial Surgery*. 2000; 20: 131–5.
5. Venta I, Turtola I, Ylipaavalniemi P. Radiographic follow-up of impacted mandibular third molars from age 2–32 year. *Interantional Journal of Oral and Maxillofacial Surgery*. 2001; 30: 54–7.
6. Koumaras G, What are the costs associated with management of third molars? *Journal of Oral and Maxillofacial Surgery*. 2012; 70: 8–10 suppl 1.
7. Kiesselbach JE, Chamberlain JG. Clinical and anatomic observations on the relationship of the lingual nerve to the mandibular third molar region. *Journal of Oral and Maxillofacial Surgery*. 1984; 41: 565.
8. Phillips C, White RP Jr, Shugars DA, Zhou X. Risk factors associated with prolonged recovery and delayed healing after third molar surgery. *Journal of Oral and Maxillofacial Surgery*. 61: 1436–48.
9. Miloro M (ed.). *Peterson's Principles of Oral and Maxillofacial Surgery*, 2nd edn. Decker Inc., Hamilton, Ontario BC, 2004.
10. Ren YF, Malmstrom H. Effectiveness of antibiotic prophylaxis in third molar surgery: a meta-analysis of randomized controlled clinical trials. *Journal of Oral and Maxillofacial Surgery*. 65: 1909–21.

11. Nitzan DNW. On the genesis of 'dry-socket'. *Journal of Oral and Maxillofacial Surgery*. 1983; 21: 226–31.
12. Sweet JB, Butler DP. The relationship of smoking to localized osteitis. *Journal of Oral Surgery*. 1979; 37: 732–5.
13. Bataineh BA. Sensory nerve impairment following mandibular third molar surgery. *Journal of Oral and Maxillofacial Surgery*. 2001; 59(9): 1012–7.
14. Blaeser BF, August MA, Donoff RB, *et al*. Panoramic radiographic risk factors for inferior alveolar nerve injury after 3rd molar extraction. *Journal of Oral and Maxillofacial Surgery*. 2003; 61: 417–21.
15. Koerner K (ed.). *Manual of Minor Oral Surgery for the General Dentist*. Blackwell Munskgaard, Ames IA, 2006.

CHAPTER 6

Pre-prosthetic Oral Surgery

Antonia Kolokythas, Jason Jamali, and Michael Miloro
Department of Oral and Maxillofacial Surgery, University of Illinois at Chicago, Chicago, IL, USA

Introduction

At the present time, and despite the current knowledge and advances in dental care, a significant portion of the population is in need of prosthetic dental rehabilitation, either due to partial or complete edentulism. When evaluating a patient for pre-prosthetic surgery, several factors should be considered before formulation of a treatment plan that will be successful in the long term. Among these are: the etiology of the edentulism (e.g., poor oral hygiene, dental neglect, poor oral health care instruction, physical limitations); the type of edentulism (partial or complete); the associated functional and cosmetic deficits and, more importantly, their significance to the patient; and the presence of systemic health conditions, as well as local etiologies that may play a role in, or are key contributors to, the current oral-dental condition.

Alveolar bone loss is a natural sequence of the aging process and tooth loss, which occurs with variable rates in both the upper and lower jaw among individuals. The rate of bone loss depends on local factors such as the upper or lower jaw, peri-extraction events (simultaneous alveoplasty or simple "atraumatic" tooth removal), the presence of opposing teeth and their periodontal status, the use of denture prostheses as well as systemic conditions, such as endocrine dysfunction, or bone homeostasis or nutritional imbalances. The loss of alveolar bone will eventually adversely affect the stability and retention of a removable prosthesis, the health and appearance of surrounding soft tissues, and the interocclusal distance (vertical dimension of occlusion [VDO]), leading to functional and esthetic compromises. Therefore, the main objective of any pre-prosthetic

surgery is to create, or in some cases recreate, support structures (including both the hard and soft tissues) that will allow for placement of a functional, comfortable, and esthetic prosthetic appliance. The practitioner involved in the care of the edentulous patient should be familiar with the indications, advantages, disadvantages, and limitations of the commonly used pre-prosthetic surgical procedures.

Patient evaluation and treatment planning

The initial patient evaluation is critical in assessing the "chief complaint," the main reason(s) why the patient is seeking consultation, so the treatment plan can be tailored accordingly to address the patient's concern(s). A detailed medical history should be obtained as well as a list of all prescription and over-the-counter (OTC) medications that the patient is currently taking. Any medication allergies or reactions should be documented as well as information regarding previous surgical procedures (non-dental and dental) and relevant perioperative or postoperative complications with emphasis on bleeding, infection, and wound healing problems. A social history should be obtained, with emphasis on the use of tobacco (in pack-years) as well as smokeless tobacco, alcohol, and illicit drugs. A detailed dental history with emphasis on the etiology of tooth loss, history of trauma to the facial skeleton and/or dental structures, as well as previous and current dental rehabilitation success or failure treatments is a critical component of the history of

Manual of Minor Oral Surgery for the General Dentist, Second Edition. Edited by Pushkar Mehra and Richard D'Innocenzo.
© 2016 John Wiley & Sons, Inc. Published 2016 by John Wiley & Sons, Inc.

the present illness. A consultation with the patient's primary care provider should be sought when deemed necessary or when questions and concerns about the overall health status of the patient arise based on the medical history and physical examination.

Close communication between the health care providers involved in the dental rehabilitation of the edentulous patient is mandatory so that the most predictable treatment plan may be formulated. The patient's wishes and expectations should be carefully considered, all concerns should be addressed before determination of the final treatment plan, and adjustments should be made as deemed necessary. The goal of treatment remains the provision of a functional and esthetically pleasing dental prosthesis. Specifically, pre-prosthetic surgery aims to achieve the goals shown in Table 6.1.

As with all dental patients, a thorough head and neck examination should be performed that includes palpation of the cervical lymph nodes and thyroid gland with emphasis on evaluation for (pathologic) enlargement, asymmetries, or the presence of any "lumps" or irregularities. Palpation of the major salivary glands and evaluation of salivary flow, including the quality and quantity of saliva, should be included in the examination, especially in elderly patients and those with systemic conditions or those patients who may be taking medications that may cause xerostomia. Finally, examination of the temporomandibular joint and evaluation for pain, crepitus, subluxation, and dislocation should be done.

Evaluation of maxillomandibular relationships

The relationship of the maxillomandibular complex becomes altered with the atrophy of (alveolar) bone that follows tooth loss. The rate and precise pattern of

bone loss is unique to each individual patient and depends on several local and systemic factors as stated earlier, but the general skeletal appearance is that of mandibular pseudoprognathism (skeletal class III pattern), which is more evident with advanced bone loss. This is manifested as maxillary retrusion with mandibular protrusion due to the resorptive pattern of the jaws, with the maxilla resorbing superiorly and posteriorly, and the mandible resorbing anteriorly and inferiorly (Figure 6.1A–C). Some common oral findings in the completely edentulous patient include mandibular overclosure (loss of VDO), severe anterior maxillary ridge resorption with soft tissue redundancy when the natural opposing anterior mandibular dentition is present (combination syndrome), increased interarch distance in complete edentulism with severe bone resorption, or decreased interarch distance in partial edentulism with opposing teeth and dentoalveolar supereruption. Radiographic examination with either plain films (anteroposterior and lateral cephalometric radiograph), tomograms (panoramic radiograph), or with the current use of office-based three-dimensional imaging with cone beam computed tomography (CBCT), is essential for development of a comprehensive treatment plan. Three-dimensional imaging allows for a comprehensive assessment of maxillomandibular relationships, as well as an evaluation of both hard and soft tissues.

Evaluation of soft tissues

The ideal soft tissue covering the edentulous areas that will be reconstructed with a removable prosthesis should be thick keratinized tissue, free of inflammation, firmly attached to the underlying alveolar ridge. Therefore, examination of the soft tissues should focus on identification of any loose, inflamed, irregular, or excessive soft tissue on the alveolar ridge, at the depth of the maxillary or mandibular vestibule, or on the palate or below the tongue. These findings are very common under ill-fitting dentures and interfere with stability of the prosthesis (Figures 6.2 and 6.3). The presence of frenum (labial and lingual) and muscle (mylohyoid, genioglossus) attachments on the residual alveolar bone require careful examination because they may contribute to displacement of the prosthesis or loss of a denture seal.

Table 6.1 Goals of pre-prosthetic surgery

Provide a bony foundation for the prosthesis
Eliminate hard and soft tissue pathology
Provide proper interarch relationships
Achieve properly contoured alveolar ridges (tall, broad, u-shaped)
Eliminate bony and soft tissue undercuts and protuberances
Ensure adequate keratinized attached gingiva in denture-bearing areas
Ensure adequate vestibular depth
Plan for possible dental implants

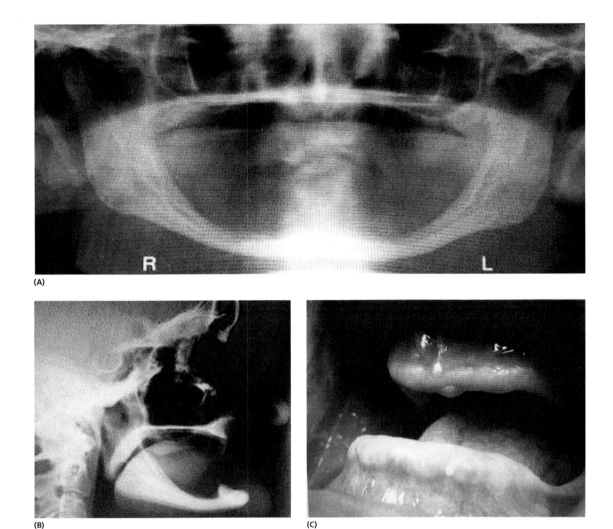

Figure 6.1 (A) Panoramic radiograph of an edentulous patient showing severe mandibular atrophy. (B) Lateral cephalometric radiograph demonstrating a Class III skeletal pattern in an edentulous patient. (C) Clinical intraoral photograph of an edentulous patient demonstrating a Class III skeletal pattern of bone resorption.

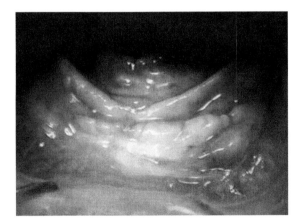

Figure 6.2 Epulis fissuratum.

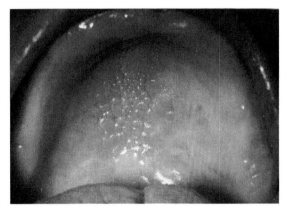

Figure 6.3 Inflammatory papillary hyperplasia of the palate.

Evaluation of hard tissues

The remaining alveolar ridge should be assessed by visual inspection and tactile examination for the presence of irregularities, such as undercuts or sharp bony edges, and prominent canine eminences that will interfere with the function of the prosthesis due to trauma to overlying soft tissues and resultant pain and inflammation. Exostoses and tori may interfere with the insertion of a denture prosthesis or cause trauma to the thin overlying soft tissues when the prosthesis is used. A decrease in the interocclusal clearance due to maxillary tuberosity enlargement will prevent the appropriate denture flange extension necessary to create the soft palate seal or may cause denture displacement (Figure 6.4).

Armamentarium

As with every surgical procedure, appropriate instrumentation is required to execute the necessary steps properly. A basic surgical instrument tray that includes the following instruments should be available for pre-prosthetic surgical procedures: a blade(s) (#15) and blade handle(s), a periosteal elevator, tongue and cheek retractors, end- and side-cutting ronguers, a bone file, tissue forceps, needle holders, and tissue and suture scissors. If extraction of teeth is planned at the time of the pre-prosthetic surgical procedure, appropriate

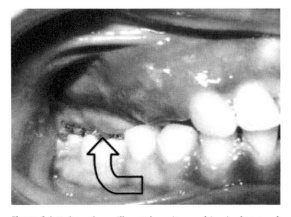

Figure 6.4 Enlarged maxillary tuberosity resulting in decreased interocclusal space and thus inadequate space to restore the edentulous span. The arrow in the picture shows a severe loss of inter-ridge distance. There is no space to restore the edentulous span.

dental elevators and forceps should be included in the surgical tray. A slow-speed handpiece with appropriate burs (large round, oval, and cross-cut fissure burs) should be readily available as well as a method of providing irrigation during the drilling process. Cooled normal saline solution irrigation is important during the use of rotary instruments to maintain bone temperature below 47°C and avoid bony necrosis, and to remove debris and bone dust at the conclusion of the procedure and before wound closure in order to minimize postoperative wound complications.

Hard tissue (bone) surgery

Alveolar ridge recontouring

The main objective of these hard tissue procedures is to recontour the alveolar ridges and remove any bony irregularities that will interfere with insertion, retention, and/or function of the final denture prosthesis. The following procedures are included in this category.

Alveoplasty with extractions/alveoplasty of the edentulous ridge

Extraction of teeth and immediate placement of a denture prosthesis is highly desirable as this saves the patient from doing without a prosthesis. This approach allows for minimal alterations of dietary intake and more importantly eliminates the social and esthetic concerns of edentulism. The treating team should carefully coordinate the sequence of appointments to allow for all necessary procedures to be performed and appropriate timely follow-up visits to be planned. The specific steps for immediate denture fabrication and the proper extraction sequence for immediate rehabilitation is beyond the scope of this chapter.

The alveolar ridges are examined before the extractions, and the areas that will require recontouring or that will interfere with insertion of the denture prosthesis are marked on the dental casts. These dental casts should be available at the time of surgery for perioperative consultation and accurate execution of the treatment plan. It must be emphasized that conservative bone recontouring should be performed to avoid over-reduction of the ridges and future issues with poor denture fit. The physiologic bone resorption that follows extractions should be taken into consideration as well as the need for future denture relining of the immediate prosthesis.

Profound anesthesia for the proposed extractions and immediate alveoplasty is achieved with a combination of nerve blocks and infiltration to cover the entire surgical field while remaining aware of the maximum local anesthetic dosage limitations. Infiltration of a local anesthetic with a vasoconstrictor may facilitate soft tissue flap elevation via hydrodissection and will also assist with hemostasis. Sulcular incisions around the necks of the teeth and alveolar crestal incisions in keratinized tissue in edentulous regions are performed with a #15 blade before the dental extractions. Releasing incisions are planned and placed when necessary to avoid tearing the mucosa upon flap elevation or during tooth extractions or bone reduction, and full thickness mucoperiosteal flaps are elevated in a subperiosteal plane. The periosteum is protected to prevent wound-healing problems (dehiscence) and minimize postoperative edema. Flap elevation should be kept to a minimum depth toward the vestibule, the floor of mouth, or palate, to allow adequate access for execution of the proposed bony reduction and avoid excessive flap reflection that will add to postoperative discomfort and wound-healing problems. Extending the incisions into the depths of the vestibule would also involve the muscles used for facial expressions, which, when activated postoperatively, could lead to flap dehiscence. Iatrogenic flap tears should be avoided with careful surgical technique, planning, and appropriate use of surgical instruments. Flap tears (or buttonholes) will also contribute to postoperative discomfort and wound-healing delays, and may lead to wound dehiscence. Once retracted, the mucosal flaps are protected during the remaining portions of the surgical procedure with appropriate instruments, such as a Seldin, Austin, or Minnesota retractor. It is advisable to protect the patient's lips and cheeks throughout the procedure, and self-retaining lip/cheek retractors offer excellent protection, access, and visibility, and should be included in the armamentarium (Figure 6.5).

The extractions are performed next, as atraumatically as possible to avoid tearing of the mucosa or inducing fractures of the buccal or lingual alveolar plates. Bone recontouring with hand-held instruments, such as end- or side-cutting ronguers and bone files (Figure 6.6), or rotary instruments, such as large round or oval burs on a handpiece under copious irrigation, is performed next, addressing the areas previously marked on the dental casts. After all planned irregularities are contoured, the

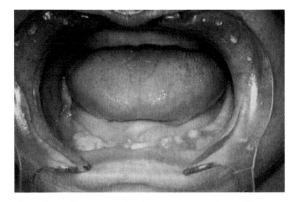

Figure 6.5 Self-retaining cheek retractors provide excellent access and visibility for pre-prosthetic surgery.

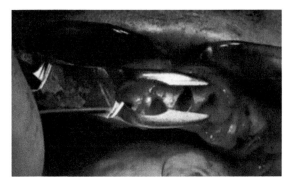

Figure 6.6 Following extraction(s), a side-cutting ronguer is used to remove sharp bone edges to relieve undercuts on the labial and buccal surfaces. A bone file may be subsequently used to smooth out any bony irregularities.

mucosal flap is repositioned over the bone, and the alveolar ridge is palpated for any remaining sharp bony edges; these are then reduced as necessary. A clear stent fabricated on a stone cast on which the bony irregularities are removed can be very helpful at this stage to ensure that all irregularities are adequately treated and to help detect areas that require additional bony reduction. At the completion of the procedure, copious amounts of normal saline are irrigated under all reflected flaps to ensure removal of any bone dust and other debris to prevent postoperative infection. Any areas of bleeding should also be controlled to prevent a postoperative hematoma that could result in flap dehiscence and/or wound infection.

After bone reduction, excess soft tissues may be present in some areas and will require conservative trimming at this point. The dental papillae are trimmed as well or alternatively may be used to achieve primary closure over the extraction sockets if they are not excessively long. Care should be taken to preserve as much keratinized tissue as possible as a future denture base. The immediate denture is inserted, and the patient is usually instructed not to remove the denture until the follow-up appointment with the restorative dentist within 24 to 48 hours after the procedure. It is important to check at the time of the insertion for gross interferences or areas of pressure from the denture flanges that will interfere with stability or cause trauma to the tissues as these issues require immediate correction. The immediate denture will serve as a pressure dressing to limit edema and also prevent hematoma formation, but some postoperative edema will invariably occur and may result in an unpleasant sensation for the patient for the first few days; this may make removal of the immediate denture difficult if there are undercuts and extensive edema has occurred. It is helpful to communicate this information to both the patient and the restorative dentist, and it may be best for the surgeon to see the patient in 3 to 5 days for removal of the immediate denture and assessment of the surgical site(s).

The main difference between the above described procedure (alveoplasty with extractions) and alveoplasty in edentulous areas, is, of course, the dental extractions. All other steps are performed in a similar manner. When teeth have been removed well in advance of the alveoplasty procedure, usually several weeks before, the physiologic alveolar bone resorption is near complete, and areas of irregularity may require more aggressive reduction. Because no teeth are remaining at this time, all incisions are planned in a mid-crestal location in attached keratinized tissue. It is critical to ensure that keratinized tissue is retained on either side of the incision to assist with wound closure and limit wound-healing complications. Keratinized tissue may be limited, especially in cases of prolonged edentulism or denture use, and various vestibuloplasty techniques may be considered to increase attached tissue.

Interseptal alveoplasty is a procedure that involves the removal of the interseptal bone only at the time of dental extraction(s). For this procedure to be considered, the height of the alveolar ridge should be adequate. The soft tissues are retained on the bone, no flaps are elevated, and the teeth are extracted as atraumatically as possible. Following the extraction(s), the interseptal bone is removed with a ronguer, and the alveolar process is

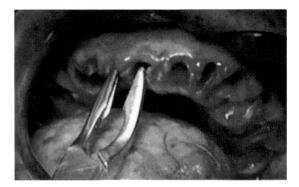

Figure 6.7 If an interseptal alveoloplasty is planned, an end-cutting rongeur is used to remove the interradicular bony septum. The labial/buccal cortical plates are then compressed manually to remove undercuts.

compressed with manual digital pressure (Figure 6.7). The main, clear disadvantage of this technique is the reduction of the alveolar width that may actually prevent denture accommodation and interfere with future dental implant rehabilitation. This approach, however, may be needed in selected areas of excess alveolar width, such as the maxillary molar region when extensively divergent roots are present, because it allows for preservation of the buccal plate.

Soft tissue closure after alveoplasty procedures is best performed with slowly resorbable sutures (chromic gut or Vicryl) that are placed in a running interlocking fashion. This method avoids the presence of multiple knots under the denture and is less irritating for the patient during the postoperative healing period.

Maxillary bony tuberosity reduction

Excessive height and width of the maxillary tuberosity may interfere with denture insertion, stability, and function and often requires appropriate reduction before denture fabrication. Both the hard and soft tissues of the tuberosity may contribute to this excess, and it is important to determine which component should be addressed. Often, both hard and soft tissue reduction is needed to varying degrees. Radiographic examination of the area with a panoramic radiograph is important to evaluate the extent of the maxillary sinus in the area. Often the sinus is pneumatized extensively and may even extend into the hard tissue tuberosity region. In such cases, the surgeon should be prepared to manage an oroantral communication that may occur at the time of the tuberosity reduction.

The technique for reduction of a maxillary bony tuberosity begins after infiltration of a local anesthetic solution with a vasoconstrictor via blocks (posterior superior alveolar and descending palatine blocks) and infiltration, and a full-thickness mid-crestal incision is made to the bone with a #15 blade on the alveolar ridge over the hypertrophic tuberosity. The local anesthetic can be used before the incision for hydrodissection, although the tissues in this area are usually thick enough and elevation of flaps is usually not problematic, with little chance of flap tearing. Releasing incisions may be required, but care should be taken to adequately extend the crestal incision anteriorly and posteriorly in order to avoid tearing the mucosal flaps. Full thickness mucoperiosteal flaps are elevated buccally and palatally enough to expose the portion of the bony tuberosity that requires surgical reduction. A stone model with the area requiring reduction marked on it and a clear stent fabricated on a stone model with the tuberosity reduced are very helpful perioperatively to ensure adequate reduction of the bone is achieved, based on the prosthesis plan. Either hand-held instruments, side- or end-cutting ronguers, and bone files or rotary instruments (large round or oval burs on a slow-speed handpiece under copious irrigation) can be used for the actual reduction of the bone. It is important to protect the soft tissues while using rotary instruments with appropriate retractors (Seldin or Minnesota retractors) to avoid accidental injury and tears that will interfere with wound healing. Conservative bone removal and perioperative use of a clear stent or evaluation of the stone model, if available, are key to adequate tuberosity reduction and to avoid over-reduction. After the bone reduction is completed, the surgical wound is irrigated thoroughly and the buccal and palatal soft tissues are re-draped over the bone so any sharp or irregular bony edges can be detected on palpation. The soft tissues in the area will require some degree of trimming after bony tuberosity reduction, and this can be done with simple excision of the excess tissue with a scalpel or scissors upon re-approximation of the flaps. Wound closure is performed with resorbable sutures in a locking fashion similar to that used in the alveoplasty procedure. Figure 6.8(A–F) depicts the steps involved in maxillary tuberosity reductions while Figure 6.4 and Figure 6.8G show a clinical case with pre-operative and postoperative photos.

Buccal–palatal exostosis and undercut correction

Often following extractions after physiologic bone remodeling has occurred, irregularities such as exostosis or undercuts remain on the buccal surface of the remaining alveolar ridges and may interfere with insertion of a removable denture prosthesis. Conversely, buccal and/or palatal exostoses that are not the result of irregular bone resorption after extractions may be present in a significant percentage of the population (Figure 6.9). The etiology of this excessive bone formation is not clearly understood; it is thought to be multifactorial, including habits such as bruxism, but these habits occur more commonly in women than men. The exostoses are more commonly found in the maxilla than the mandible, and in the maxilla they may occupy more extensive regions of the jaw. A midline maxillary exostosis is a torus palatinus. Exostoses are often found on the palatal aspect of the maxillary alveolus as well, while on the lingual aspect of the mandible they usually represent, or are associated with, mandibular lingual tori. In any case, the overlying tissue covering the excess bone is usually very thin, with the exception of the palatal tissue that is inherently thick toward the alveolar ridge.

When intervention is needed, usually to facilitate insertion of the denture prosthesis, perhaps the most important part of the surgery is to avoid trauma to the thin overlying tissue. Hydrodissection when infiltrating with a local anesthetic solution over the area of the exostosis will assist with flap elevation in addition to patient comfort and surgical site hemostasis. It is important to keep in mind that the local anesthetic solution should be administered close to the bone in a subperiosteal plane for effective hydrodissection. Deposition of the anesthetic solution close to bone is very painful so regional anesthesia should be administered before this procedure.

The incision design is based on the presence or absence of teeth similar to the alveoplasty procedure. Sulcular incisions in dentate areas and mid-crestal incisions in edentulous regions are carried out with a #15 blade and extended well beyond the length of the exostosis. As a general rule, the incisions should extend one to two teeth or 1.0–1.5 cm beyond the anteroposterior extent of the exostosis. In cases of large, wide exostoses, these distances may need to be

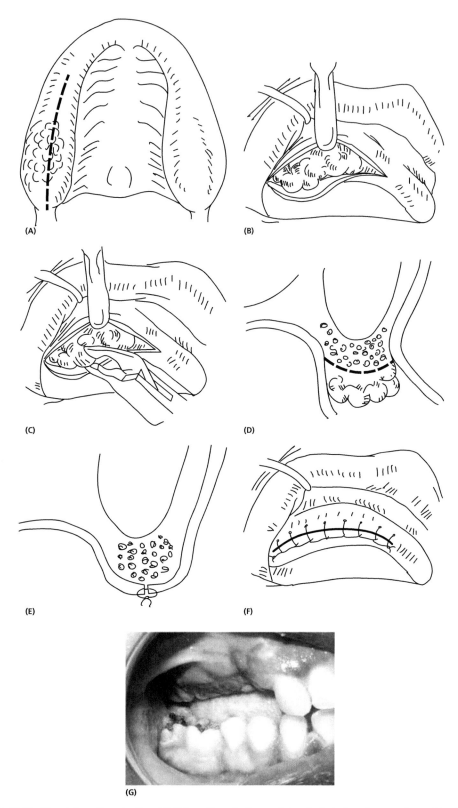

Figure 6.8 (A–F) Maxillary tuberosity reduction. (G) Tuberosity reduction and alveoloplasty have been performed to obtain an adequate inter-arch distance.

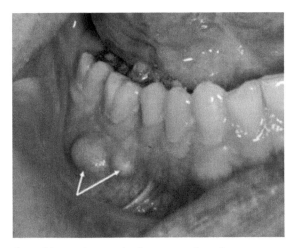

Figure 6.9 Buccal exostosis. The arrows point to bony exostoses. Exostoses are usually found buccally, in contrast to tori, which are located lingually.

increased, or releasing incisions may be required, to avoid tension and potential tears of the mucosal flaps. The soft tissue flaps are elevated beyond the occlusal-apical extent of the exostosis for several millimeters to ensure adequate exposure, and, again, to avoid damage to the tissues at the "base" of the exostosis. Rongeurs, bone files, or a bur on a slow-speed hand-piece may be used for the actual bone removal. Occasionally, sharp chisels and a mallet can be used for buccal exostosis removal in select cases, but caution should be exercised, especially for the novice surgeon, to avoid causing trauma to the surrounding soft tissues and structures (e.g., vessels, nerves, teeth). Careful palpation of the area over the mucosa to ensure smooth underlying bone is performed before wound closure with resorbable sutures in a running interlocking fashion.

Tori reduction

The presence of maxillary (palatal) and mandibular (lingual) tori may interfere significantly with the fabrication, retention, and function of a removable denture prosthesis, and surgical reduction procedures for tori are commonly performed. Another reason for removal of tori is that the soft tissue mucosa covering the tori, especially the maxillary torus, is often very thin and easily traumatized during mastication.

Maxillary torus palatinus reduction

Bilateral descending palatine nerve blocks are required for maxillary torus palatinus reduction, along with additional anesthesia administered to the anterior portion of the palate, either with a nasopalatine incisive canal block or local infiltration. Additional infiltration of the overlying mucosa with local anesthetic containing a vasoconstrictor will assist with hemostasis and with flap elevation via hydrodissection. The incision may be a midline incision, directly over the middle of the torus with anterior and posterior vertical releases in a double-Y fashion. Alternatively, palatal degloving can be performed to expose the torus by designing a U-shaped incision with the base posteriorly. Care should be taken when using the latter approach to protect the greater palatine neurovascular bundles as they will provide the blood supply to the U-shaped palatal flap. The incisive neurovascular bundle is sacrificed with this U-shaped design and will not provide blood supply to the palatal flap. Full-thickness mucoperiosteal flaps are elevated with care so as not to create any tears of the soft tissues, especially in areas where it is very thin, as this will increase postoperative discomfort and delay wound healing. The manner in which the torus is reduced largely depends on the size. For a small torus, a large round or oval bur can be used to "smooth down" the bone until it is flat, while for larger tori, serial sectioning with a fine cross-cut fissure bur allows for segmental removal with thin chisels or osteotomes or ronguers. It is extremely important to ensure that the floor of the nose is not violated when the torus palatinus is removed. This is best avoided if curved chisels or osteotomes are used and are directed away from the nasal cavity. Also, it is best to under-reduce the torus with chisels and then finish smoothing irregularities with a bone file or rotary instruments. Copious irrigation during the use of rotary instruments and at the completion of the procedure is important to avoid bone necrosis and wound-healing delays. For maxillary torus palatinus reduction, having a clear stent fabricated on a stone model on which the torus is reduced can help to ensure that adequate reduction is accomplished, and also, the stent can be used postoperatively to help maintain the closure and prevent hematoma formation. After maxillary torus reduction, there will be soft tissue that appears redundant over the area of the torus. It is best not to trim these tissues too aggressively but rather close the incisions with resorbable sutures and place the clear stent over the wound closure. The stent will help eliminate dead space and hematoma formation in this area.

It is important that the stent does not apply any pressure on the surgical site to avoid tissue necrosis. The stent is kept in place for 10 to 14 days, or longer if necessary, for the soft tissues to heal. It is not uncommon to encounter tissue breakdown in the mid-palatal region after torus palatinus reduction. A conservative treatment approach with good oral hygiene, prevention of additional trauma, and the use of a stent will assist with healing and improve patient comfort. Figures 6.10 (A–J) shows the common clinical steps involved in a torus palatinus reduction procedure.

Mandibular lingual torus reduction

Bilateral lingual nerve blocks and additional infiltration along the soft tissues covering the mandibular torus is accomplished with a local anesthetic solution containing a vasoconstrictor. Similar to the soft tissues covering the maxillary palatal torus, the lingual mucosa covering the mandibular torus is exceptionally thin and easily injured. Hydrodissection with injection of the local anesthetic solution in this area is critical to assist with flap elevation. If teeth are present, gingival sulcular incisions are designed, extending at least one to two teeth beyond the torus. In edentulous ridges, a mid-crestal incision, favoring the buccal aspect, is performed with a #15 blade. Incisions placed directly over the torus should be avoided so that the wound closure is not directly over the operative site. It is essential to maintain the lingual frenal attachment at the midline in order to limit postoperative floor of mouth edema that may compromise the airway. As mentioned earlier, when designing incisions over the ridge of the atrophic mandible, the mental nerve should be identified and keratinized tissue should be maintained on either side of the incision to ensure adequate closure and presence of attached tissue for a denture base. Full-thickness mucoperiosteal flaps are elevated until the tori are completely exposed. It is critical to protect the soft tissues of the floor of the mouth throughout the procedure with appropriate retractors (Seldin or Weider) to avoid trauma to the soft tissue flaps and adjacent vital structures. If the tori are relatively small, they can be reduced with burs on a slow-speed handpiece under copious irrigation. For medium-sized tori, a cross-cutting fissure bur is used to outline the occlusal, mesial, and distal aspects of the torus/mandible interface first, and thin chisels of osteotomes are used to sharply remove the bone by "fracturing it off" the mandibular lingual cortex. For larger mandibular tori (Figure 6.11A), sagittal sectioning may be best accomplished first with a thin cross-cutting fissure bur so that removal in smaller sections can be easily performed using chisels or osteotomes. It is important when removing mandibular tori to use curved chisels or osteotomes and place their convex surfaces toward the mandible to avoid directing the fracture toward the mandible, which might result in a mandible fracture, especially in an atrophic jaw. An essential step is the initial outline of the torus/mandible interface, which needs to be deep enough to ensure a clean, sharp removal of the torus. Once the wounds are irrigated and adequate hemostasis is achieved, the incision is reapproximated with resorbable sutures. Close postoperative follow up is critical in cases of bilateral large mandibular tori reduction due to the high risk for floor of mouth edema and/or hematoma formation that may be life threatening. The use of dentures immediately postoperatively may help to minimize the discomfort or hematoma formation, but meticulous surgical technique and gentle tissue handling is of utmost importance here. In some cases it may be best to stage the procedures and perform one torus reduction at a time. Figure 6.11(B–E) demonstrates the classic steps involved in a mandibular torus reduction procedure.

Soft tissue surgery

With the physiologic alveolar bone loss that follows tooth loss, soft tissue changes and muscle attachment alterations can be encountered that may interfere with the fabrication of a removable denture prosthesis. In addition, with the long-term use of a removable denture prosthesis, bone loss occurs in some areas at a more rapid rate than others, and this can result in a less than ideal fit of the denture prosthesis, causing trauma during function and chronic inflammation of the tissues overlying the ridge. In addition, frenal insertion changes occur after alveolar height reduction that can also interfere with the insertion or functional stability of the prosthesis. It is generally advised that any soft tissues removed from the patient should be submitted to histopathologic confirmation to rule out pathology.

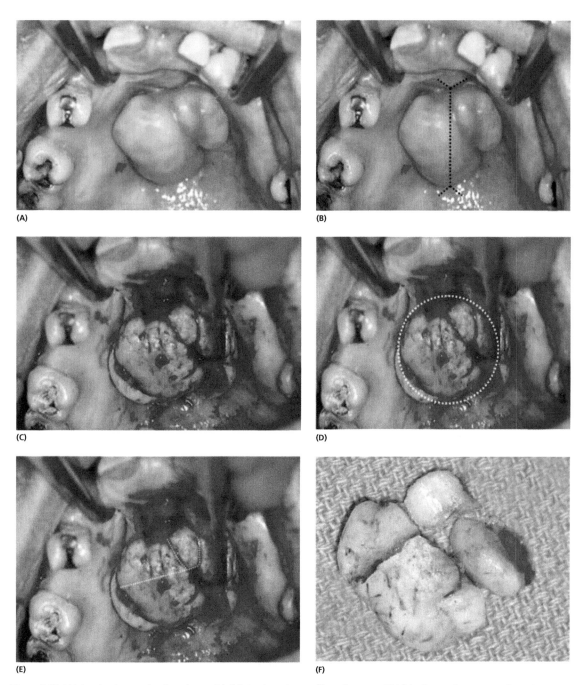

(A)   (B)   (C)   (D)   (E)   (F)

Figure 6.10 (A) A palatal torus that interferes with fabrication of a maxillary denture. (B) This picture shows an outline of a surgical incision for torus removal. The incision is placed over the torus and extended beyond its anterior/posterior borders. The typical incision looks like two Ys joined in the midline. (C) Flaps are reflected and the torus is exposed. (D) The bony torus is outlined in the picture. (E) Tori are surgically removed in small segments. An attempt to remove a palatal torus in one piece could lead to a perforation to the nasal cavity. The outline shows the surgeon's choice to section the torus before its removal. (F) The excised bony torus is shown.

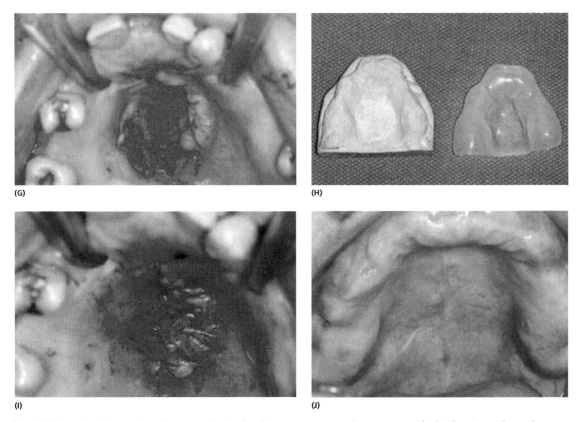

(G)

(H)

(I)

(J)

Figure 6.10 (*Continued*) (G) Tori can be removed using hand instruments, rotary instruments, or both. The picture shows the appearance of the site after surgery. It is not necessary to completely remove the bony growth. The extent of removal can be assessed by frequent closing of the flaps and feeling the area for sharp edges of bone. (H) Surgical templates can be used to create pressure for hemostasis and provide a method of delivering soft tissue liners as a surgical dressing. In this case, because the patient was also scheduled for full arch extractions, a complete upper clear surgical template was fabricated. An immediate denture could also have been used. (I) Flaps are then closed with sutures. (J) This eight weeks postoperative picture shows healthy mucosa and excellent healing.

Maxillary soft tissue tuberosity reduction

Earlier in this chapter, the reduction of a maxillary bony tuberosity was discussed, but as mentioned, occasionally, the excess may be confined solely to soft tissues of the tuberosity. The clinical assessment of soft tissue excess is easily confirmed with radiographic examination of the area using panoramic radiographs or 3D imaging. The area is best anesthetized with regional administration of a local anesthetic solution as an infiltration of a local anesthetic solution over the redundant soft tissues will cause tissue distortion and improper excision. A wedge excision of the excess tissue is performed, with incisions carried down to the periosteum. It is important to be conservative at the initial design of the "wedge" to avoid over-reduction. After the initial excision is done, the buccal and palatal flaps (one on either side of the incision) may be "thinned out" with submucosal resection of fibrous tissue to allow for passive approximation of the flaps over the alveolar ridge (Figure 6.12A–C).

Hypermobile soft tissue reduction/epulis fissuratum reduction

Hypermobile soft tissue is often found over the edentulous alveolar ridge in the anterior maxillary region when the opposing natural dentition is present (combination syndrome). It represents the soft tissue remaining after (rapid) resorption of the underlying alveolar bone, which results in an ill-fitting denture prosthesis. An epulis fissuratum, on the other hand,

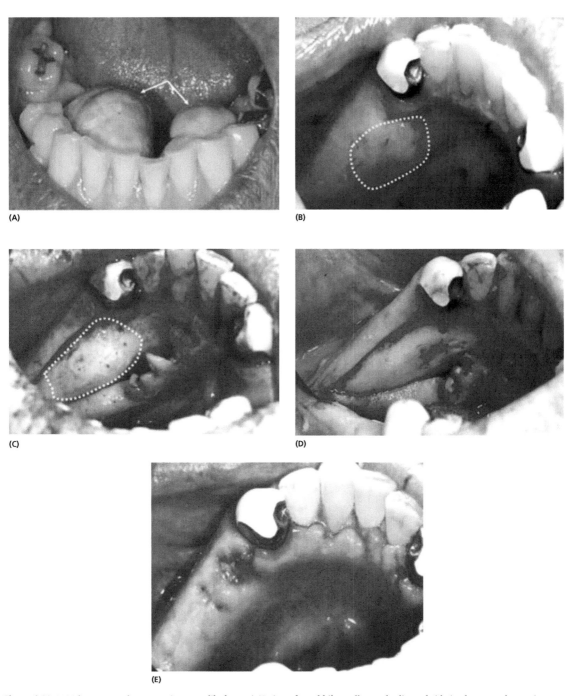

Figure 6.11 (A) The arrows show massive mandibular tori. Tori are found bilaterally on the lingual side in the premolar canine area. (B) Outline of a mandibular torus. Mandibular tori can create undercuts, thereby making denture fabrication and insertion cumbersome. The mucosa covering the torus is thin and prone to pressure ulceration from dentures. (C) Mandibular torus after surgical exposure. An incision was made over the crest of the ridge, extending the equivalent of two teeth beyond the torus on each end. (D) The torus is removed and the surface smoothed. The smoothness can be checked by replacing the flaps and then feeling for rough bony areas. (E) This postsurgical result shows a great improvement in the shape of the mandibular ridge and absence of any undercuts.

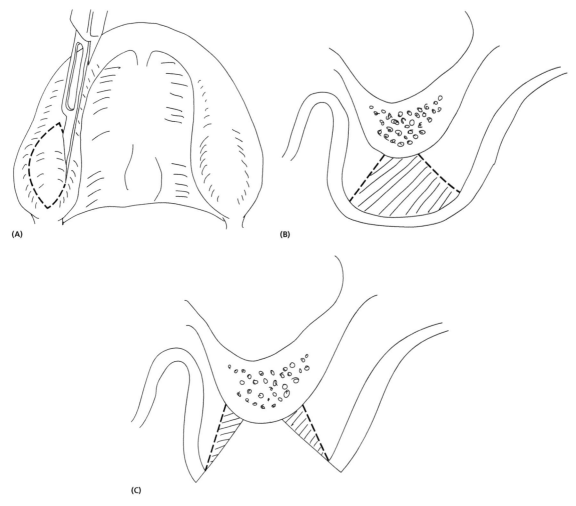

(A)

(B)

(C)

Figure 6.12 (A–C) Soft tissue maxillary tuberosity reduction.

represents an overgrowth of previously traumatized soft tissues from a denture flange overextension, and it is generally found in the buccal vestibule (Figure 6.2). Surgical excision can be performed with sharp dissection using a #15 blade, CO_2 (carbon dioxide) laser, or electrocautery. As with all delicate soft tissue surgery, infiltration of a local anesthetic solution should be avoided as it may cause distortion of the tissues. The excess tissue is held with tissue forceps, and excision is performed at the supraperiosteal level. Closure is not needed, and healing may occur by secondary intention (granulation tissue formation). An appropriately trimmed, newly relined denture or a clear surgical acrylic stent may be inserted at the time of surgery to assist with healing and patient comfort. It is imperative that the dentures are replaced or appropriately modified, or the epulis lesion will likely recur.

Inflammatory papillary hyperplasia

Inflammatory papillary hyperplasia (Figure 6.3) is commonly the result of poor oral hygiene and candida superinfection under an old, ill-fitting denture prosthesis. The process is benign, but if not reversed with antifungal treatment and denture replacement, it will require surgical correction. This can be performed by several methods, but usually a CO_2 (carbon dioxide) laser ablation is easily tolerated by the patient and causes less bleeding than using a scalpel or rotary instruments.

Labial frenectomy and lingual frenectomy

The tissue of the maxillary labial frenum includes thin bands of fibrous connective tissue extensions covered with mucosa and may contain muscle fibers. The composition of the lingual frenum may vary somewhat with regard to the presence of muscle fibers in addition to fibrous connective tissue. Regardless of the type of tissue(s) present, frenal attachments may interfere with the functional stability of removable denture prostheses when these attachments are located high on the alveolar ridge. In addition, the mucosa may be easily injured during use of the prosthesis and cause patient discomfort.

For maxillary labial frenectomy, a simple elliptical excision to the depth of the vestibule can be easily made while remaining within the confines of the abnormal tissue. The frenum can be defined by adequate lip retraction and held with a forceps before the excision. A supraperiosteal resection is performed at the alveolar side of the frenum, and the excision is carried down to the muscle layer on the labial aspect of the anterior maxilla. Wound closure should start at the depth of the vestibule, with resorbable sutures placed in an interrupted fashion. Figure 6.13(A,B) shows a classic frenectomy procedure via a simple excision technique. For a wide-based labial frenum, the incision may be allowed to heal by secondary intention. Occasionally a Z-plasty may be employed to ensure the depth of the vestibule is maintained after the frenum excision (Figure 6.13C–E).

When excision of the mandibular lingual frenum is planned, care should be taken to avoid injury to the Warthin's ducts of the submandibular gland, which may be in close proximity to the surgical site. A #15 blade or CO_2 laser can be used to excise the frenum. Curved mosquito hemostats are very helpful to "isolate" the frenum. The convex sides of the hemostats are placed on the frenum, one toward the ventral side of the tongue and the other toward the lingual surface of the mandible. This placement allows for maximum exposure and will assist with adequate soft tissue removal. The #15 blade is used when the forceps are in place to excise the frenum following the convex surface of the forceps. The frenum is excised, and, if needed, minimal submucosal dissection on the ventral surface of the tongue can be performed to assist with tissue closure. Interrupted sutures using resorbable material are used

for wound closure starting at the depth of the defect. Alternatively, the CO_2 laser may be used for the frenectomy procedure, and the wound is allowed to heal by secondary intention. Figure 6.14(A,B) shows preoperative and postoperative results following a lingual frenectomy procedure.

Vestibuloplasty

The goal of a vestibulopasty is to remove unwanted muscle insertions into the alveolar ridge. This is done by exposing bone at the place where these muscles formerly attached. The surgical technique requires an adequate amount (height) of alveolar bone (the minimum is at least 10 mm). The basic problem here is usually not the lack of bone but rather that the shallow vestibule prevents the denture flange from extending to provide adequate stability and retention. If the patient does not have enough bone height, then a ridge augmentation procedure might need to be done before a vestibuloplasty.

During the presurgical evaluation, it is important to evaluate the proximity of anatomical structures such as nerves and the location of muscle insertions. A panoramic radiograph or cone beam CT scan will help to evaluate the bone height and identify structures such as the mental foramen. Nerve blocks and infiltration should be used to obtain profound anesthesia and hemostasis. The incision is placed at the junction of attached and unattached mucosa with a #15 blade. A partial-thickness flap is raised with the blade or fine-tip scissors supraperiosteally, thereby preserving the periosteum. Any muscle fibers attached to the periosteum should be removed. Small perforations of the periosteum will not likely cause complications but should be avoided. The mucosal edge of the split-thickness flap is sutured to the apical end of the dissected area.

The resulting denuded periosteum may be handled in different ways. If the operator decides to let it heal by secondary intention, the relapse rate is about 50%. Another method is to graft the area with palatal mucosa, collagen membrane, or cadaveric mucosal membrane. Grafts should be perforated with the tip of a #11 blade after suturing in order to prevent blood clots from forming between the graft and the periosteum. Light pressure on a graft is desirable to prevent blood clot formation, and also to immobilize the graft. This can be accomplished with the patient's denture after it has been relieved and a soft tissue relining material placed

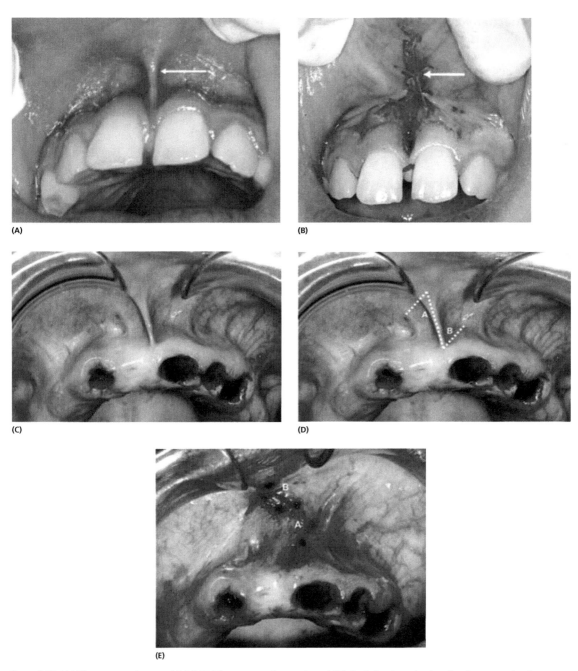

Figure 6.13 (A) The arrow points to a high labial frenum attachment in a child. Such freni can lead to development of a diastema between the central incisors. (B) The frenal attachment is corrected by a simple excision technique. The arrow points to the part of the wound that was sutured. Below this area, sutures could not be placed because the soft tissue could not be closed. It is left to heal by secondary intention. It is important to remove the fibrotic tissue between the centrals. (C) The labial frenum in the picture interferes with denture border extension and stability. (D) The lines represent a Z-plasty technique. Areas marked as A and B indicate two flaps that will be surgically repositioned, thereby eliminating the frenum. (E) Surgical correction of this prominent frenum attachment shows the dramatic improvement.

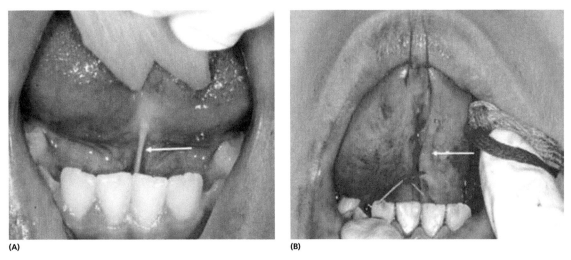

Figure 6.14 (A) An abnormal position of a lingual frenum close to the tip of the tongue, called tongue-tie, can restrict its movement. The arrow shows this condition. (B) The tongue is corrected surgically by a procedure called a lingual frenectomy. The arrow shows an immediate postsurgical improvement in the range of tongue movement.

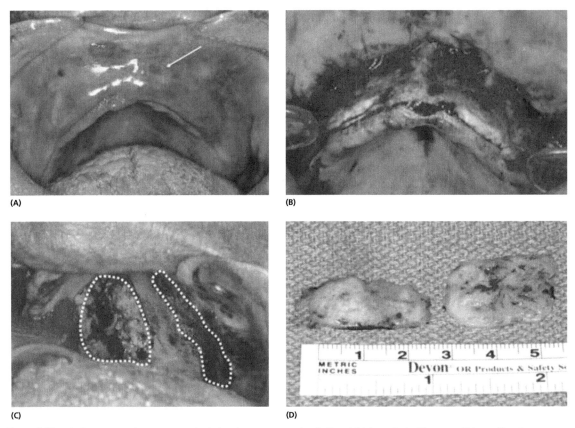

Figure 6.15 (A) The arrow points to unattached alveolar mucosa and a shallow labial vestibule. These conditions affect denture stability and retention. (B) The recipient site is prepared with a partial-thickness flap. The periosteum is preserved, but any muscle or fatty tissue is removed in order to have a non-movable graft after healing. (C) Outlined areas represent a palatal graft donor site. (D) Palatal grafts of the required size are obtained from the donor site. Yellowish areas in the graft represent fatty tissue, which should be removed before adapting the grafts to the recipient site.

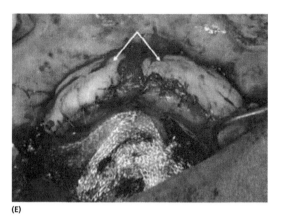

(E)

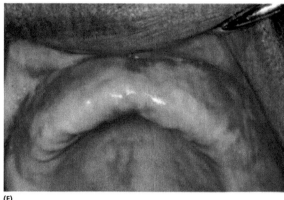

(F)

Figure 6.15 (*Continued*) (E) The arrows show palatal grafts sutured in place. There is a corresponding increased depth of the labial vestibule. (F) This three months postsurgical picture shows excellent vestibular depth and healthy keratinized tissue.

inside. One should be careful that the soft tissue relining material does not get lodged under the graft. Another alternative is to use a soft clear splint kept in place with two titanium screws or wires. Screws are simple to place and to remove. The denture or splint should not be removed for approximately 2 to 4 weeks. When the splint is removed, the grafted tissue will often look white and avascular. This is normal. It usually means that the superficial layer of the graft has been lost, but one should not worry because the rest of the graft will be vital. Angiogenesis into the graft occurs within 48 hours, and healing takes up to 5 to 6 weeks. Figure 6.15 shows a vestibuloplasty procedure where keratinized tissue was harvested from the palate and placed in the maxillary anterior region.

Further reading

Barrett GD. A simplified surgical guide stent technique for the reduction of the impinging maxillary tuberosity. *Compendium of Continuing Education in Dentistry*. 1988; 9(3): 196–202.

Bell RA, Richardson A. Prosthodontic treatment of pendulous maxillary tuberosities. *Journal of the American Dental Association*. 1981; 103(6): 894–5.

Bullock N, Jr. The use of the CO2 laser for lingual frenectomy and excisional biopsy. *Compendium of Continuing Education in Dentistry*. 1995; 16(11): 1118, 1120, 1122–3.

Costello BJ, Betts NJ, Barber HD, Fonseca RJ. Preprosthetic surgery for the edentulous patients. *Dental Clinics of North America*. 1996; 40(1): 19–38.

Freedman AL, Stein MD, Schneider DB. A modified maxillary labial frenectomy. *Quintessence International Dental Digest*. 1982; 13(6): 675–8.

Hamilton WS. Letter: Interseptal alveoplasty. *Dental Journal*. 1975; 41(10): 534.

Hernandez A. Maxillary tuberosity ridge reduction. *Dental Surveys*. 1978; 54(3): 43–4.

Hopkins R, Stafford GD, Gregory MC. Pre-prosthetic surgery of the edentulous mandible. *British Dental Journal*. 1980; 148(7): 183–8.

Khosla VM. Labial and lingual frenectomy. *Dental Assistant*. 1972; 41(7): 22–5.

Leonard M. The maxillary tuberosity: indications and simple technique for reduction. *Dentistry Today*. 2001; 20(2): 52–5.

Spagnoli D, Nale JC. Pre-prosthetic and reconstructive surgery. In: Miloro M, Ghali GE, Larsen P, Waite P, eds. *Peterson's Principles of Oral and Maxillofacial Surgery*, 3rd edn. Vol. 1. PMPH-USA, Shelton, CT, 2012, pp. 123–157.

Tucker MR, Farrell BB, Farrell BC. Pre-prosthetic surgery. In: Hupp J, Ellis E, Tucker MR, eds. *Contemporary Oral and Maxillofacial Surgery*, 5th edn, Vol. 1. Elsevier, St. Louis, MO, 2008, pp. 213–252.

Vyloppilli S, Prathap A. Lingual frenectomy using multiple series Z-plasty. *Journal of Oral and Maxillofacial Surgery*. 2010; 9(2): 195–7.

Yang HM, Woo YJ, Won SY, Kim DH, Hu KS, Kin HJ. Course and distribution of the lingual nerve in the ventral tongue region: anatomical considerations for frenectomy. *Journal of Craniofacial Surgery*. 2009; 20(5): 1359–63.

CHAPTER 7

Evaluation and Biopsy Technique for Oral Lesions

Marianela Gonzalez[1], Thomas C. Bourland[1], and Cesar A. Guerrero[2]

[1] Department of Oral and Maxillofacial Surgery, Texas A & M Baylor College of Dentistry, Dallas, TX, USA
[2] Division of Oral and Maxillofacial Surgery, Department of Surgery, University of Texas Medical Branch, Galveston, TX, USA

Introduction

Oral cancer is a vast and proliferative disease that plagues the world with an estimated incidence of 275,000 cases per year with two-thirds of cases occurring in developing nations.[1] No other clinician spends more time in the oral cavity or has a better chance of early detection and diagnosis than the general dentist. This chapter will help guide the clinician to properly evaluate, diagnose, document, and manage a lesion within the oral cavity—malignant or benign. The guidelines provided will help outline and discuss the indications for biopsy and materials for early detection of any suspicious area of the oral cavity as well as the indications for referral for higher level of care. Instructions for the different type of biopsy techniques will also be provided for the clinician to utilize. Careful application of sound principles, adequate skill and keen judgment will aid in the practitioners ability for early detection and diagnosis of any intraoral lesion allowing for more favorable outcomes for the patient.

Patient evaluation

In order to establish a diagnosis, the dentist should obtain a thorough history specific to the lesion, besides the patient's medical and dental health history. This information must be combined with findings from a clinical exam in order to put the questionable lesion into proper context. Often, the clinician will have to rely

upon experience and judgment to determine if the lesion is reactive or pathologic. Thorough investigation of a patient's past health history, including medications, trauma, diet, previous surgeries and habits are a necessity. Answers to many of these questions will often reveal the probable cause of the lesion and may help direct the clinician down an obvious path of treatment.

Health history

The dentist should be in possession of a written health history that is verified and reviewed at all appointments. Included in the health history should be an updated and accurate list of all medications the patient is taking. The patient's answers on the form should only be used as the initial point of evaluation and should allow the dentist to gather other information for a more complete picture of the patient's health. The health history informs the clinician about situations that might cause or predispose to development of a lesion. The history can also alert the clinician to various systemic conditions that could influence a decision regarding a proposed biopsy or other treatment. In these instances, it may be appropriate to investigate these issues further through a physician consultation. Other conditions may, at the very least, require special precautions, such as hypertension, uncontrolled diabetes, heart defects, coagulopathies, and pregnancy. The clinician must take into account that many oral lesions are manifestations of systemic conditions. Indeed, it is true that the oral cavity is a good barometer of overall health. Common examples of this include, but certainly are not limited to, Crohn's disease,

Manual of Minor Oral Surgery for the General Dentist, Second Edition. Edited by Pushkar Mehra and Richard D'Innocenzo.

human immunodeficiency virus, lupus, Sjögren's syndrome, diabetes, and many different viral, bacterial, and fungal infections.

Being aware of the patient's systemic conditions and how they may present is part of the puzzle in helping the clinician determine a differential diagnosis.

Lesion history

In order to assess a lesion appropriately, accurate and definitive questions should be answered and documented. The following questions can assist the practitioner:

1. *Time*: How long has the lesion been present? The patient should be asked when the lesion was originally felt and visualized. Oral lesions that have been present more than several weeks with no provoking habitus are highly suspicious. The dentist should look for signs or symptoms of trauma such as denture irritation if applicable, sharp cusps or fractured dentition. These possible causes should be eliminated.

2. *Metamorphosis*: Has the lesion changed in size, shape or color since detection? An easy depiction for documentation is noting the ABC's of the lesion—architecture, borders and color.

3. *Pain*: Is the lesion causing discomfort? It is important to note the duration and frequency of the pain. The clinician should also discern if the lesion is the source of discomfort or if the pain is referred. A quantitative level of pain should also be noted.

4. *Sensation*: Has the lesion caused anesthesia or paresthesia of surrounding tissues? If no lesion is present then a systemic implication could likely be the cause such as diabetic neuropathy. However, if a lesion is present then malignancy can be placed higher on the differential diagnosis.

5. *Nodes*: Are there any palpable lymph nodes? Malignancies metastasize hematogenously and through the lymphatic system. Reactive nodes are often tender to palpation and are freely movable. Lymph nodes that are cancerous have a correlation with enlargement and firmness with no mobility.

6. *Symptoms*: Does the patient have any constitutional symptoms? Does the patient appear frail? Has the patient had unexpected weight loss? Does the patient experience fatigue and malaise? It is important for the evaluating clinician not to focus only on the affected area but also to see the patient's entire appearance for the appropriate diagnosis.

7. *Genetics*: Has the patient or anyone in the patient's family had oral cancer diagnoses previously? Some oral cancers are not just factors of environmental influence but have a genetic component as well. Some syndromes like Gardener's or basal cell nevus syndrome have a high rate of malignancy. The more information one can gather during investigation will allow for a more comprehensive diagnosis.

Examination

Proper inspection and depiction of a lesion should be documented in the patient's chart. If the clinician is still using paper charting, a hand-drawn description with appropriate terminology should be made. If the clinician is using an electronic medical record, the lesion should be accurately described and charted on an accepted template prior to submission from biopsy. Pictorial documentation should be printed out and placed in the paper chart with size calibration or attached to the digital record. The lesion should be measured at each appointment and compared to previous history or documentation if applicable. Accurate documentation will allow the dentist to submit the information to the pathologist or aid in referral to a surgeon if warranted.

During initial examination, it is important to have careful description and documentation prior to manipulation. The edges of epithelium can be easily torn and vesicular lesions are friable and may rupture. The dentist can change the color and size of the lesion by drying it with the air/water syringe. Appropriate documentation should be completed prior to aggressive handling.

When referring the lesion to a specialist for biopsy or second opinion, or submitting the lesion to an oral pathologist for evaluation, accepted medical and dental terminology is required. Not only will the correct terminology aid in the communication and diagnosis of the lesion, but also help in the billing process for the clinician. By using the right descriptors, the multi-disciplinary specialists involved can obtain the right *International Classification of Diseases*, 9th edition (ICD-9) and CPT codes which will aid all parties the submission of dental and medical claims. A list of such terms are provided in Table 7.1.

Table 7.1 Examples of some common CPT codes which are required for billing biopsy procedures to a patient's medical (not dental) insurance.

Treatment	CPT Code
Excision, lesion/tumor w/simple repair	41826
Excision, lesion/tumor w/complex repair	41827
Excision, hyperplastic alveolar mucosa, each quadrant (specify)	41828
Biopsy lip, excisional	40490
Excision, lesion, palate, uvula; w/simple primary closure	42106
Biopsy, palate, uvula	42100
Biopsy, oropharynx	42800
Biopsy, tongue; anterior two-thirds	41100
Biopsy, tongue; posterior one-third	41105
Biopsy, mouth, floor	41108
Excision, lesion, tongue w/closure; anterior two-thirds	41112
Excision, lesion, tongue w/closure; posterior one-third	41113
Excision, lesion, mouth floor	41116

Clinical judgment

After the specimen is evaluated and the clinical picture is pieced together with an appropriate differential diagnosis, it is imperative a working diagnosis is made prior to treatment. Extended observation with no diagnosis is below the standard of care.[2] If the clinician feels the area in question is beyond his/her scope of care then accurate referral and documentation will aid in favorable diagnosis and outcome for the patient.

For example, if the clinician suspects the hyperkeratosis in evaluating a white lesion on the lateral border of the tongue due to a sharp cusp tip adjacent to the area or trauma, then it is more than appropriate to smooth the cusp tip and then follow the patient for a short period of time to see if the lesion resolves. However, if the patient has multiple risk factors for malignancy, such as extended tobacco use, and clinical signs, such as palpable lymph nodes, then immediate biopsy is warranted. Delineating between watching and waiting and biopsy is the essence of clinical judgment.

In the United States, 50,000 head and neck cancers are diagnosed annually.[3] In a clinical study by Holmes *et al.*, referral patterns were evaluated for patient with head and neck cancer lesions. 90% of those lesions were in the oral cavity and 80% were diagnosed and referred by a general dentist.[4]

Most oral cancers are asymptomatic at an early stage, and symptoms develop as the depth of invasion increases. The consequence of the lack of early symptoms is usually a later stage diagnosis. The classic sign of oral cancer is an indurated lesion with raised, asymmetric borders. Paresthesia or neuropathies can develop as the depth of the penetration increases.

Often, the more difficult lesion to treat is the precancerous lesion with atypical and dysmorphic cellular components that reside in superficial layers. The authors recommend close follow-up and a wide variety of treatment modalities, including laser removal wider excisional biopsy. The most important treatment is for the clinician to have an accurate diagnosis and recognizing one's limitation in treating the area in question.

Biopsy

Biopsy is the sampling or removal of cells and tissue from the body for examination and evaluation to establish or confirm a diagnosis. Biopsy comes from Greek origin of the words *bio* meaning life and *opsia* meaning to see. Most often, a scalpel is used to remove or shave cells from living tissue to submit a specimen for microscopic inspection. A blade-removed specimen is considered the gold standard for providing tissue for diagnosis. Other methods are available, such as brush biopsy or needle biopsy, and are less invasive but also not without limitation.

Five techniques are useful to the general dentist for biopsy. These five procedures are: (1) oral brush biopsy, (2) needle aspiration biopsy, (3) incisional biopsy, (4) excisional biopsy, and (5) oral speculoscopy. A description of the most useful methods will be discussed including suggestions on how to perform each type.

Brush biopsy
The brush biopsy was designed to screen oral epithelial abnormalities for cellular atypia.[5] The specimen obtained from a brush submits cells for computer analysis at OralCDx (OralCDx Laboratories, Suffern, NY). Efficacy of the value of oral brush biopsy has been debated in the literature. OralCDx Laboratories reports the probability of a patient with an atypical OralCDx report having a cancerous or precancerous lesion between 30 and 40% (Figure 7.1).

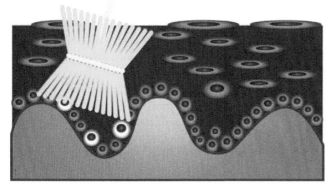
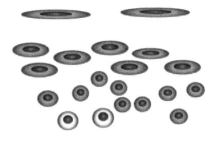

Figure 7.1 The brush biopsy was designed to screen oral epithelial abnormalities for cellular atypia. The specimen obtained from a brush is submitted for computer analysis.

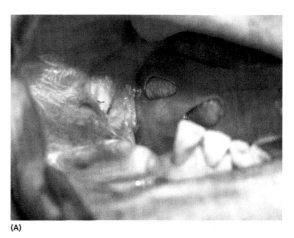

(A)

Figure 7.3 (A) A posterior mandible lesion, with no apparent clinical signs of malignancy.

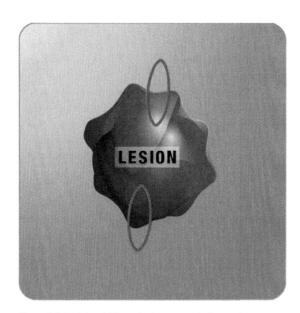

Figure 7.2 Incisional biopsy is the removal of a portion or sample of tissue. If a lesion has different characteristics, individual biopsy specimens of these areas should be obtained.

Incisional biopsy

Incisional biopsy is the removal of a minor portion of tissue for sampling. It is the most common biopsy procedure and aims to establish a definitive diagnosis before treatment. If the differential diagnosis includes as the four most realistic possibilities lesions that are curable by removal, then excisional biopsy is recommended (Figures 7.2, 7.3A, B and C, 7.4).

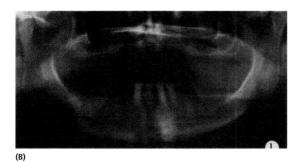

(B)

Figure 7.3 (B) Panoramic radiograph showing signs of irregular bone configuration of the right mandibular angle, exactly underneath the lesion on the soft tissue.

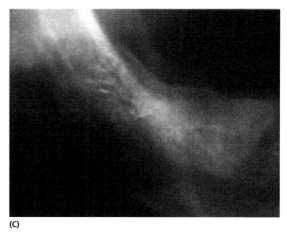

(C)

Figure 7.3 (C) A closer view, showing an irregular bony configuration.

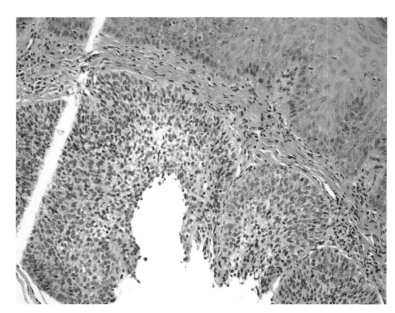

Figure 7.4 Hematoxylin and eosin histology shows signs of malignancy, nuclear hyperchromatism, irregular cells, and divided nucleus, leading toward squamous cell carcinoma. In this clinical stage, surgical resection and reconstruction followed by radiotherapy is the standard care of treatment to rehabilitate the patient.

Excisional biopsy

Excisional biopsy is the removal of the entire lesion, including at least 2 mm of normal tissue all around and deep into the tissue to make sure the entire lesion and normal tissue are included. The most common benign lesions to be encountered in a routine oral evaluation, that can be easily completely excised, are mucoceles and fibromas. Improper tissue handling during any step of the biopsy procedure can compromise the diagnosis. The most common mistakes are: inadequate size of the specimen, improper or insufficient fixative (always use formalin, not water and the ratio should be 10:1), desiccation with the use of laser or electrocautery, crush injuries to the cells when handling the specimen, improper labeling or mailing. Figures 7.5 A–C, 7.6 A–H, and 7.7 A–D demonstrate important principles which should be applied during intraoral biopsy procedures.

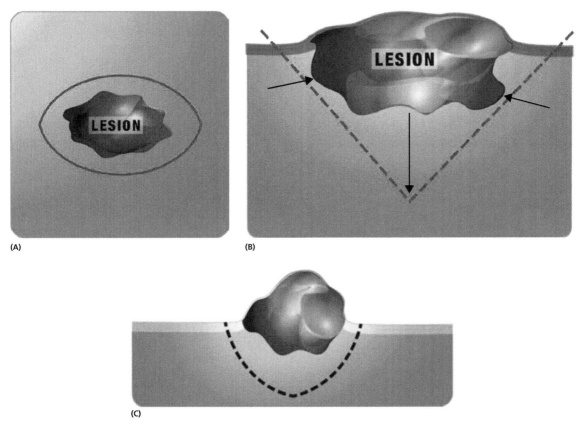

(A)

(B)

(C)

Figure 7.5 (A–C) Excisional biopsy is the removal of the entire lesion including at least 2 mm of normal tissue all around and deep into the tissue to make sure lesion and normal deep tissue are included with the lesion. Although the excisional biopsy seems symmetrical in (A), it is clearly seen in (B) that the depth of excision is excessive at the base (arrow), and the margins at the lower edges are closer than at the superficial edges (arrows). (C) shows the proper biopsy technique with relatively proportional margins all around the specimen.

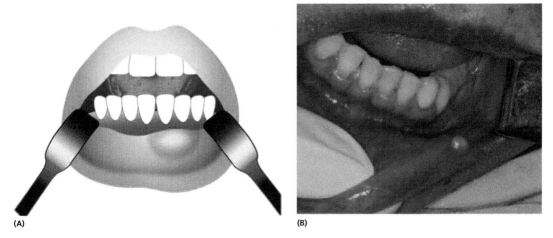

(A)

(B)

Figure 7.6 (A) Complete history and laboratory exams are reviewed before the surgery is scheduled. (B) Plan for an excisional biopsy of a fibroma in the lower lip.

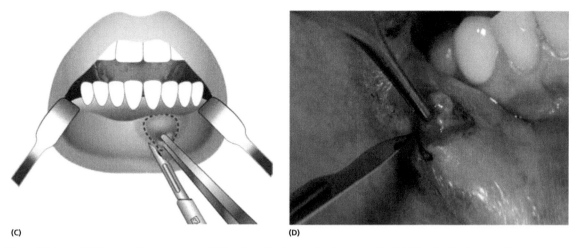

(C)　　　　　　　　　　　　　　　　　　　　(D)

Figure 7.6 (C and D) Pre-marking the mucosa. Wait at least 7 minutes after local anesthetic infiltration for hemostasis and meticulous surgery are important.

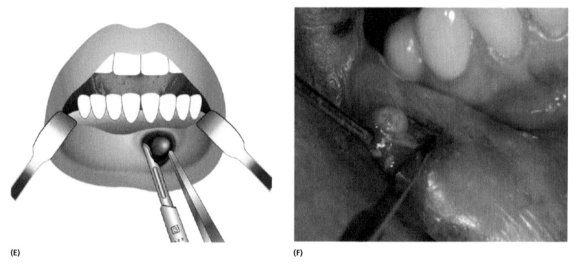

(E)　　　　　　　　　　　　　　　　　　　　(F)

Figure 7.6 (E and F) The entire lesion is eliminated with a 2 mm margin.

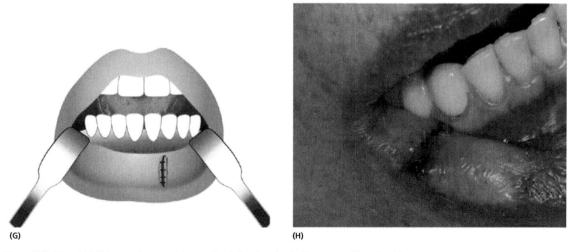

(G)　　　　　　　　　　　　　　　　　　　　(H)

Figure 7.6 (G and H) Primary closure with suturing following the lip lines to avoid noticeable scars.

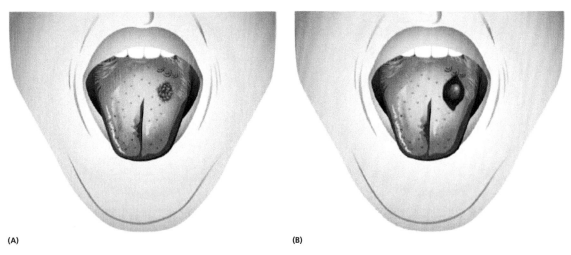

(A) (B)

Figure 7.7 (A) Lesion on the dorsal aspect of the tongue. (B) Excisional biopsy of the tongue.

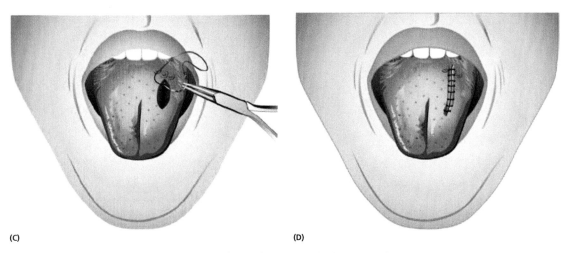

(C) (D)

Figure 7.7 (C) Deep sutures with Vicryl to approximate the muscle. (D) Superficial closure with Vicryl or silk sutures to avoid postoperative bleeding.

Instrumentation

The basic instrumentation for an incisional or excisional biopsy should contain: local anesthetic with epinephrine for local hemostasis, #15 blade with a handle, Adson pickups to avoid tissue crush damage, marking pen to delineate the margins of the incision in an ovoid fashion for better closure, a ruler to measure the lesion after removal for pathology and chart records. Choice of sutures may vary with the type of oral tissue one is working on. The sutures commonly used for oral mucosa in the wet area of the lip or the inner part of the cheeks is resorbable 4–0 chromic gut; when taking a biopsy from the tongue, special consideration should be taken to use deeper sutures for the musculature of the tongue (4–0 Vicryl) and superficial closure with 3–0 Vicryl. Use of a layered closure technique decreases the incidence of bleeding postoperatively. A labeled, adequately sized container with formalin should be available before the procedure starts, and the assistant should be ready to handle the container with the specimen inside (Figures 7.8, 7.9, 7.10, and 7.11).

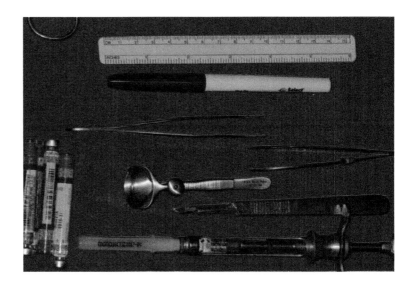

Figure 7.8 Basic instrumentation.

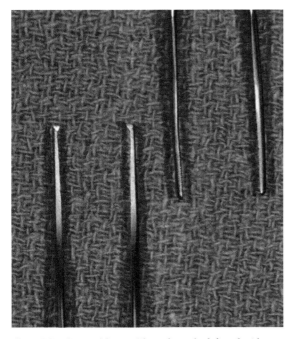

Figure 7.9 Adson's pickups with teeth on the left and without teeth on the right.

Hemostasis

Bleeding is a common problem when dealing with soft tissue lesions; the clinician needs to be aware of the importance and caliber of the vessels involved, which usually depends on the size and location of the lesion.

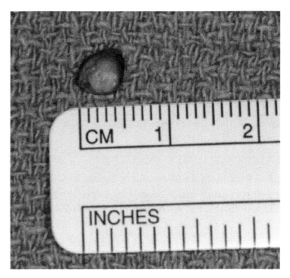

Figure 7.10 Photographing the specimen with a ruler and marking the sample to identify positioning are important steps.

Utilizing local anesthesia with vasoconstrictors is fundamental, especially, peripheral infiltration. If a biopsy of the lip is indicated, the assistant needs to use both hands on either side of the lip to compress the labial arteries with the fingers and avoid active bleeding; placing an initial suture next to the biopsy area helps in closing the wound much faster, running a continuous locked suture to avoid postoperative bleeding.

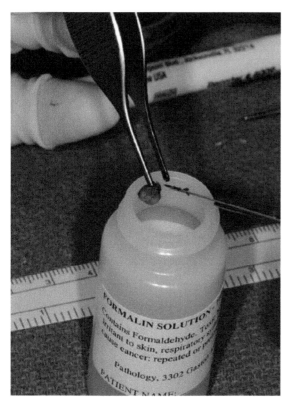

Figure 7.11 The specimen's handling, labeling and mailing are managed carefully.

Knowledge of local anatomy helps the clinician prevent injuring major vessels or nerves, which are adjacent to the lesion; if it is necessary to section a major vessel it is better to slowly identify and dissect it, continuing with tight suture knots on either side and sectioning the vessel; it may be indicated to use electrocautery to coagulate small vessels. The wound must be carefully sutured and compressing gauzes placed for at least an hour.

Postsurgical bleeding is a stressful event for the patient and family that needs to be avoided by applying cold compresses allowing vasoconstriction in the area, avoiding high pressure events (related to pain, lifting weights, etc.), not disturbing the wound and sutures with the fingers or tongue and maintain communication with the clinician in case of an emergency event.

References

1. Warnakulasuriya S. Living with oral cancer: Epidemiology with particular reference to prevalence and life-style changes that influence survival. *Oral Oncology.* 2010; 46: 407.
2. Golden DP, Hooley JR. Oral mucosal biopsy procedures. *Dental Clinics of North America.* 1994; 38(2): 279–300.
3. SEER Stat Fact Sheets. 2009. Available at: <http://seer.cancer.gov/statfacts/html/oralcav.html>, accessed January 12, 2015.
4. Holmes JD, Martin RA, Gutta R. Characteristics of head and neck cancer patients referred to an oral and maxillofacial surgeon in the United States for management. *Journal of Oral and Maxillofacial Surgery.* 2010; 68(3): 555–61.
5. Sciubba JJ. Improving detection or precancerous and cancerous oral lesions: Computer-assisted analysis of the oral brush biopsy. *Journal of the American Dental Association.* 1999; 130: 1445.

CHAPTER 8

Surgical Implantology

Alfonso Caiazzo[1] and Frederico Brugnami[2]

[1] Department of Oral and Maxillofacial Surgery, Boston University Henry M. Goldman School of Dental Medicine, Boston, MA, USA; Private Practice of Oral Surgery and Implantology, Salerno, Italy
[2] Private Practice of Periodontology and Implantology, Rome, Italy

Introduction and terminology

Implant dentistry is one of the most popular office-based dental procedures today. Since the introduction of the original two-staged threaded titanium root-form implant in the United States by Branemark in 1978, oral implantology has undergone a complete metamorphosis. Today, most clinicians realize that for a result to be categorized as successful in terms of function and esthetics, both hard- and soft-tissue harmony must be achieved. Contemporary surgical implantology involves placement of implants to fulfill precise restorative goals. Thus, development of surgical sites is prosthetically driven, and the patient's and restorative dentist's needs determine the surgical strategy.

A careful and detailed preoperative evaluation is mandatory even if implant placement does not require hard and/or soft tissue augmentation. Treatment planning is, in fact, germane for successful implant treatment and will decrease the incidence of adverse outcomes (Table 8.1). This preoperative preparation and evaluation includes obtaining an accurate patient medical history, comprehensive extra- and intraoral examinations, study casts with diagnostic wax-ups, and laboratory or chair-side fabrication of surgical stents to guide implant positioning (Figure 8.1A–D).

Historically speaking, for most situations, a good-quality panoramic radiograph or a full-mouth periapical dental X-ray series can be considered an adequate radiological work-up. However, more recently, three-dimensional radiographic evaluation with cone beam computerized tomography (CBCT) is now being accepted as the standard of care. It has many advantages, including in-office availability, low cost, and minimal radiation. A custom-made stent with radiopaque markings should be used during CBCT examination; besides allowing for an accurate preoperative evaluation of the anatomic bony structures and dimensions of the alveolus at the planned implant site, it can also be used later as a surgical guide for precise implant placement (Figure 8.2).

Once treatment planning has been completed, the next step is to choose the type of implants and to know the surgical armamentarium. Irrespective of any implant system choice, there must be biocompatibility between the host tissue and the implant, for functional longevity. A material is considered to be biocompatible when it is non-toxic and non-carcinogenic, does not interfere with the healing of the host tissue, and when its mechanical properties are well tolerated by the host tissues. The materials used for the implants should be bioinert (react to bone only with direct contact) and bioactive (create an osteogenic bond between the implant surface and the surrounding bone).

Knowing the anatomy and topography of the implant system of choice is paramount for success. The clinician can choose between multiple manufacturers, and each system further offers different type of implants. Implants can be made of commercially pure titanium or variable titanium alloys; they come in tapered or cylindrical shapes and are usually self-tapping and threaded, with a roughened surface. Fixtures can be classified according to the connection with the prosthetic abutment in internal or external connection or with the abutment seating inside the fixture platform, creating the so-called platform switching that will prevent bone resorption at the crown–implant interface. The field of implantology

Manual of Minor Oral Surgery for the General Dentist, Second Edition. Edited by Pushkar Mehra and Richard D'Innocenzo.
© 2016 John Wiley & Sons, Inc. Published 2016 by John Wiley & Sons, Inc.

Table 8.1 Flowchart of implant positioning

1.	Medical history
2.	Extraoral examination:
	Face harmony
	Midline
	Smile line
3.	Intraoral examination: Interarch space
4.	Soft-tissue quality and quantity
5.	Hard tissues
6.	Oral hygiene
7.	Periodontal health
8.	Impressions
9.	X-ray evaluation: OPT or periapical series
10.	CBCT (when required) with radiological stent
11.	Evaluate diagnostic wax-up
12.	Decide number and type of implants
13.	Perform surgery

is an ever-evolving discipline, and with advances in biotechnology, newer implant types and coatings will likely continue to develop at a rapid pace.

Nomenclature and terminology

Timing of placement or loading can be variable. In the earlier phases, during the initial development of dental implantology, it was customary to insert the surgical fixtures 6 to 9 months after extraction of teeth. Similarly, loading of osseointegrated implants was usually done during the 4- to 6-month interval after the insertion. More recently, there has been a paradigm shift in the thought process, and there is much greater emphasis on early placement or loading.

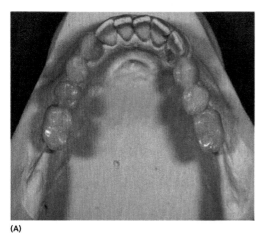

(A)

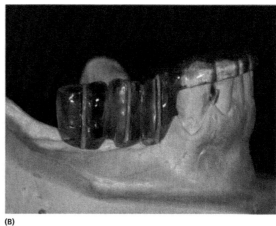

(B)

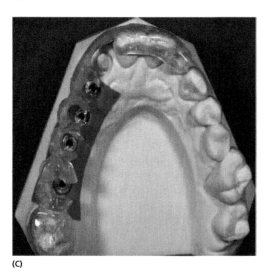

(C)

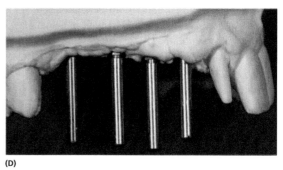

(D)

Figure 8.1 (A) Diagnostic wax up on study cast. (B) Surgical and radiologic stent with radiopaque material inserted at the tooth long axis. (C) Correct implant positioning as guided by a surgical stent (occlusal view). (D) Lateral view. Note parallelism of implants.

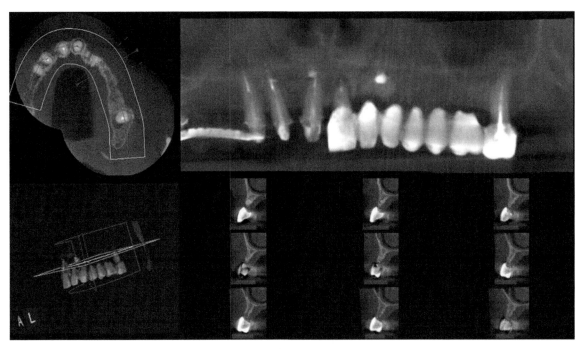

Figure 8.2 A CBCT taken with a radiopaque stent inserted in place in the oral cavity.

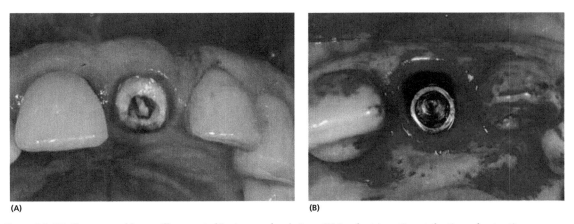

(A)   (B)

Figure 8.3 (A) Non-restorable maxillary central incisor: occlusal view. (B) Implant insertion at the time of extraction (immediate implant).

Depending on the time of placement, one can categorize the procedure of implant placement as *immediate* (implant is placed immediately following extraction of tooth in the same setting) or *delayed* placement (after healing of extraction site as a separate procedure) (Figure 8.3A, B). Similarly, placed implants can be termed as immediately loaded or not, depending on the timing of loading.

Other common terminology used for describing the surgical aspect of the treatment includes descriptions such as one- or two-stage surgery, depending on the practitioner's decision to connect a temporary healing abutment, which rests above the soft tissues at the time of implant placement (one-stage), versus submerging the implant under the soft tissues (two-stage) for a 4- to 6-month period before connecting the temporary healing abutment. In the two-stage surgical technique, an implant is placed during the first stage and allowed to integrate under the gingival mucoperiosteum. It requires surgical re-entry to expose the implant and connect the temporary healing abutment.

Management of extraction socket

Alveolar ridge resorption following tooth extraction is a frequently observed phenomenon that may either decrease the predictability of dental implant placement or impair the final esthetic results. Better understanding of the biologic process behind extraction socket healing has led to the development of techniques to preserve the natural architecture of the alveolus after extraction, such as immediate implant placement in fresh sockets and the use of osseous graft materials.

It is now known that resorption will especially target the buccal plate if the socket is not grafted immediately after dental extraction, thereby increasing the risk for facial soft-tissue recession. Even when minimal, such resorption usually has significant adverse clinical effects, particularly esthetic ones. Despite successful osseointegration of a dental implant, an anterior implant restoration may be judged a failure if the soft-tissue appearance is poor. Surgical techniques meant to preserve natural bone and soft-tissue contours after tooth extraction are thus of great interest to contemporary clinicians. This is especially true if an implant is placed and provisionalized immediately after tooth extraction.

Numerous authors have focused on immediate functional loading of dental implants in order to minimize the delay between the surgical and prosthetic treatment phases. This technique is increasingly being applied when replacing teeth in the maxillary anterior region, where esthetic outcomes are important. However, recent studies have reported that recession of the marginal peri-implant mucosa may occur after even immediate implant placement. This, in turn, may adversely affect the final esthetic outcome.

Factors that have been reported to influence the frequency and extent of marginal mucosal recession include the tissue biotype, the condition and thickness of the facial bone, and the orofacial position of the implant shoulder. Connecting a provisional crown immediately after implant insertion and grafting of the facial peri-implant marginal defect with bone or bone substitutes also have been cited as factors. In addition to these parameters, a recent experimental study showed that the facial socket wall, which is composed almost entirely of bundle bone, might be susceptible to resorption in the vertical and horizontal planes. Such crestal bone resorption may lead to intermediate- and long-term recession of the facial marginal mucosa.

Any alteration of the soft or hard tissues may impair the final esthetic outcome of immediately loaded implants in the anterior area. Thus, the clinician must decide whether to perform an immediate implant or not, and this decision must be individualized and customized based on surgeon experience, patient preference, and a thorough knowledge and understanding of the anatomy, morphology, and topography of the hard- and soft-tissue structures of the alveolus and jaws.

Contrary to what was thought earlier, placement of immediate implants by themselves may not always be the best treatment choice for preventing labial/buccal plate resorption in an extraction socket. This may be especially true in anterior esthetic zone cases where the labial cortical plate thickness is less than 2 mm. In such cases, either bony augmentation of the extraction socket (commonly known as *socket preservation*) and/or labial alveolar cortex (known as *buccal plate preservation* [BPP]) may be indicated with delayed implant placement. Socket preservation includes placement of a particulate bone graft, which is most commonly derived from bovine or human sources (allogeneic bone graft), within the socket. Depending on the type of bone graft material used, implant placement is usually delayed by approximately 6 to 12 months in order to allow for bone consolidation within the socket. An alternative new technique is BPP. This surgical technique aims to prevent recession of the facial wall of the extraction socket without interfering with the healing process. It involves placement of a slowly resorbing particulate bone-graft material underneath the soft tissues into a surgically created gingival pouch adjoining the buccal plate. It has been shown to maintain optimal soft-tissue contours and predictably provides a solid base for optimal esthetics and functional replacement of a missing tooth (Figure 8.4A, B). Because the extraction socket by itself is not grafted, after BPP, dental implants can be placed either immediately or in a delayed fashion; even with delayed placement, the time interval is shorter than that required for socket preservation as the socket heals with natural bone-healing mechanisms rather than incorporation of an implanted allogeneic or alloplastic graft material.

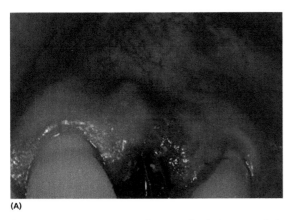

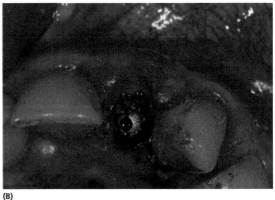

(A)   (B)

Figure 8.4 (A) BPP: creating a subperiosteal soft-tissue pouch that allows for insertion of a slow resorbing grafting material. This technique is used to counteract buccal plate resorption after tooth removal. (B) Clinical appearance: occlusal view.

Surgical procedure and clinical management

Preoperative preparation

According to the most recent literature, prophylactic anti-biotics are advisable (penicillin or clindamycin are accept-able), and the route of administration is oral, approximately 1 hour before the procedure. Chlorhexidine oral rinses before surgery are also recommended. Anesthesia with an appropriate vasoconstrictor-containing local anesthetic (if not medically contraindicated) is all that is required for anesthesia.

Incision and exposure

When planning an incision, there are at least three anatomic factors to be considered: (1) proximity of vital structures; (2) periodontal health of contiguous teeth, if any; and (3) quantity of the attached keratinized gingiva present. The incision can be made crestally or slightly lingual/palatal to the crest with a #15 Bard–Parker blade; the exact buccolingual placement is dependent on the amount of keratinized, attached gingiva present locally in the area. A #9 Molts periosteal elevator is then used to elevate a full-thickness mucoperiosteal flap. A vertical incision may or not be necessary, and should perhaps be avoided in anterior esthetic zone areas.

Osteotomy

The implant site preparation includes the development of an appropriately sized osteotomy using surgical implant drill bits (burs) of progressively increasing diameter,

sequentially, as per the specific recommendations of the manufacturer. For most implant systems, the osteotomy site is "under-prepared" compared to the actual diameter of the chosen implant, normally by 0.5 to 0.75 mm. The implant drill bits should be used under continuous irrigation with a sterile saline solution. Use of a custom-made surgical stent is highly recommended to guide and accurately position the osteotomy. Once the site is fully prepared, an endosseous implant can be inserted with or without saline irrigation (this often depends on the recommendations of the manufacturer and preference of the surgeon) at the recommended drill speed (usually from 20 to 35 rpm) (Figure 8.5A–E).

After insertion of the fixture, the surgeon must decide between a one- or two-stage procedure. If a one-stage procedure is chosen, a temporary healing abutment should be connected to the fixture. This abutment usually extends 1 to 3 mm above the gingival level and may promote optimal soft-tissue healing. For a two-stage procedure, a cover screw is attached to the implant, and this cover screw is buried subgingivally under the flap. Closure of the surgical incision is commonly performed with 3–0 or 4–0 size resorbable, or non-resorbable, sutures. At the end of the procedure, a postoperative X-ray (preferably a peri-apical radiograph) must be taken to control the correct implant positioning and also to ensure that the cover screw/healing abutment is properly seated (Figure 8.6).

Surgical trauma must be minimized during all aspects of implant surgery to maximize success. Overzealous instrumentation and surgical trauma can lead to fibrous encapsulation of the fixture within the osteotomy

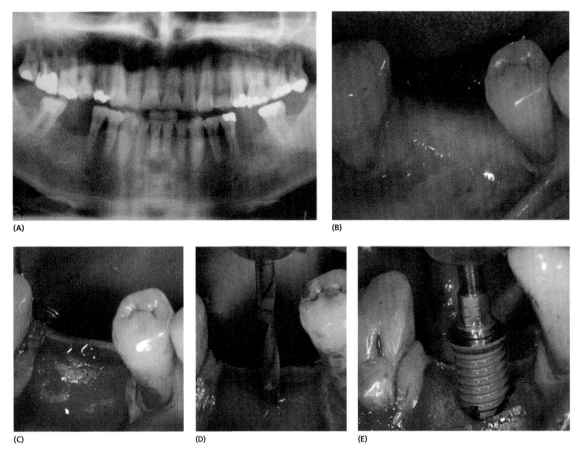

(A)   (B)

(C)   (D)   (E)

Figure 8.5 (A) Radiographic examination. (B) Clinical appearance of the site showing an adequate vertical and lateral thickness of the edentulous ridge. The attached keratinized gingival (AKG) tissue is sufficient, but the clinician must make plans to preserve it. (C) The incision is made slightly lingual to the crest to preserve AKG, and the clinician takes care to avoid including the papillae of the contiguous teeth. (D) After the perforation of the cortex with a round bur, preparation of the implant site is started with a pilot drill at the desired length. (E) Implant positioning.

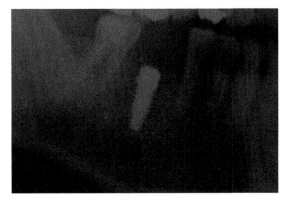

Figure 8.6 Postoperative X-ray taken to verify optimal implant positioning.

instead of complete osteointegration. Similarly, there is minimal, if any, margin for error in implant surgery. Thus, the surgeon should always consider taking intra-operative X-rays to verify proper implant site pre-paration. Recently, computer-guided implant insertion (Figure 8.7A–C) has been introduced, and it is gaining in popularity. Proponents of this technique claim that it allows for a safer and more accurate implant placement. Computer-based planning and surgery requires that the treatment has been suitably planned "virtually" on a computer preoperatively by an experienced clinician. The clinician uses CT scan data to identify all vital struc-tures around the surgical area, measure the quantity of bone available at each implant site, and then choose an

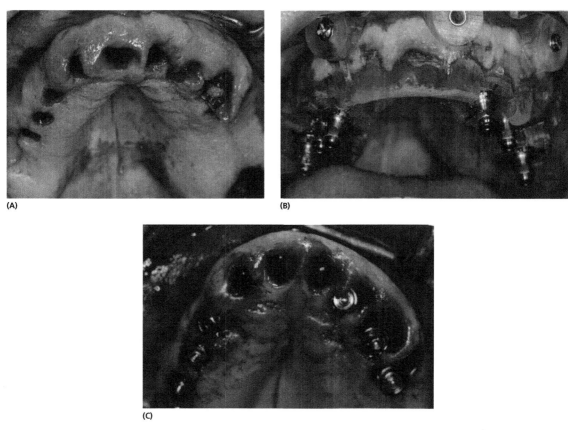

(A)

(B)

(C)

Figure 8.7 (A) Flapless guided surgery after extractions. (B) The prefabricated surgical stent following a computer-guided plan has been secured in place. (C) After the implants are inserted, the surgical guide is removed, and, if immediate loading is planned, the prosthesis is concomitantly delivered.

appropriately sized implant. The scan data is electronically sent back to the manufacturing company where a custom stent (guide) is fabricated. This guide is used intraoperatively to dictate implant placement, many times in a flapless manner where there is no need for an incision and flap elevation. The authors recommend that computer-guided surgery be reserved for dentists who already possess advanced experience in implant surgery.

Postoperative considerations

Postoperative instructions include the use of ice packs to minimize swelling, a soft diet for approximately a week, and the use of chlorhexidine 0.2% rinses bid for 7 to 10 days. Postsurgical follow-up and suture removal are usually scheduled for the 1-week postoperative interval. Over-the-counter pain medications are prescribed, and the preoperative antibiotic, if indicated, might be continued for 7 to 10 days.

Optimal implant positioning

Proper positioning of implant fixture and restoration are important prerequisites for functionally and esthetically successful implant rehabilitation. The prosthetically driven implant placement concept necessitates implant insertion in an optimal three-dimensional position that correlates with the final restorative phase of treatment.

Mesiodistal positioning

Spacing is primarily influenced by the span of the edentulous area and the periodontal width of the adjacent teeth. It is recommended to maintain a distance of 2 mm between the cervical implant face and a natural tooth and greater than 3 mm cervical distance between two adjacent implants. Following these guidelines will minimize crestal bone loss, allow for better soft tissue fill, and ensure proper bone support for interproximal papillae. If these critical distances are compromised, there is greater likelihood of resorption of the interproximal alveolar crest down to the level of the implants. This loss of interproximal bone will result in reduction of papillary soft tissue height, adversely affect the emergence profile, and lead to compromised clinical outcomes.

Buccolingual positioning

Precise planning and construction of the surgical template dictates proper buccolingual positioning of implants. It has been proposed that there must be a minimum bone thickness of approximately 2 mm around the implant. This is critical to maintain an optimal esthetic outcome. However, this may be difficult to always obtain in certain areas, especially in the maxillary anterior regions, where there is pre-existing buccal plate resorption or thinness. Clinicians may often encounter the necessity to place the implants more buccally, but the bone quantity precludes such positioning. Although it may be difficult to achieve a good subgingival emergence profile and the correct crown height in such cases without bone grafting, an acceptable alternative is to orient the implant fixtures by approximately five degrees palatally and place the implants at a site closer to the palatal cortical areas.

Apicocoronal positioning

The implant collar should be located 2 mm apical to the cement–enamel junction (CEJ) of the adjacent teeth, if no gingival recession is present, and 3 mm from the free gingival margin when there is pre-existing recession. This will allow for optimal emergence profile maintenance and a superior esthetic result (Figure 8.8A–C).

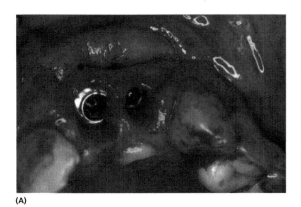

(A)

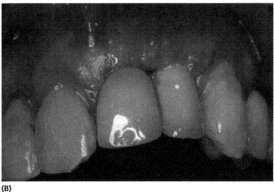

(B)

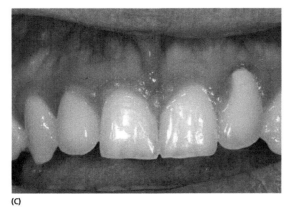

(C)

Figure 8.8 Implant positioning mistakes. (A, B) Mesiodistal mistake: Two implants have been placed too close to each other; this will significantly affect the esthetic outcome adversely. (C) Buccal–lingual mistake: The implant has been placed too buccally, and soft tissue resorption will occur, thereby showing the implant collar.

Implant loading

The modern-day surgeon must be aware of current concepts relating to loading protocols, even if he/she does not perform the prosthetic phase. Loading of implants is another key factor that may influence the final outcome. Usually three different stages of loading are classified: (1) *immediate* (at the time of placement), (2) *early* (4 to 6 weeks after placement), or (3) *standard* (3 months or more after placement). If the clinician decides to connect a temporary restoration at the time of insertion (a form of immediate loading), a torque of insertion of at least 35 N/cm^2 is required as it indicates that there is adequate primary stability of the fixture to withstand such loading.

Mucogingival and soft-tissue considerations

Soft-tissue grafting procedures have been used successfully for many years in periodontal surgery to resolve recession defects around natural teeth and augment alveolar ridge contours. Specific techniques and strategies for soft-tissue grafting in implantology are discussed elsewhere in this book. There are, however, some soft tissue deficiencies that may need to be identified and addressed at the time of implant placement. Attached keratinized gingiva (AKG) tissue can be sufficient, insufficient, or totally absent in an area for which an implant-supported restoration is planned. If inadequate in terms of quality or quantity, a decision must be made about whether to increase AKG, either at the time of implant insertion or at a secondary stage. It is not clear if AKG is required for long-term survival and maintenance of implants. However, there are least two clinical indications to preserve or augment AKG: (1) A good quantity of such tissue around the neck of the implants may help with prosthetic procedures, such as impressions, change of abutments, and so on; and (2) it is easier for the patient to perform and maintain good oral hygiene because it is much less sensitive and relatively more immovable as compared to oral mucosa. There are two surgical options to improve AKG: relocating it from an adjacent site (Figure 8.9A–D) or transplanting it from a remote site (usually the palate) (Figure 8.10A–C).

First, all clinicians should keep in mind that it is prudent to, at least, preserve existing AKG. Thus, unless a surplus of such tissue is present at the site, it is perhaps not advisable to use a tissue punch to expose implants. Second, in implant surgery, one must always try to improve peri-implant tissues, and so a slightly lingual-placed horizontal incision may help in apically re-positioning the existing AKG in some cases (Figure 8.9). The preferred method for AKG augmentation involves a partial-thickness flap, but it can be also done with a full-thickness approach (Figure 8.10).

Complications

The best method of managing complications in implant dentistry is to prevent them! However, despite good planning and surgical execution, complications may occur and must be managed accordingly. Complications in implant dentistry can broadly be classified as *surgical* or *prosthetic*. Surgical complications can further be subdivided into *intraoperative* or *postoperative* categories. Next is a summary of some of the complications that may occur in implant surgery. For greater details regarding management of common surgical complications in intraoral minor oral surgery, please refer to other chapters of this book.

The most common intraoperative complications include bleeding, violation of vital structures, poor implant positioning, and lack of primary stability. Intraoperative bleeding can be controlled in most cases with pressure. If the hemorrhage is a slow, generalized ooze from the implant osteotomy (this is often related to bleeding of the vascular medullary bone rather than an injury to a major vessel), insertion of the implant fixture will often stop the bleeding. Appropriate treatment planning and careful surgical execution will prevent violation of vital structures. Care should be taken while placing implants in the anterior mandible, especially in atrophic mandible cases. If the implants are positioned too lingually, violation of the lingual cortex is likely, and there is a high risk of injuring vasculature in the floor of the mouth region, which can cause a serious, life-threatening hemorrhage.

In the mandible, two anatomic structures can be violated when placing implants: the floor of the mouth and the inferior alveolar canal. Violation of the canal (Figure 8.11) will result in significant neurosensory

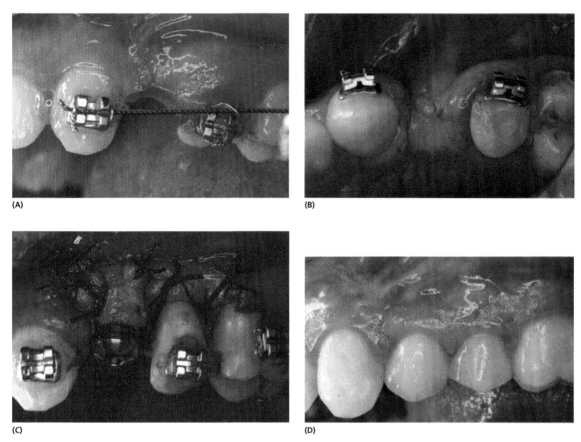

(A)

(B)

(C)

(D)

Figure 8.9 (A) Lack of attached keratinized gingiva and soft tissue deficiency is evident in the upper first premolar area, where an implant and guided bone regeneration procedures were performed 6 months earlier. (B) A horizontal incision has been placed palatally. This allows for AKG to be relocated labially/buccally and will restore the mucogingival line and the soft-tissue thickness. (C) Keratinized gingiva has been apically positioned and secured with 4–0 sutures. Crown lengthening on the distal tooth has also been performed. (D) Final result: note the restored mucogingival line and the mimetic effect of both restorations and soft-tissue appearance.

impairment for the patient in the V3 nerve distribution and may be indicated by excessive bleeding from the implant osteotomy. The impairment could be temporary or permanent, depending on the damage caused to the inferior alveolar nerve. If the patient complains of extended postoperative numbness beyond the time expected due to local anesthetic, the implant fixture should be immediately backed-off or removed. A low-dose oral steroid can be prescribed for short-term therapy, and immediate referral to a specialist oral and maxillofacial surgeon is mandated. As previously mentioned, violation of the floor of the mouth, either in the anterior or posterior mandible, can result in massive bleeding and airway compromise that may require hospitalization. In the maxilla, the surgeon must give special consideration to the maxillary sinuses and nasal cavity. Violation of these

structures can result in infection, bleeding, and implant failure. Displacement of implant fixtures during insertion into the sinus cavity (Figure 8.12) requires surgical intervention to retrieve the foreign body from the maxillary sinus by a surgeon experienced in this type of surgery with adequate postoperative follow-up.

Inadequate positioning complications can be minimized by proper planning and use of a surgical stent fabricated according to the diagnostic wax-up obtained from study models (Figure 8.13). A poorly positioned implant is usually not restorable prosthetically and, even if restorable, usually results in a very unesthetic prosthetic restoration. Common mistakes in positioning can include improper placement relative to depth, resulting in an unnatural emergence profile of the crown; mesiodistal, resulting in loss of papilla or an unnatural emergence

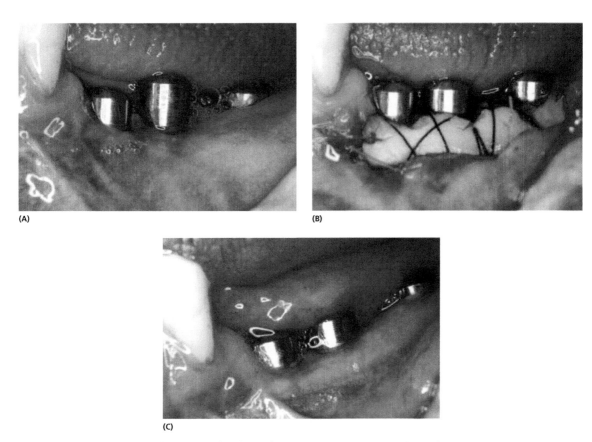

(A)

(B)

(C)

Figure 8.10 (A) Complete lack of AKG. Note that the implants are surrounded by moveable oral mucosa. Also note the malpositioned frenum attachment. (B) A free gingival graft harvested from the palate and secured on the vestibular aspect of the implants. (C) Attached keratinized tissue has been restored, and the frenum attachment surgically corrected.

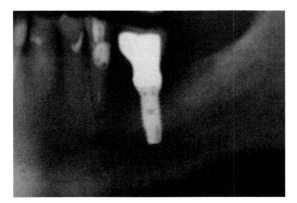

Figure 8.11 Violation of the mandibular canal.

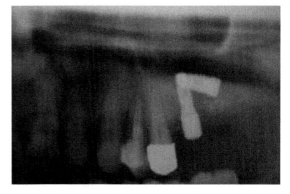

Figure 8.12 Displacement of an implant into the left maxillary sinus.

profile; and buccolingual, resulting in an exposure of prosthetic abutment or an unnatural emergence profile.

Lack of primary stability will often result in an implant failure with lack of osseointegration. It is usually related

to the stage of healing of the extraction socket and may be due to an error in judgment (too early placement) or surgical execution (inadequate, wider implant site preparation). When primary stability is not achieved,

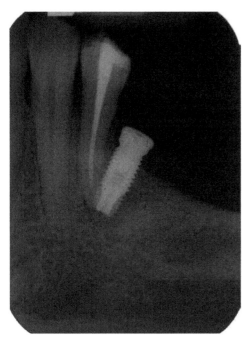

Figure 8.13 Insertion of an implant without a surgical stent: amputation of the root of the adjacent tooth.

the operator should either abort the procedure or consider inserting a wider diameter implant without enlarging the prepared implant site.

The two most common postoperative complications are infection and lack of osseointegration. Both could be considered short-term postoperative complications. Infections can be minimized by the use of antibiotics, chlorhexidine rinses, and instruction in a meticulous oral hygiene maintenance and home-care regimen. If a postoperative infection occurs, it should be managed using standard principles employed for management of infections in intraoral surgery. If an implant does not integrate, it must be removed and then reinserted after the bone is completely healed. Consideration should be given to cleaning out the socket with curettage and grafting. Long-term fractures of the implant fixture have been reported, and these require removal of the fixture (Figure 8.14A–C) and replacement, if indicated at a later stage. It is recommended that all implant surgery patients be monitored for long-term loss of peri-implant bone and/or osseointegration by enrollment in a periodic recall program after prosthetic delivery.

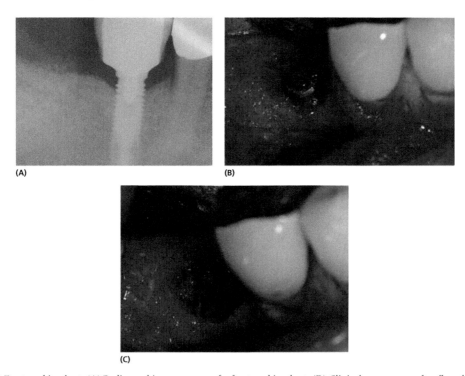

(A)

(B)

(C)

Figure 8.14 Fractured implant. (A) Radiographic appearance of a fractured implant. (B) Clinical appearance after flap elevation. (C) Surgical site after implant removal with a trephine bur.

Further reading

Adell R, Eriksson B, Lekholm U, Branemark PI, Jemt T. Long term follow up study of osseointegrated implants in the treatment of totally edentulous jaws. *International Journal of Oral and Maxillofacial Implants.* 1990; 5: 347–59.

Albreksson T, Lekholm U. Osseointegration. Current state of art. *Dental Clinics of North America.* 1989; 33: 537–42.

Albreksson T, Jansson T, Lekholm U. Osseointegrated dental implants. *Dental Clinics of North America.* 1986; 30: 151–65.

Albreksson T, Zarb G, Worthington P, et al. The long-term efficiency of currently used dental implants: A review and proposed criteria of success. *International Journal of Oral and Maxillofacial Implants.* 1986; 1: 11–7.

Bahat O, Daftary F. Surgical reconstruction. A prerequisite for long term implant success. A philosophic approach. *Practical Periodontics and Aesthetic Dentistry.* 1995; 9: 21–9.

Beagle J. Surgical reconstruction of the interdetal papilla: case report. *International Journal of Periodontics and Restorative Dentistry.* 1992; 12: 145–51.

Bernimoulin JP, Luscher B, Muhlemann HR. Coronally repositioned periodontal flap. Clinical evaluation after one year. *Journal of Clinical Periodontology.* 1975; 2: 1–8.

Block MS. De-epithelialized connective tissue pedicle graft, the palatal roll. *Atlas of Oral and Maxillofacial Surgery Clinics of North America.* 1999; 7: 109–15.

Bowers GM, Chanroff B, Carnevale R, Mellonig J, Corio R, Emerson J, et al. Histologic evaluation of new attachment apparatus formation in humans. Part III. *Journal of Periodontology.* 1989; 60: 683–93.

Branemark PI, Hannson BO, Adell R, Breine U, Lindström J, Hallén O, et al. Osseointegrated implants in the treatment of edentulous jaw. *Scandinavian Journal of Plastic and Reconstructive Surgery.* 1977; 11: 234–7.

Branemark PI, Zarb GA, Alberktson T. *Tissue integrated prosthesis: Osseointegration in clinical dentistry.* Quintessence Publishing, Chicago, 1985, pp. 12–8.

Brugnami F, Caiazzo A, Leone C. Review of intraoral harvesting for bone augmentation: selection criteria, alternative sites, and case report. *Compendium of Continuing Education in Dentistry.* 2010; 31(7).

Brugnami F, Caiazzo A. Efficacy evaluation of a new buccal bone plate preservation technique: a pilot study. *International Journal of Periodontics and Restorative Dentistry.* 2011; 31: 67–73.

Brugnami F, Caiazzo A. Immediate placement and provisionalization with buccal plate preservation: a case report of a new technique. *Journal of Oral Implantology.* 2013; 39(3): 380–5. doi: 10.1563/AAID-JOI-D-11–00154.

Brugnami F, Then P, Moroi H, Leone WC. Histological evaluation of human extraction sockets treated with demineralized freeze-dried bone allograft (DFDBA) and a cell occlusive membrane. *Journal of Periodontology.* 1996; 67: 821–5.

Brugnami F, Then P, Moroi H, Kabani S, Leone WC. Guided bone regeneration with DFDBA prior to implant placement.

Clinical evaluation and histologic evidence of osteoblastic and osteoclastic activities in demineralized freeze-dried bone allograft. *International Journal of Periodontics and Restorative Dentistry.* 1999; 19(3): 259–67.

Buser D, Martin W, Besler U. Optimizing esthetics for implant restorations in the anterior maxilla. Anatomic and surgical considerations. *International Journal of Oral and Maxillofacial Implants.* 2004; 19: 43–61.

Caiazzo A, Brugnami F, Mehra P. Buccal plate augmentation: a new alternative to socket preservation. *Journal of Oral and Maxillofacial Surgery.* 2010; 68: 2503–6.

Caiazzo A, Casavecchia P, Barone A, Brugnami F. A pilot study to determine the effectiveness of different amoxicillin regimens in implant surgery. *Journal of Oral Implantology.* 2011; 37(6): 691–6.

Caiazzo A, Brugnami F, Mehra P. Buccal plate preservation with immediate post-extraction implant placement and provisionalization: preliminary result of a new technique. *International Journal of Oral and Maxillofacial Surgery.* 2013; 42: 666–70.

Carlos EF, Laércio WV. *Metal-Free Esthetic Restorations.* Quintessence Publishing, Brazil, 2003, pp. 52–68.

Christopher EK, Misch CE, Khalaf AS, David PS, Wang HL. Implant plastic surgery. A review and rationale. *Journal of Oral Implantology.* 2004; 30: 242–53.

Cohen DW, Rose SE. The double papillae repositioned flap in periodontal therapy. *Journal of Periodontology.* 1968; 39: 65–74.

Daftary F. Natural aesthetics with implant prosthesis. *Journal of Aesthetic Dentistry.* 1995; 1: 10–9.

Duncan JM, Westwood RM. Ridge widening for the thin maxilla: a clinical report. *International Journal of Oral and Maxillofacial Implants.* 1997; 12: 224–32.

Garber DA, Belser UC. Restoration driven implant placement with restoration generated site development. *Compendium of Continuing Education in Dentistry.* 1995; 15: 796, 798, 802–9.

Grunder U, Speilmann HP, Gaderthuel T. Implant supported single tooth replacement in the aesthetic region: a complex challenge. *Practical Periodontics and Aesthetic Dentistry.* 1996; 8: 830–8.

Grupe HE. Modified technique for the sliding flap operation. *Journal of Periodontology.* 1966; 37: 491–501.

Jarcho M. Biomaterial aspect of calcium phosphates. *Dental Clinics of North America.* 1986; 30: 2547–56.

Jarcho M. Calcium phosphate as hard tissue prosthetics. *Clinical Orthopedics.* 1981; 157: 259–68.

Jemt T. Failures and complications in 391 consecutively inserted fixed prosthesis supported by Branemark implants in edentulous jaws: A study of treatment from the time of prosthesis placement to the first annual check up. *International Journal of Oral and Maxillofacial Implants.* 1991; 6: 270–9.

Jemt T, Linden B, Lekholm U. Failures and complications in 127 consecutively placed fixed partial prosthesis supported by Branemark implants: From prosthetic treatment to first annual check up. *International Journal of Oral and Maxillofacial Implants.* 1992; 7: 40–8.

Langer B, Calagna J. The subepithelial connective tissue graft, a new approach to enhancement of anterior cosmetics. *International Journal of Periodontics and Restorative Dentistry.* 1982; 2: 22–8.

Langer B, Calagna L. The sub-epithelial connective tissue graft. *Journal of Prosthetic Dentistry.* 1980; 44: 363–7.

Langer B, Langer L. Subepithelial connective tissue graft technique for root coverage. *Journal of Periodontology.* 1985; 56: 715–20.

Leois S, Beumer J, Hornburg W, May P. The UCLA abutment. *International Journal of Oral and Maxillofacial Implants.* 1988; 3: 183–90.

Mellonig JT, Bowers GM, Cotton W. Comparison of bone graft materials. Part I. New bone formation with autografts and allografts determined by strontium-85. *Journal of Periodontology.* 1981; 52: 291–6.

Mellonig JT, Bowers GM, Cotton W. Comparison of bone graft materials. Part II. New bone formation with autografts and allografts determined: a histological evaluation. *Journal of Periodontology.* 1981; 52: 297–306.

Schwarz MS, Rothman SL, Chafetz N, Rhodes M. Computed tomography in dental implantation surgery. *Dental Clinics of North America.* 1989; 33: 555–96.

Nevins M, Mellonig J. Advantages of local crest augmentation before implant placement. *International Journal of Periodontics and Restorative Dentistry.* 1994; 2: 96–106.

Pepas NA, Langer R. New challenges in biomaterials. *Science.* 1994; 263: 1715–22.

Philips K, Kois JC. Aesthetic peri-implant site development, the restorative connection. *Dental Clinics of North America.* 1998; 42: 57–67.

Rissolo AR, Bennet J. Bone grafting and its essential role in implant dentistry. *Dental Clinics of North America.* 1998; 42: 91–108.

Saadoun AP, Le Gall M, Touati B. Selection and ideal tri dimensional implant position for soft tissue aesthetics. *Practical Periodontics and Aesthetic Dentistry.* 1999; 11: 1063–73.

Saadoun AP, Le Gall M. Implant positioning for periodontal, functional and aesthetic results. *Practical Periodontics and Aesthetic Dentistry.* 1992; 4: 43–53.

Saadoun AP. Single tooth implant restoration. Surgical management for esthetic results. *International Journal of Dentistry Symposium.* 1995; 3: 30–8.

Salama H, Salama M, Graber D, Adar P. Developing optimal peri-implant papillae within the aesthetic zone. *Journal of Aesthetic Dentistry.* 1995; 7: 125–33.

Scarf D, Tarnow D. Modified roll technique for localized alveolar ridge augmentation. *International Journal of Periodontics and Restorative Dentistry.* 1992; 12: 415–22.

Seibert J. Reconstruction of deformed, partially edentulous ridges, using full thickness onlay grafts. Part I. Technique and wound healing. *Compendium of Continuing Education in Dentistry.* 1983; 5: 437–42.

Silverstein LH, Leflkove M, Gamick J. The use of free gingival soft tissue to improve the implant/soft tissue interface. *Journal of Oral Implantology.* 1994; 20: 36–44.

Spray JR, Black CG, Moris HF, Ochi S. The influence of bone thickness on facial marginal bone: stage I placement through stage II uncovering. *Annals of Periodontology.* 2000; 5: 199–208.

Sullivan HC, Atkins JH. Free autogenous gingival grafts. I. Principle of successful grafting. *Periodontics.* 1968; 6: 121–9.

Tarnow D, Eskow R. Considerations for single-unit esthetic implant restorations. *Compendium of Continuing Education in Dentistry.* 1995; 16: 778–84.

Tarnow D, Magner AW, Fletcher P. The effect of the distance from the contact point to the crest of bone on the presence or absence of inter-proximal papilla. *Journal of Periodontology.* 992; 63: 995–1003.

Tarnow DP, Chow SC, Wallace SS. The effect of inter implant distance on the height of inter implant bone crest. *Journal of Periodontology.* 2000; 71: 546–9.

Touti B. Custom guided tissue healing for improved aesthetics in implant supported restorations. *International Journal of Dentistry Symposium.* 1995; 3: 36–9.

Touti B. Improving aesthetics of implant supported restorations. *Practical Periodontics and Aesthetic Dentistry.* 1995; 7: 81–92.

Touti B. Double guidance approach for the improvement of the single tooth implant replacement. *Dental Implantology Update.* 1997; 8: 89–93.

Touti B. The double guidance concept. *International Journal of Dentistry Symposium.* 1997; 4: 4–12.

Touti B. The double guidance concept. *Practical Periodontics and Aesthetic Dentistry.* 1997; 9: 1089–94.

Urist MR, Silverman BF, Büring K, Dubuc FL, Rosenberg JM. The bone induction principle. *Clinical Orthopedics.* 1967; 53: 243–52.

Urist MR, Strates BS. Bone formation in implants of partially and wholly demineralized bone matrix. *Clinical Orthopedics.* 1970; 71: 271–6.

Urist MR, Strates BS. Bone morphogenic protein. *Journal of Dental Research.* 1971; 50: 1392–1406.

Wohrle PS. The synergy of taper and diameter: enhancing the art and science of implant dentistry with the Replace™ implant system. *International Journal of Dentistry Symposium.* 1997; 4: 48–52.

CHAPTER 9

Hard-Tissue Augmentation for Dental Implants

Pamela Hughes

Department of Oral and Maxillofacial Surgery, Oregon Health & Science University, Portland, OR, USA

Bone healing principles

Before one can undertake hard-tissue augmentation procedures, the clinician must understand bone healing principles in order to properly plan treatment and choose the best option for each individual patient. No one option is the only option in a majority of cases; thus, understanding the healing process, and the advantages or disadvantages of each process, is important.

Primary vs. secondary bone healing

Much like soft tissues, bone heals via primary or secondary intent. Primary bone healing refers to the healing of two segments of bone that are in close proximity to each other, for example, across a fracture line. Osteoclasts work in groups to create a cutting cone, then osteoblasts follow closely behind, laying down osteoid that becomes mineralized. Secondary bone healing requires the formation of a callus that produces osteoid, which is then mineralized. The best example of this would be the bone healing that occurs in an extraction site. There are three phases that encompass secondary bone healing: (1) the inflammatory phase, (2) the recruitment or repair phase, and (3) then the remodeling phase. During the inflammatory phase, inflammatory cells invade the wound, followed by fibroblasts, which then recruit osteoblasts to lay down osteoid that eventually becomes a vascularized callus. After the callus is mineralized, the remodeling phase begins, which takes many months. During the remodeling phase, bone, unlike soft tissue, is restored to its original strength.

Bone graft healing

Bone grafts will take on one of these types of bone healing, depending on the type of graft used. Cortical block grafts will heal similarly to primary bone healing where the osteoclasts will resorb the graft and osteoblasts will follow behind and lay down osteoid that will become mineralized. This is commonly referred to as "creeping substitution."[1] Cortical block grafts will take longer to heal than cancellous or cortical particulate grafts that heal by secondary intent because the particulate grafts do not need to undergo resorption before vascularization occurs. These grafts provide a scaffold that induces apposition of bone. In addition, if cancellous bone is used, there are far more osteoprogenitor cells in the defect that contain several growth factors that are chemotactic, mitogenic, and angiogenic. This type of graft affords a more predictable healing process than cortical block grafts alone, and they sometimes are placed along with cortical block grafts.

There are several factors that can affect bone graft healing. Patient factors such as age, immunocompromise, smoking, and radiation are red flags. As one ages, the number of osteoprogenitor cells present in the bone marrow decreases significantly. Bone grafts rely on good vascularity, usually from surrounding soft tissues (periosteum); so if there is significant scarring or damage (e.g., radiation) to the surrounding soft tissues, bone graft healing will be compromised. Mobility will also compromise healing. If there is gross movement of a graft, fibrocartilage formation will lead to non-union of the graft; this is especially the case with the cortical block graft or onlay graft. Cancellous or particulate grafts can

Manual of Minor Oral Surgery for the General Dentist, Second Edition. Edited by Pushkar Mehra and Richard D'Innocenzo.
© 2016 John Wiley & Sons, Inc. Published 2016 by John Wiley & Sons, Inc.

withstand more mobility due to the nature of the secondary healing process, which does not require intimate proximity of native bone to the bone graft.

Before a discussion of procedures, it is also important for the clinician to understand the classification of bone grafts, based on where they are obtained. It is not always necessary to use bone that is harvested from the patient.

There are four types of bone grafts commonly used in contemporary dentistry. Autografts, or autogenous bone grafts, are grafts that are harvested from and implanted into the same patient. The advantages of autografts are that they have no possibility of disease transmission and contain osteoinductive properties. The disadvantage is that it requires that the patient has a donor site, which carries a potential for additional morbidity. Allografts are bone grafts that are taken from a donor of the same species, but implanted in a recipient who is not the donor. An example of this would be a human cadaveric graft. These grafts have some osteoinductive properties but not as much as autogenous grafts. The advantage is that the patient does not experience any morbidity associated with a donor site. Xenografts are grafts that are taken from a different species; most commonly, a bovine or porcine species. An alloplast, or synthetic graft, is a graft that is synthesized from non-living tissue (Table 9.1). Both xenografts and alloplasts have osteoconductive properties that are inferior to autogenous and allogeneic grafts, but the advantage is that the patient does not experience any donor-site morbidity.

Hard-tissue augmentation procedures for implant reconstruction

There are two primary issues to consider when determining if the bony alveolus is adequate for implant placement: adequate width and adequate height. If either of these are inadequate, hard-tissue augmentation will be necessary.

When considering width, whether in the maxilla or mandible, onlay cortical bone block grafting typically is the most predictable. Most commonly, the cortical graft is an autogenous graft harvested from the patient's mandibular ramus or chin, if the area of grafting is at maximum 2 to 4 edentulous areas. In situations where there is a need for significant grafting, for example, an entire edentulous maxilla, there may be a need for more significant grafting from distant donor sites; this is beyond the scope of this text. Onlay bone grafting is most predictable when used for augmenting width. Although some height can be gained from onlay procedures, this is fairly technical and requires significant expertise to gain height, especially in the posterior mandible.

When treatment planning before alveolar width augmentation procedures, one must consider the following: adequacy of soft tissue, frenal attachments, and the adjacent dentition. If there is significant scarring of the soft tissue, inadequate keratinized tissue, or periodontal defects on adjacent teeth, these soft-tissue issues should

Table 9.1 Classification of bone grafts

Type	Definition	Examples	Properties	Advantages	Disadvantages
Autogenous graft (autograft)	Harvested from and implanted into the same person	Anterior iliac crest Mandibular ramus Menton	Osteoinductive and osteoconductive	No chance of disease transmission Osteoinductive	Donor-site morbidity
Allogenic graft (allograft)	Harvested from the same species	Human cadaver-harvested (mineralized or demineralized freeze-dried bone)	Osteoinductive and osteoconductive	No donor-site morbidity Osteoinductive	Small chance of disease transmission
Xenograft	Harvested from a different species	Bovine bone, red algae	Osteoconductive	No donor-site morbidity	Small chance of disease transmission Osteoconductive
Synthetic graft (alloplast)	Derived from synthetic material	Bioactive glass, calcium sulfate	Osteoconductive	No donor-site morbidity No chance of disease transmission	Osteoconductive

Adapted from Deatherage 2012.[2]

be dealt with first. There also should be no significant risk for infection in the area of the grafting procedure, for example, teeth that are in need of endodontic therapy, periodontal therapy, or restorative therapy.

Onlay bone grafting

Ramus bone graft harvest

The ramus is a very good source of cortical bone and easily accessible in the posterior mandible. After the recipient site is exposed, and the size of the needed graft is identified, an incision is made along the external oblique ridge of the mandible (Figure 9.1). This incision is similar to an incision made for third molar extraction. Once the external oblique ridge is identified, two vertical osteotomies are made distal to the most terminal tooth in the quadrant, taking into consideration the width of the graft needed. Next, the two vertical incisions are connected by

a sagittal osteotomy along the external oblique ridge (Figure 9.2). After this is accomplished, osteotomes are used to outfracture the graft and free the graft (Figures 9.3 and 9.4). The recipient site is then prepared to receive the graft, which should be mortised in place as much as possible. The more bone contact that the graft has with the native bone, the more predictable the integration. The graft should be secured with a bone screw (Figure 9.5), and the soft tissue closed without tension over the graft. If there is tension, or if vertical height is desired, there may be an issue with the graft becoming exposed. If a graft is exposed, there is potential for the entire graft to be lost. The clinician should wait approximately 15 to 20 weeks before implant placement in the area of an onlay graft. There are inherent potential complications associated with the ramus graft, including any potential complications associated with surgery: bleeding, pain, swelling, infection, damage to adjacent teeth/roots, and specifically numbness of the lips, chin, or tongue.

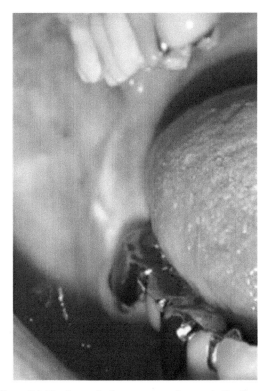

Figure 9.1 The donor site for a ramus graft extends distally along the external oblique ridge of the mandible distal to the most posterior tooth.

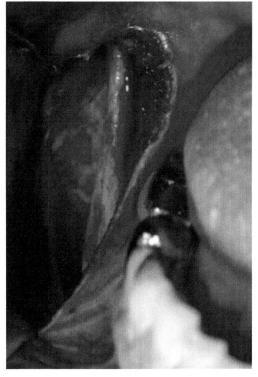

Figure 9.2 A sagittal osteotomy is created along the external oblique ridge connecting the vertical osteotomies at the superior and inferior extents of the graft.

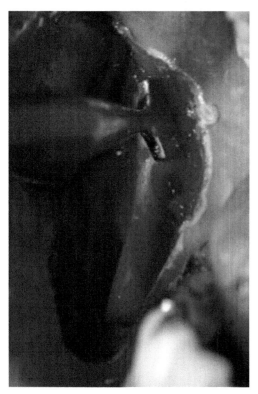

Figure 9.3 An osteotome is used to outfracture and deliver the graft.

Menton bone harvest

The menton bone harvest is, in principle, similar to the ramus graft, in that it is a unicortical onlay graft. The chin is exposed through a transoral incision, either a sulcular incision or a vestibular incision. After the chin is exposed, a drill is used to create a unicortical osteotomy in the shape and size of the needed graft. Once the osteotomy is created, osteotomes are used to free the graft from the facial aspect of the chin. The graft is then mortised into place and secured as described above. One should take care to resuspend the mentalis muscle upon closing to avoid a cosmetic defect of the chin. Given the approximation of the mental nerves to the harvest site, the potential complications are the same as the ramus harvest.

Osteotome technique for width augmentation

If a single-tooth, maxillary edentulous area requires only 1 to 3 mm of augmentation, ridge-widening osteotomes may be considered.[3,4] This procedure takes advantage of

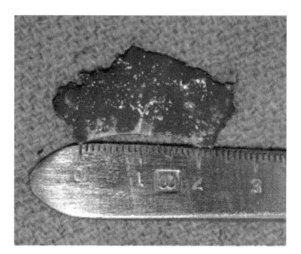

Figure 9.4 The harvested graft.

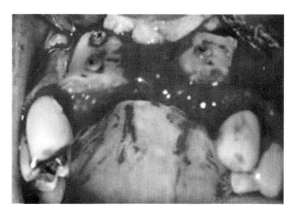

Figure 9.5 The graft is separated, placed into the recipient site, and secured with bone screws to ensure immobility.

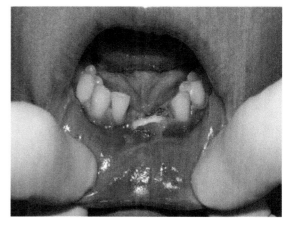

Figure 9.6 An example of an exposed ramus graft due to wound tension upon closure. Note the shallow, scarred vestibule.

the malleable nature of the maxillary bone and is done at the time of implant placement. No grafting is necessary with this technique. An implant pilot drill is used to begin the osteotomy, then sequentially larger-sized osteotomes (Figure 9.7) are tapped to depth to gradually widen the ridge without removing bone (Figures 9.8, 9.9, 9.10, 9.11, 9.12, and 9.13). After the osteotomy has reached its appropriate size, the implant is placed.

There are other ridge-splitting techniques available that are similar to this technique and may or may not require grafting as well.

Maxillary posterior vertical augmentation (sinus lift)

Maxillary sinus augmentation has become a predictable, widely recognized pre-implant reconstructive procedure that has taken on several procedural nuances over the past three decades. In the infancy of sinus grafting procedures, autogenous bone (mostly from the anterior iliac crest) was the preferred graft of choice. Since that time, most allogenic and xenogenic materials on the market today have been shown to provide good outcomes without the need for bone harvest, thus negating donor-site morbidity. Furthermore, new

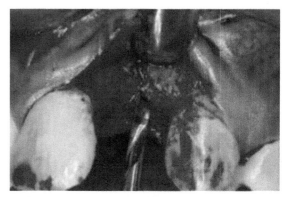

Figure 9.9 A pilot drill is used to create the initial osteotomy.

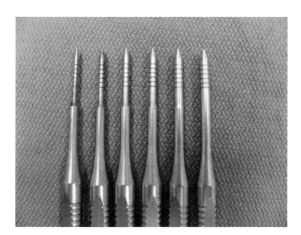

Figure 9.7 Ridge-widening osteotomes. Note the progressively larger diameter of the osteotomes and the pointed tips.

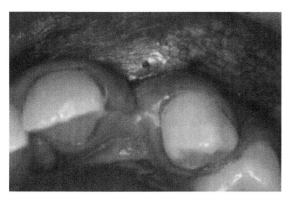

Figure 9.8 Labial bone defect at site #10.

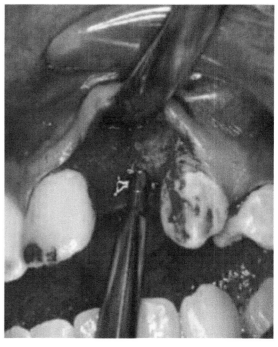

Figure 9.10 A smaller sized osteotome is initially inserted into the implant osteotomy site and tapped to the required depth.

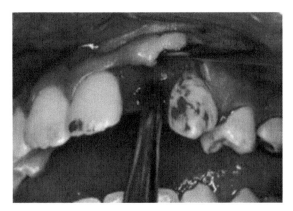

Figure 9.11 A larger osteotome is next used to further widen the alveolus.

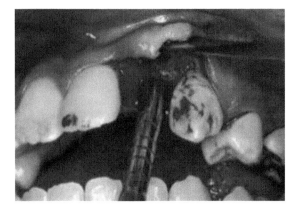

Figure 9.12 Sequentially larger osteotomes are used to expand the alveolus to the desired width.

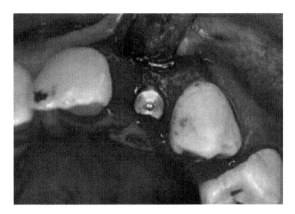

Figure 9.13 The implant fixture in place after preparing the implant osteotomy with ridge-widening osteotomes.

techniques involving a bone morphogenic protein (BMP-2) have been approved for use in the maxillary sinus by the Food and Drug Administration. Whatever material the clinician prefers, the most widely used approach for placing sinus augmentation materials is the lateral antrostomy, sometimes referred to as the Caldwell–Luc approach.

Before a discussion of the sinus lifting procedure, it is critical to understand that a diseased sinus is not a good host for successful grafting. The clinician must understand how to properly assess the health of the sinus and treat chronic or acute sinusitis (or refer the patient to be treated) before commencing with treatment.

Clinical evaluation for sinus augmentation

The clinical evaluation begins similarly to any other oral exam to rule out any pathoses unrelated to the area of interest. Next, the alveolar ridge in question is inspected. The alveolar width, interocclusal space, and soft tissues are inspected, keeping in mind that if there is a significant width discrepancy, lateral augmentation may also be needed in conjunction with the sinus lift procedure. A panoramic radiograph or cone beam computerized tomography (CT) scan should be acquired to assess the amount of residual alveolar height inferior to the floor of the maxillary sinus. Typically, bone height of less than 8 to 10 mm will require some type of augmentation procedure. The clinician should also perform a diagnostic wax-up to determine the prosthodonic plan and the position of the proposed implants.

Sinus augmentation procedures

Direct sinus lift

As mentioned previously in this chapter, the most commonly used approach to the sinus is the lateral antrostomy. A crestal inicision is made and the mucosa reflected to expose the lateral wall of the maxilla. The clinician many times can identify the vertical position of the sinus floor given the bluish hue that is sometimes recognizable through the thin bone of the lateral maxillary wall. Carefully, a rectangular or circular osteotomy is created, taking care not to penetrate the very thin sinus membrane. Curettes are then used to reflect the sinus membrane off the sinus floor, and the bone window that was created is then gently pushed medially and superiorly. This segment will become the new sinus floor. The clinician's grafting material is then placed and the mucosa re-approximated. Depending on the material placed, the implants are placed 3 to 5 months after the sinus lift.

In some instances, where there is enough residual bone for initial stabilization of the implants, this procedure can be done at the same time as placement of the implants (Figures 9.14, 9.15, and 9.16).

Indirect sinus lifting procedure (osteotome technique)

Just as with maxillary alveolar widening, a sinus lift can be performed using sinus lift osteotomes (commonly referred to as Summer's Osteotomes).[3] These circular, progressively widening osteotomes have a cupped end to capture and push bone superiorly (Figure 9.17). The procedure is similar to that previously described with the widening technique, except that particulate bone graft material is placed into the osteotomy site each time a new osteotome is introduced to push grafting material up into the sinus cavity. Studies have shown that, realistically, 3 to 5 mm of bone can be gained from this technique.[3,4] However, there needs to be enough residual bone to allow for stability of the implant fixture (Figures 9.18 and 9.19).[3,4]

Postoperative course

No matter what augmentation procedure is performed, the patient should be advised of the potential complications. Infection and dehiscence of the graft are the most commonly encountered problems that can lead to failure of the augmentation. The clinician should consider that perioperative antibiotics may be warranted for these procedures, especially for patients who may be somewhat immunocompromised. Careful preoperative medical assessment, clinical assessment, and treatment planning play a crucial role in the success of these procedures. When handled correctly, they have a high rate of success and can positively impact the patient's overall function and esthetics.

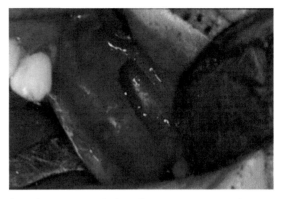

Figure 9.14 Creation of a lateral antrostomy to access the maxillary sinus. Note the amount of alveolar bone, enough to provide initial stabilization of the implants.

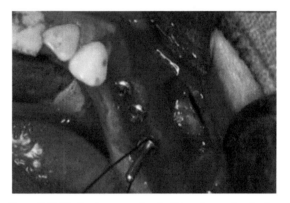

Figure 9.15 The implants are placed. Although not visualized in this picture, the apical two-thirds of the implants protrude into the maxillary sinus. The coronal one-third is supported by the alveolar bone that is present.

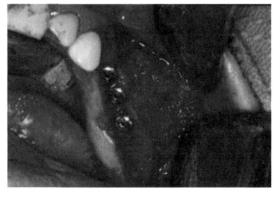

Figure 9.16 Particulate bone graft is placed into the maxillary sinus and around the implant that is protruding into the maxillary sinus.

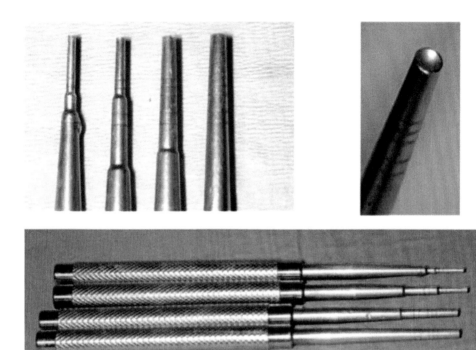

Figure 9.17 Sinus lift osteotomes (Summer's Osteotomes). Note the cupped shape at the end of the osteotome.

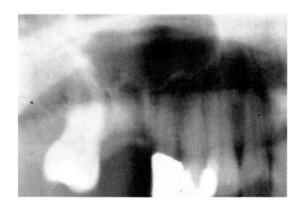

Figure 9.18 Radiographic representation of an edentulous area before an indirect sinus-lifting procedure.

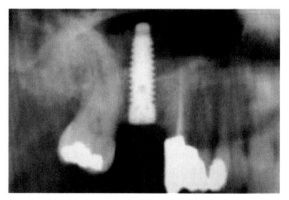

Figure 9.19 Radiographic representation of the postprocedure result. Note the bone surrounding the portion of the implant that is in the sinus cavity.

References

1. Roden D. Principles of bone grafting. *Oral and Maxillofacial Surgery Clinics of North America.* 2010; 22: 295–300.
2. Deatherage J. Bone materials available for alveolar grafting. *Oral and Maxillofacial Surgery Clinics of North America.* 2012; 22: 347–52.
3. Summers RB. A new concept in maxillary implant surgery: the osteotome technique. *Compendium.* 1994; 15(2): 152, 154–6.
4. Rake A, Andreasen K, Rake S, Swift J. A retrospective analysis of osteointegration in the maxilla utilizing an osteotome technique versus a sequential drilling technique. 1999, AAOMS. Abstract.

Further reading

Moy P (ed.). Dental Implant Site Preservation and Development. *Oral Maxillofacial Surgery Clinics of North America.* 2004; 16(1).
Ness G. Maxillary sinus grafts and implants. In: Fonseca RJ, ed. *Oral and Maxillofacial Surgery*, 1st edn, Vol 7. WB Saunders Co., New York, 2000.

CHAPTER 10

Soft Tissue Surgery for Dental Implants

Hussam Batal

Department of Oral and Maxillofacial Surgery, Boston University Henry M. Goldman School of Dental Medicine, Boston, MA, USA

Introduction

Over the past 20 years, there has been a paradigm shift in implant dentistry relative to concepts, especially for the anterior esthetic zone. The objective of such surgery has shifted from obtaining a functional restoration to obtaining a functional esthetetic restoration that fully blends with the surrounding. It has been shown that an adequate quality and quantity of soft tissue provides the best peri-implant environment. Attached tissue around dental implants increases soft tissue stability and decreases the incidence dentition of peri-implant mucositis. Additionally, an adequate band and thickness of soft tissue in the esthetic zone is needed to provide the desired optimal esthetic outcome that allows the final restoration to seamlessly blend with the surrounding dentition.

When evaluating surgical results for soft-tissue grafting and implant surgery, it is important to perform an objective evaluation that allows for quantitative and qualitative assessment. The pink esthetic score (PES) is an example of a good objective scoring system to evaluate treatment outcome.[1] This system of classification has a maximum of 14 points that rate seven distinct variables in relation to gingival esthetics. The variables include mesial papilla, distal papilla, level of gingival margin, soft tissue color, soft tissue texture, alveolar process contour, and marginal tissue contour. Each of these factors can be assigned an individual score on a scale of 0–2 (Figure 10.1 and Table 10.1).

Gingival biotype

Esthetic outcomes in implant dentistry strongly correlate with the patient's gingival biotype. There are two distinct gingival biotypes: thin scalloped and thick flat biotype.[2–4] There are three key areas of variation between the two biotypes: soft tissue, bone, and tooth morphology. Determination of biotypes on occasion is controversial and also, at the same time, can be quite challenging. Thus, use of objective criteria is recommended, and for example, combining the direct measurement of soft-tissue thickness and tooth morphology can aid in the determination and classification of the biotype.

Thin scalloped gingival biotype

For the thin scalloped biotype, the bony and soft-tissue architecture tends to be highly scalloped; the soft tissue is thin (Figure 10.2). The underlying buccal plate tends to be thin with frequent fenestration and dehiscence types of defects. The bony architecture tends to undergo extensive remodeling after extraction of teeth, including increased loss of height of the buccal plate and socket dimension compared to patients with a thicker buccal plate. The teeth tend to be more triangular in shape with narrow contact areas located in the incisal one-third, and the crowns at the cervical area are either flat or have a subtle convexity with a flat emergence profile.

Manual of Minor Oral Surgery for the General Dentist, Second Edition. Edited by Pushkar Mehra and Richard D'Innocenzo.

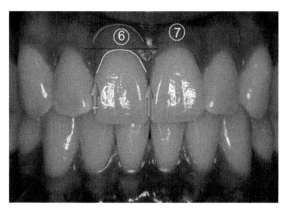

Figure 10.1 PES score: gray arrows are mesial and distal papillae, white line is soft tissue contour, red line is soft-tissue level, green line is alveolar convexity, 6 is soft tissue color, and 7 is soft-tissue texture. Each category is assigned a score of 0–2.

Table 10.1 PES score

Variable	Score 0	Score 1	Score 2
Mesial papilla	Missing	Incomplete	Complete
Distal papilla	Missing	Incomplete	Complete
Soft tissue contour	Unnatural	Virtually natural	Natural
Soft tissue level	Discrepancy > 2 mm	Discrepancy 1–2 mm	Discrepancy < 1 mm
Alveolar process	Clearly resorbed	Slightly resorbed	No difference
Soft tissue coloring	Clear difference	Slight difference	No difference
Soft tissue texture	Clear difference	Slight difference	No difference

Thick flat gingival biotype

For the thick flat biotype, the bony and soft tissue architecture tends to be flat with short interdental papillae, supported further by a dense and thick band of attached tissue (Figure 10.3). The underlying bony architecture is thick and rarely has dehiscences or fenestrations. The thick plate tends to undergo less remodeling after surgical procedures. The teeth tend to be squarer in shape with long contact areas extending to the cervical one-third. The emergence profile tends to be pronounced.

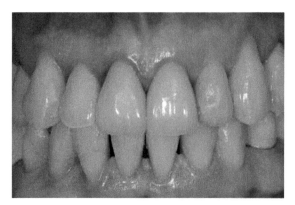

Figure 10.2 Thin scalloped gingival biotype with triangular-shaped teeth.

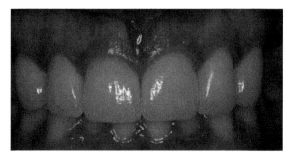

Figure 10.3 Thick flat gingival biotype with square-shaped teeth.

There is general consensus that the addition of a soft-tissue graft to the surgical implant protocol in patients with a thin scalloped biotype will increase gingival thickness and improve esthetic outcomes, especially at the buccal gingival margin level. It is likely to even improve long-term soft-tissue stability.

Healing of soft-tissue grafts

The subepithelial graft is ideal for reconstruction of most soft-tissue defects. This graft is mostly composed of a connective tissue matrix that allows for ingrowth of new fibroblasts, which is in addition to the fibroblasts that are already transported with the graft. The initial healing depends on plasmatic imbibition or diffusion for the first 24 to 48 hours. The initial hypoxic gradient between the graft and the recipient site is responsible for initiating this process. This initial plasmatic diffusion is responsible for the initial metabolite influx to the graft. Inflammatory mediators stimulate neovascularization of new capillaries from the recipient site into the graft. Anastomosis between the vessels of the recipient site and graft is established, and the graft will have adequate blood supply by the eighth postoperative day. During the revascularization process, connective tissue reattachment between the graft and the recipient bed occurs. This process is complete by the tenth postoperative day. Upon final healing, the graft will undergo secondary contraction.

General principles of soft-tissue grafting

When performing soft-tissue grafting, there are general principles that will increase the chances of success and decrease the incidence of complications. These principles are divided into recipient site preparation and donor site management guidelines. These general principles are derived from the physiological healing process and the local and systemic conditions needed to achieve them. In brief, they are:

1. Creation of a large recipient bed
2. Adequate hemostasis at the recipient site
3. Intimate adaptation of the graft
4. Immobilization of the graft
5. Primary closure, when feasible (dual blood supply)

Soft-tissue graft healing depends on adequate preparation and the vascularity of the recipient site. Grafts initially survive by plasmatic diffusion and then by revascularization. Good adaptation and immobility of the graft are critical for these processes to occur effectively. Increased mobility could disrupt the revascularization process and increase the chance of necrosis of the graft. Intimate adaptation to the recipient site is imperative to success and decreases the diffusion and capillary travel distance by providing early nutrition to the graft. Also, adequate hemostasis at the recipient site will decrease capillary bleeding or large clot formation, both of which could impair the nutrient supply. In cases where there is decreased vascularity at the recipient site (scarring, implant abutment, root surface), use of a pedicled graft with contiguous blood supply should be considered as opposed to free grafts. If a pedicled graft is not feasible, care should be taken so that the recipient site and graft are wide enough to allow for peripheral circulation, which will support the graft over the poorly vascularized area.[5] When preparing the recipient site, clinicians should ensure that the surface is uniform and will allow for adequate immobilization of the grafted tissue. Adequate hemostasis is mandatory to permit the graft to sufficiently adapt to the recipient bed.

Generally speaking, intact and viable periosteum is considered an ideal coverage layer. Periosteum has an excellent blood supply, is non-movable, and will allow for adequate immobilization and suturing of the graft. The graft should be of uniform thickness as this allows for better adaptation of the graft to the recipient site. The thickness of the graft plays a role in the healing process and could also determine the amount of secondary contracture of the graft. Thin and intermediate-thickness grafts have a higher percentage of survival. Contrastingly, thicker grafts yield better clinical outcomes, with less secondary contracture, but are more technique sensitive. Finally, whenever possible, creation of a flap at the recipient site that permits primary closure is likely to improve outcomes and decrease the possibility of graft necrosis.

Timing of soft-tissue grafting

Soft-tissue grafting can be performed at a variety of times during implant therapy. It can be performed before, at the same time, or after bone grafting, at the time of implant placement, at the time of second-stage abutment placement, and after prosthetic crown connection. The predictability of stable and successful outcomes decreases when soft-tissue grafting is performed after crown connection (Figure 10.4).

Connective tissue autografts

A variety of intraoral donor sites have been described for connective tissue grafts. The most commonly used source is the hard palate. Other possible donor sites are the maxillary tuberosity and the retromolar pad area. Although the greatest thickness of tissue is usually present in the maxillary tuberosity area, the maximum volume of tissue obtainable is from the palate. The amount of tissue available tends to be limited in the fully dentate patient.

Types of connective tissue that are harvested from intraoral sites can be divided into subepithelial connective tissue grafts and epithelial connective tissue grafts (Figure 10.5A, B, C).

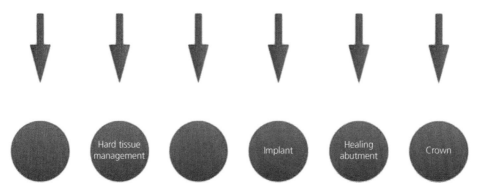

Figure 10.4 Timing of soft-tissue grafts.

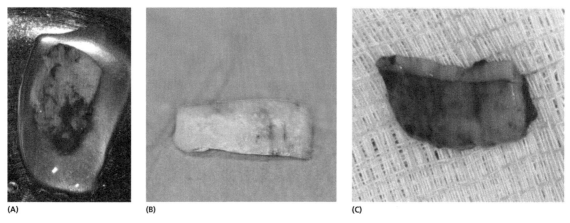

(A) (B) (C)

Figure 10.5 (A) Subepithelial connective tissue graft. (B) Epithelial connective tissue graft. (C) Subepithelial connective tissue graft with epithelial collar.

Epithelialized palatal graft

Epithelialized palatal grafts have been widely used for correction of mucogingival defects for many years. Bjorn[6] and Sullivan and Atkins[7] were the first to describe the free gingival autograft. Sullivan *et al.* classified gingival grafts based on their thickness as either full-thickness or split-thickness grafts. Thicker gingival grafts are ideal for cases in which the main purpose is to increase the zone of attached tissue. Thicker grafts are more technique sensitive but provide better outcomes. These grafts undergo less secondary graft contraction compared to split-thickness grafts.

Technique

Using a #15 C blade, an incision of the desired length is made at the junction of the attached and non-attached tissue. At either end of the horizontal incision, two vertical incisions are then made. A partial thickness flap is next developed and reflected using instruments of choice (scissors and/or blades). It is critical to dissect as close to the periosteum as possible to remove epithelium, connective tissue, and muscle fibers; this minimizes the amount of movable tissue that is present. Thus, performing this step carefully will decrease the incidence of graft mobility and promote healing. The dissection is next carried out in a supraperiosteal fashion (Figure 10.6A, B). The periosteum, as mentioned above, is an ideal layer to which to suture the graft. After the flap has been developed, it can be either sutured apically or excised.

After preparation of the recipient site, the clinician must focus on the harvest site. A template is used to estimate the desired size of the graft. The graft is commonly harvested from the palate, from the distal aspect of the second premolar to the mesial aspect of the canine, avoiding the midline and paramidline rugae area. The

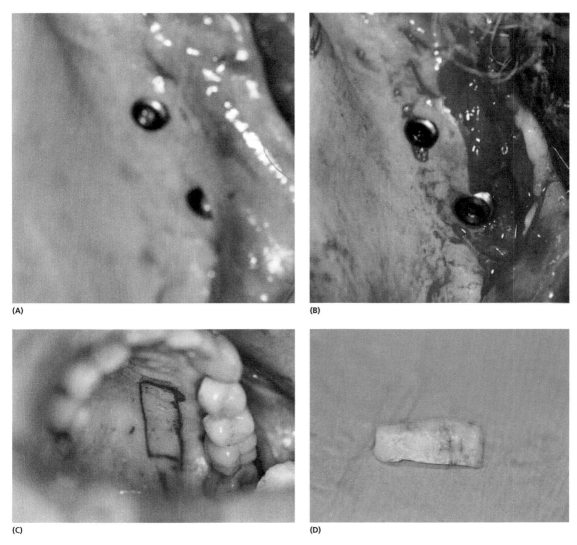

(A)   (B)

(C)   (D)

Figure 10.6 (A) Preoperative view showing no attached tissue on the buccal aspect of the posterior implant. (B) Split-thickness incision is developed buccal to the implant and sutured apically. (C) Split-thickness epithelial graft is harvested. (D) Epithelial connective tissue graft.

graft is outlined with the use of a #15C blade. The most superior aspect of the incision is then made, staying approximately 3 mm apical to the cemento–enamel junction (CEJ) of the teeth. The dissection is carried down to the desired depth throughout the graft length with either a #15C blade or a sharp scissors such as Dean scissors (Figure 10.6C). Once the graft has been harvested, it is trimmed to the desired shape and thinned out, if needed (Figure 10.6D). The graft is adapted to the recipient site and secured with several 4–0 or 5–0 resorbable sutures. The graft is initially secured at the mesial then the distal corners; this procedure ensures that the entire area is covered and that the graft is well adapted to the recipient site. Sutures are then placed in other areas to fully secure the graft (Figure 10.6E). If desired, additional sling or horizontal mattress sutures can be added to further stabilize the graft. Once suturing is complete, pressure is applied to the graft for approximately ten minutes; this aids with hemostasis and decreases the dead space between the graft and the recipient site.

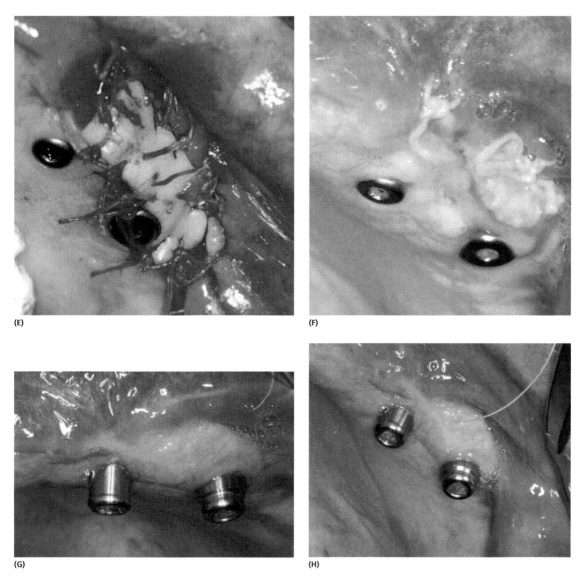

(E)

(F)

(G)

(H)

Figure 10.6 (*Continued*) (E) Graft secured and sutured in place. (F) Graft at the 4-week postoperative visit. (G and H) Graft 2 years postoperative.

Biophysiologically, during this time and beyond, plasma is converted into fibrin, and this conversion further binds the graft to the recipient site and promotes diffusion of nutrition into the graft (Figure 10.6F–H).

Harvest of subepithelial connective tissue graft

Gingival grafts are commonly harvested from the palate from an area between the palatal root of the first molar and the canine. The tissue tends to be thickest in this region. During the harvesting procedure, careful attention should be paid so as not to injure the greater palatine artery (Reiser *et al.* 1996).[8] According to Reiser's study, the greater palatine artery enters the palate in the area of the greater palatine foramen and travels across the palate anteriorly in the direction of the incisive foramen. The greater palatine foramen is most commonly located at the junction of the horizontal and vertical shelf of the palatine bone in an area corresponding

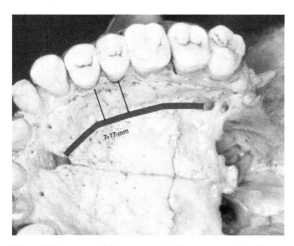

Figure 10.7 Course of the greater palatine artery exiting the greater palatine foramen and crossing the palate in the direction of the incisive canal. Crossing at the junction of the horizontal and vertical shelf of the palate. The greater palatine artery is located between 7 and 17 mm from the CEJ of the teeth, with an average distance of 12 mm.

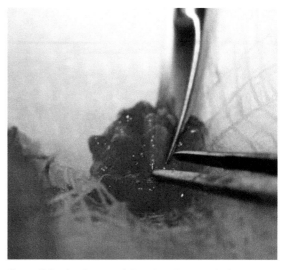

Figure 10.8 After harvest of the subepithelial graft, fat is trimmed with the use of a scissor.

to the position between the second and third molar teeth. The neurovascular bundle is located approximately 7 to 17 mm from the CEJ of the teeth, at an average distance of 12 mm (Figure 10.7). This distance is shorter in patients with a shallow palatal vault and longer in patients with a higher palatal vault. Iatrogenic injury to the greater palatine artery closer to the foramen can cause extensive bleeding compared to tissue damage in the anterior palatal area. Limiting the dissection to 8 mm in height will limit the risk of bleeding in most patients.

The palatal soft tissue is composed of three layers: epithelium, subepithelial connective tissue, and submucosa. In the anterior palatal area, especially in the area of the palatal raphae, the subepithelial layer is rich in fat. After harvesting the graft, the fat layer should be removed with scissors before suturing; this will decrease subsequent mobility of the graft (Figure 10.8). Moreover, it will allow the graft to be uniform in size and optimize its adaptation to the host recipient bed. In order to maintain vitality, it is advisable to temporarily store the harvested and prepared graft in saline-soaked sponges.

Various techniques for harvesting subepithelial connective tissue grafts have been described. The main variation is in the number and type of surface incisions.

Single-incision surgical technique: In cases where no epithelial collar is desired, the single-incision technique is recommended. After local anesthetic infiltration, a split-thickness incision is made 2 to 3 mm away from the CEJ of the teeth. The incision extends from the mesial aspect of the first molar to the canine (Figure 10.9A, B). A split-thickness flap is developed within the first incision with the use of a #15 blade. The direction of dissection is parallel to the palatal tissue (Figure 10.9C, D). The flap should be at least 1 mm thick to decrease the chances of sloughing and necrosis, which could increase postoperative pain and discomfort. This incision also determines the thickness of the tissue that will be harvested. The dissection is carried on with sharp instruments to the height of approximately 8 mm. This height usually corresponds to the cutting portion of the #15 scalpel blade. A properly carried out dissection should create a rectangular pouch (Figure 10.9E). Later, a second horizontal incision is made within the pocket all the way down to bone, about 1 to 1.5 mm apical to the initial incision (Figure 10.9F, G). This variation leaves a 1 mm ledge of connective tissue, which can be sutured to the epithelial flap to increase the potential for primary healing and decrease the chances of dehiscence and failure. Once the pouch is created, an anterior incision is made inside the pouch at the most anterior aspect, all the way down to bone to the desired depth (Figure 10.9H). Next, an incision is made in a similar

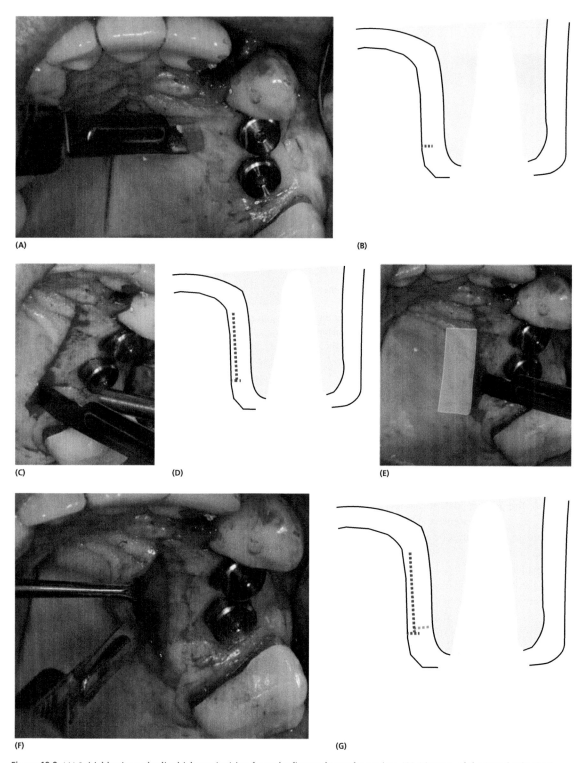

Figure 10.9 (A) Initial horizontal split-thickness incision from the first molar to the canine. (B) Diagram of the initial split-thickness incision (red dotted line). (C) Split-thickness dissection is carried to a depth of 8–10 mm. (D) Diagram showing the outline of the split-thickness flap. (E) Outline of the rectangular pouch (split-thickness dissection). (F) Second horizontal full-thickness incision 1 mm apical to the first incision. (G) Diagram of the second horizontal incision (blue dotted line).

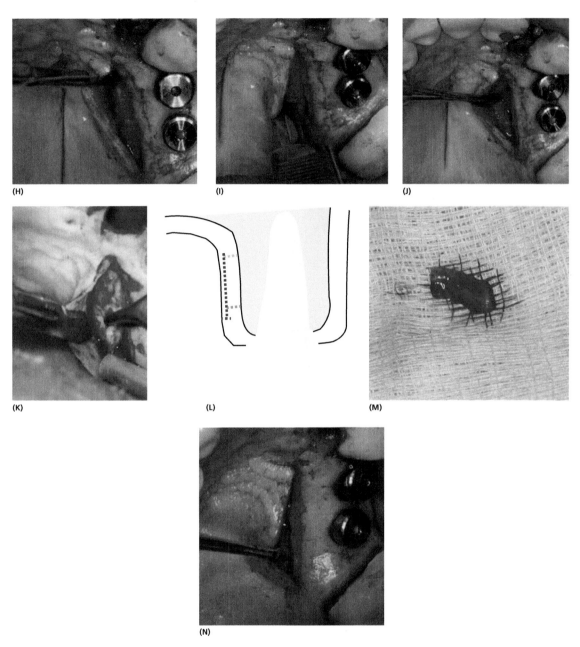

Figure 10.9 (*Continued*) (H) Anterior incision inside the pouch down to bone. (I) Posterior incision inside the pouch down to bone. (J) Dissection is carried out in a subperiosteal fashion, reflecting the graft. (K) A full-thickness incision is made along the apical aspect, and the graft is harvested. (L) Diagram of the apical incision (gray dotted line). (M) The subepithelial graft is harvested, and the fat is trimmed. (N) Stepping the incision will leave a 1 mm subepithelial collar. This will facilitate suturing and decrease dehiscence of the incision.

fashion at the posterior aspect (Figure 10.9I). A Woodson, or similar, periosteal elevator is used to elevate the graft in a subperiosteal plane (Figure 10.9J). The partially elevated graft is held with tissue pickups, an incision is made at the most apical aspect

(Figure 10.9K, L), and, using tissue forceps and gentle traction, the graft is harvested (Figure 10.9M, N).[9–11]

In another variation of the single-incision technique, an initial horizontal full-thickness incision is placed 2 to 3 mm away from the CEJ of the teeth (Figure 10.10A, B).

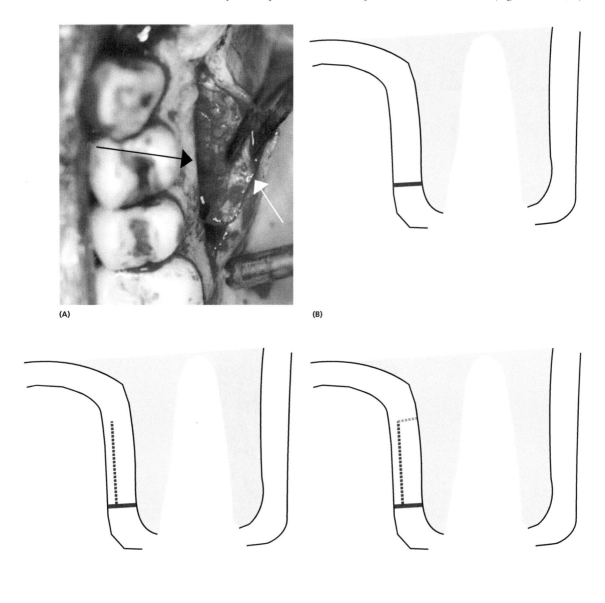

Figure 10.10 (A) The initial horizontal incision is a full-thickness incision (black arrow); the split-thickness incision is started within the first incision (white arrow). (B) Diagram of the initial full-thickness incision (red solid line). (C) Diagram showing the outline of the split-thickness flap (red dotted line). (D) Diagram of the apical incision (blue dotted line).

Next, the blade is used to start a split-thickness incision within the first horizontal incision (Figure 10.10C, D) and extended parallel to the palate. The graft is then harvested in a similar manner to the single-incision technique described above.[12]

Two-incision surgical technique: After adequate local anesthetic with a vasoconstrictor has infiltrated the area, a full-thickness horizontal incision is made 2 to 3 mm apical to the sulcular gingival margin, extending from the mesial aspect of the first molar to the canine area. A second horizontal incision is placed 1 to 2 mm apical to the first incision. The second horizontal incision is made to a depth of 1 to 1.5 mm, and, using that incision, a split-thickness flap is developed with the use of a #15 blade (Figure 10.11A–D). The direction of dissection is parallel to the palatal tissue. The flap should be at least 1 mm thick to decrease the chances of sloughing and necrosis. This incision also determines the thickness of the tissue that will be harvested. The dissection is carried on with sharp instruments to the height of approximately 8 mm. This height usually corresponds to the cutting portion of the #15 scalpel blade. A properly carried out dissection should create a rectangular pouch. Once the pouch is created, an

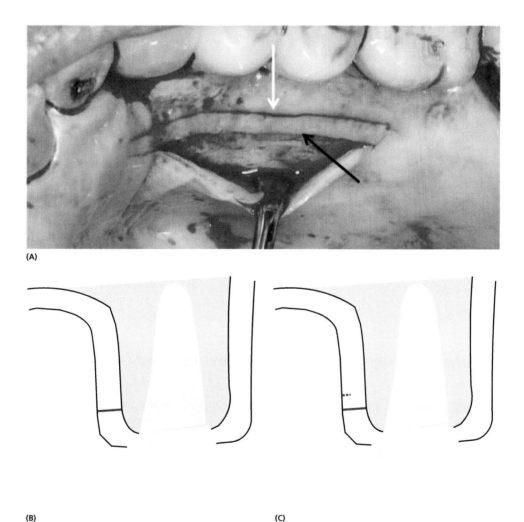

(A)

(B)   (C)

Figure 10.11 (A) In the two-incisions technique, the initial incision is a full-thickness incision (white arrow). The second incision is placed 1–1.5 mm apical and carried out in a split-thickness fashion (black arrow). (B) Diagram of the initial full-thickness incision (red solid line). (C) Diagram of the second split incision (red dotted line).

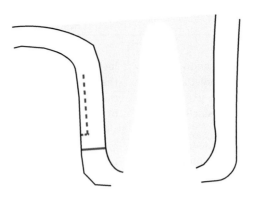

(D)

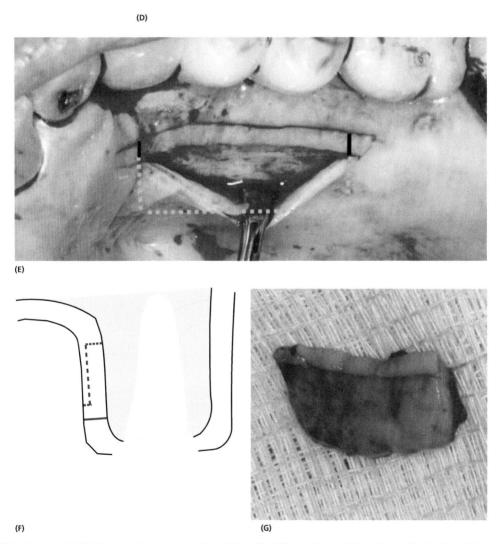

(E)

(F)

(G)

Figure 10.11 (*Continued*) (D) Diagram showing the outline of the split-thickness flap (red dotted line). (E) Outline of the anterior, posterior, and apical incisions. A solid black full-thickness incision down to bone. Incisions inside the pouch down to bone (gray dotted lines). (F) Diagram of the apical incision. (G) A subepithelial connective tissue graft with an epithelial collar.

anterior incision is made inside the pouch at the most anterior aspect all the way down to bone to the desired depth. Next, an incision is made in a similar fashion at the posterior aspect. A Woodson, or similar, periosteal elevator is used to elevate the graft in a subperiosteal plane. The partially elevated graft is held with tissue pickups, an incision is made at the most apical aspect (Figure 10.11E, F), and, using tissue forceps and gentle traction, the graft is harvested (Figure 10.11G). Pressure is applied to the recipient site, and a collagen or hemostatic dressing is placed in the harvest site and secured in place with overlying 4–0 resorbable sutures. One should always try to harvest subepithelial connective tissue grafts with attached periosteum as this makes handling easier and decreases secondary shrinkage and contraction of the graft.

Modified palatal roll technique

Abrams[13] described the original palatal roll technique. In his technique, a split-thickness palatal flap is reflected, separating the epithelium from the connective tissue. The connective tissue is reflected from the palate and rolled onto the buccal area to correct a bucco-lingual soft tissue deficiency. In 1992, Scharf and Tarnow[14] described a modification of the original palatal roll technique. In their technique, a #15 blade is used to make a full-thickness palatal incision extending from the crest of the ridge to the palatal area. This incision should avoid the papilla and be of sufficient length to allow the tissue to be rolled onto the desired area on the buccal aspect (Figure 10.12A). A similar incision is also made on the contralateral side. A partial-thickness incision connecting the two vertical incisions is made on the palatal aspect (Figure 10.12B). A partial-thickness trap door-type flap is reflected. A full-thickness incision is then carried through the connective tissue down to the periosteum at the apical extent of the two vertical incisions (Figure 10.12C). The palatal pedicle is reflected with the use of a Woodson, or similar, elevator. The pedicle is rolled and tunneled onto the buccal aspect. A horizontal mattress suture is used to stabilize the graft on the buccal aspect (Figure 10.12D). This technique can be effectively used to correct minor soft-tissue defects on the buccal aspect (Figure 10.12E). It is important to note that this technique is harder to execute in the anterior maxillary area, especially in patients with pronounced palatal rugae. The flap is much easier to develop in the premolar area because the palatal tissue is thicker and

provides better yield. A downside to this technique is decreased thickness of the palatal tissue.

The author's preference is to use a subepithelial connective tissue graft instead of the palatal roll technique for most soft-tissue deficiency cases. In his experience, the former is easier to perform and provides for more optimal and predictable clinical results.

A modification of the classic palatal roll technique can be used at the time of exposure and connection of the healing abutment. The location of the implant should be determined with the use of a periodontal probe. The gingiva occlusal to the implant is de-epithelialized with a diamond burr, laser, or #15 blade (Figure 10.13A). Then, a semicircular incision is made down to bone and the implant on the palatal aspect (Figure 10.13B). Next, the tissue is rotated and tunneled on the buccal aspect (Figure 10.13C) and secured in place with the use of a horizontal mattress suture. Finally, a healing abutment or a temporary crown is placed (Figure 10.13D).

The pouch technique

The pouch technique is commonly used to augment soft tissue in the buccal area. The technique is ideal for augmentation of buccal soft tissue at the time of immediate implant placement or correction of soft-tissue defects around a non-submerged implant or a restored implant. A horizontal incision is made with the use of keratome knives (Figure 10.14A, B). The incision is made at right angles to the epithelium, and dissection is ideally carried out in a supraperiosteal fashion to allow for a dual blood supply to the graft. The pouch must have enough thickness to decrease the incidence of flap perforation, sloughing, or tearing during tunneling of the graft. As this procedure is very technique sensitive and operator dependent, in the author's opinion, it is better to develop a thicker pouch, even if the level of dissection is subperiosteal.

The dissection should be extended laterally to allow for increased blood supply to the graft (Figure 10.14C, D). The dissection should be extended beyond the mucogingival junction as this will facilitate subsequent tunneling of the graft. After the pouch is completed, a Woodson, or similar, elevator is used to estimate the size of the pocket. The graft is harvested from the palate and trimmed to match the size of the created pouch. Appropriate suture material (e.g., 3–0 Vicryl suture on a PS2 needle) is passed from an area beyond the mucogingival junction though

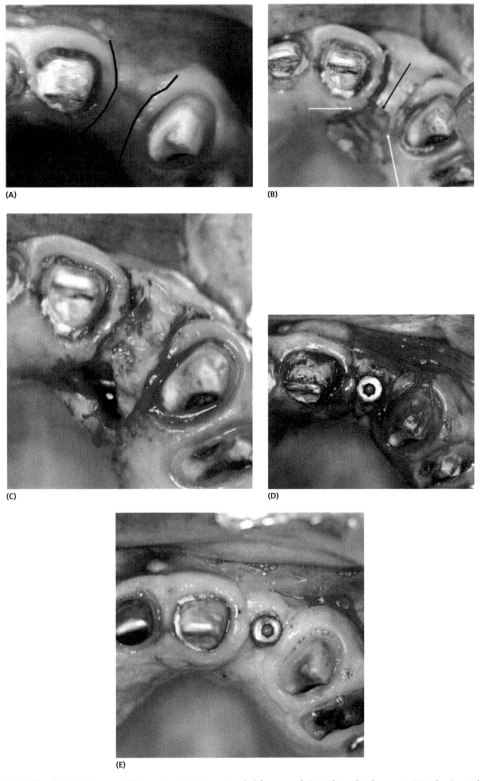

Figure 10.12 (A) Two full-thickness papilla-sparing incisions extended far enough into the palatal aspect. (B) A horizontal partial-thickness incision (black arrow) connects the two full-thickness papilla-sparing incisions (white arrows). (C) After reflection of the partial-thickness palatal flap, a full-thickness incision is made at the palatal apical area, and the tissue is reflected off the palate. (D) The palatal tissue is rolled under the buccal gingival tissue and secured with a horizontal mattress suture. (E) Area after 12 weeks of healing. Note the increased volume on the buccal aspect but the thin tissue on the palatal aspect.

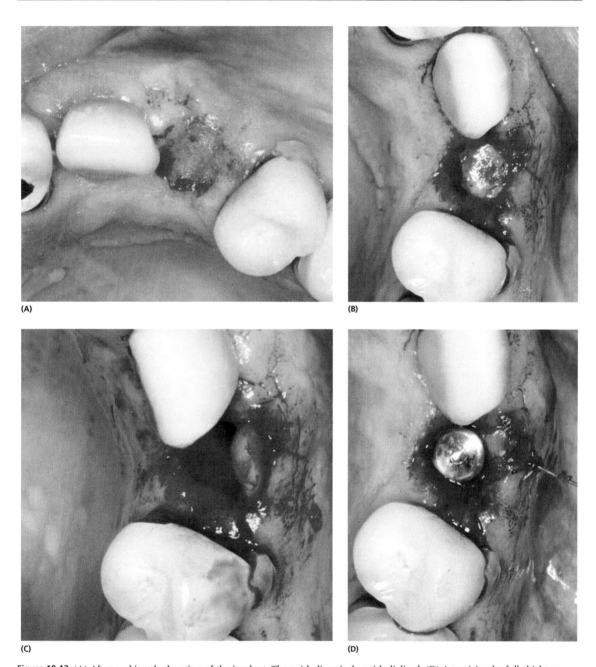

Figure 10.13 (A) After probing the location of the implant. The epithelium is de-epithelialized. (B) A semicircular full-thickness incision is made on the palatal aspect. (C) Tissue is reflected and then tunneled under the buccal flap. (D) The tissue is tunneled under the buccal tissue and secured in place with a horizontal mattress suture.

the pocket and then through the connective tissue graft, then back through the graft, through the pocket, and out through the mucogingival junction (Figure 10.14E, F). The graft is then secured manually by pulling the suture

with one hand and using a Woodson elevator to simultaneously to push the graft down into the pocket with the other hand. After the graft is positioned in the desired position, the suture is tied to prevent the graft from

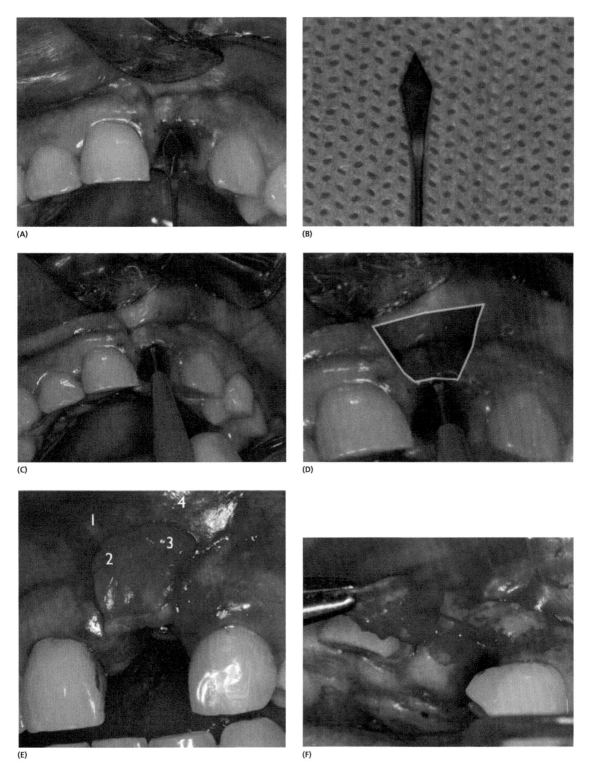

Figure 10.14 (A) A keratome knife is used to create a pouch. (B) A keratome knife. (C) During creation of the pouch, the dissection should extend beyond the mucogingival junction. (D) Outline of the pouch that will be created. (E) A graft that corresponds to the size of the pocket is harvested. Sequence in which the suture will be passed to facilitate tunneling of the graft. (F) Graft with suture in place just before tunneling the graft.

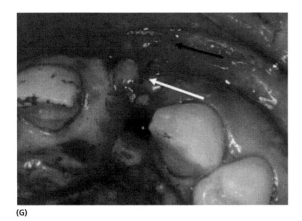

(G)

Figure 10.14 (*Continued*) (G) The graft is secured in place with the use of a horizontal mattress suture (white arrow); also, the suture that was used to tunnel the graft was tied and secured (black arrow).

being displaced apically (Figure 10.14G). The graft can be further secured with the use of a sling suture (if a crown is present) or a few horizontal mattress sutures. Pressure is applied to the area for 5 to 10 minutes.

A variation of this technique involves creating a subperiosteal pouch with the use of a Buser or Woodson elevator but making sure the pouch extends into the mucogingival junction. The graft is tunneled in a similar manner as in the technique just described (Figures 10.15, 10.16, and 10.17).

Vascularized interpositional periosteal–connective tissue (VIP-CT) flap

Schlar described the vascularized interpositional periosteal–connective tissue (VIP-CT) flap for augmentation of large soft-tissue defects.[5] This technique involves rotation of a pedicled finger flap to the anterior maxillary area. The blood supply to the flap is random-pattern blood supply. One of the main advantages of the VIP-CT flap is its effectiveness during simultaneous hard- and soft-tissue augmentation. The VIP-CT flap allows for superior soft-tissue augmentation in both vertical and horizontal directions compared to conventional free soft-tissue grafts. Practitioners can expect increased graft stability with decreased secondary shrinkage when using these flaps. It is also an ideal graft to use when the tissue bed is compromised (e.g., there is extensive scarring at the recipient site with decreased blood supply to the area).

Surgical technique

Local anesthesia with a vasoconstrictor is infiltrated in a standard manner. The initial step involves preparation of the recipient site. Generally speaking, a curvilinear, papilla-sparing incision is used. In the crestal area, the incision is placed on the palatal aspect of the ridge as this will allow for complete exposure of the alveolar ridge and also result in an increase in the vertical soft-tissue thickness at the end of the procedure. The papilla-sparing mucosal incision is next extended palatally in an exaggerated fashion, on both the mesial and distal aspects of the edentulous space (Figure 10.18A, B). A second horizontal, full-thickness palatal incision is made approximately 3 mm below the free gingival margin and extended to connect with the distal palatal incision (Figure 10.18C). Next, a split-thickness palatal incision is initiated at the first molar area and extended anteriorly in a split-thickness manner to the palatal incision area. As the dissection is carried anteriorly, the flap becomes harder to develop, especially in the palatal rugae area. Maintaining a good thickness of the flap (at least 1 mm) and starting the dissection from posterior to anterior facilitates flap development. It is recommended that the split-thickness portion of the flap be developed completely at this stage (Figure 10.18D–F).

Next, a vertical incision is made in the distal aspect of the second premolar. The incision is carried down to bone and extended as far apically as possible without damaging the greater palatine artery. A second horizontal incision is then made at the most apical aspect of the previous vertical incision. This horizontal incision is made parallel to the previous horizontal incision, extending to the mesial of the first premolar. At that point, the incision is curved toward the mid-palatal area, aiming for a line distal to the incisive papilla in order not to interrupt the blood supply to the flap (Figure 10.18G). A Buser, or similar, elevator is used to reflect in a subperiosteal plane, starting at the most distal aspect in the second premolar area and extending anteriorly to the mid-palatal area. The more anterior the desired final resting position of the VIP-CT flap, the longer is the arc of rotation of the graft and the more dissection is required. For severe cases, a reverse cutback may be needed. After releasing the pedicled finger flap, it is secured to the recipient site with 4–0 chromic gut sutures (Figure 10.18H–J). It is usually beneficial to keep the periosteal aspect of the graft facing the bone as this takes advantage of the osteoblastic potential of the flap. On occasion, when increased height of the

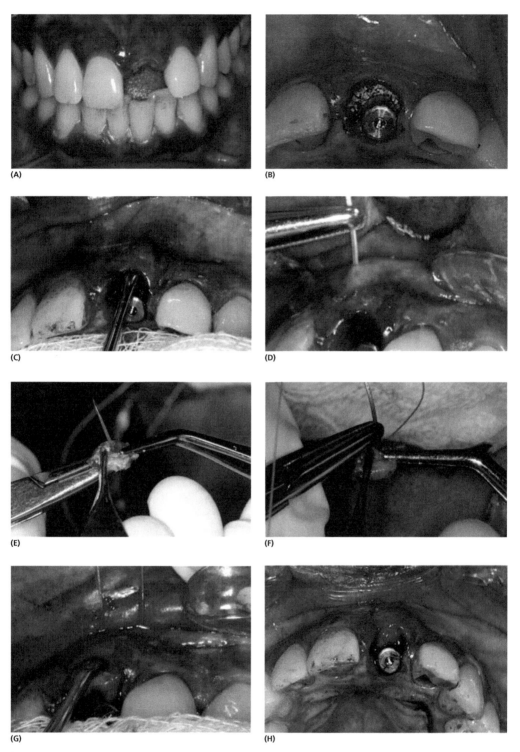

Figure 10.15 (A) Patient with non-restorable tooth #9; also, a long-ago restored implant in the area of tooth #8. (B) After extraction of tooth #9, an immediate implant is placed, and the gap between the implant and the buccal plate is grafted with a xenograft. (C) A pouch is created with the use of a Woodson elevator, and the pouch is extended beyond the mucogingival junction. (D) A needle is passed through the mucogingival junction, exiting under the gingival margin on the buccal aspect. (E) The suture is passed through the connective tissue graft on the inferior aspect (periosteal side). (F) The suture is again passed through the connective tissue graft from the superior aspect of the graft. (G) The graft is tunneled by pulling the graft with the suture and pushing the graft with a Woodson elevator inside the pouch. (H) Graft tunneled in the pouch before final suturing.

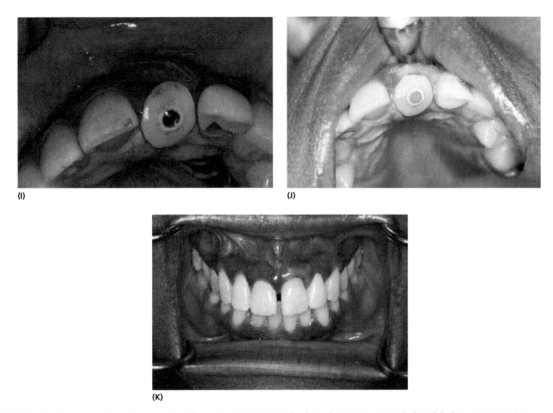

(I)　　　　　　　　　　　　　　**(J)**

(K)

Figure 10.15 *(Continued)* (I) Graft in place with a custom temporary healing abutment. (J) Healed graft before temporization. (K) Frontal view 1 year after implant placement with a graft.

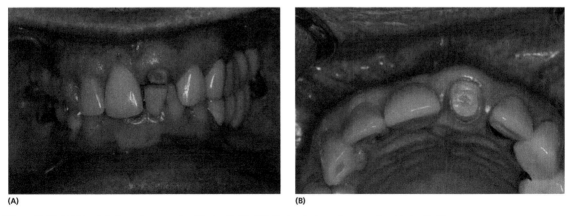

(A)　　　　　　　　　　　　　　**(B)**

Figure 10.16 (A) Frontal view of non-restorable tooth #9. (B) Occlusal view of non-restorable tooth #9.

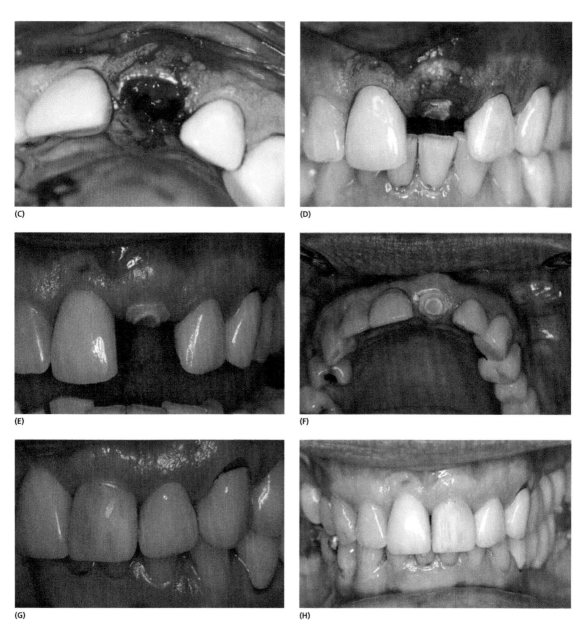

(C)

(D)

(E)

(F)

(G)

(H)

Figure 10.16 (*Continued*) (C) Occlusal view of the implant placed in the area of tooth #9 with a soft-tissue graft using the pouch technique before placing a custom temporary healing abutment. (D) Implant placed in the area of tooth #9 with a soft-tissue graft using the pouch technique with a custom temporary healing abutment. (E) Frontal view after 4 months of healing; note preservation of root prominence. (F) Occlusal view after 4 months of healing; note preservation of root prominence. (G) Lateral view with a temporary crown in place. (H) Frontal view with a temporary crown in place.

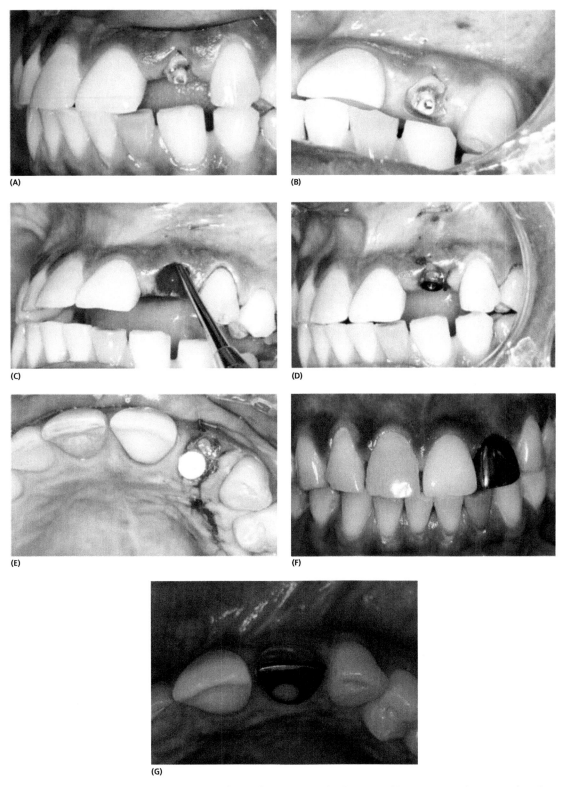

Figure 10.17 (A) Frontal view of non-restorable tooth #10; the patient has the thin gingival biotype. (B) Occlusal view of tooth #10. (C) A pouch is created with the use of a Woodson elevator. (D) Frontal view of an immediate implant in place with a tunneled soft-tissue graft. (E) Occlusal view of an immediate implant in place with a tunneled soft-tissue graft. (F) Frontal view of a final crown, with a stable facial margin. (G) Occlusal view of a final crown; note preservation of the root prominence.

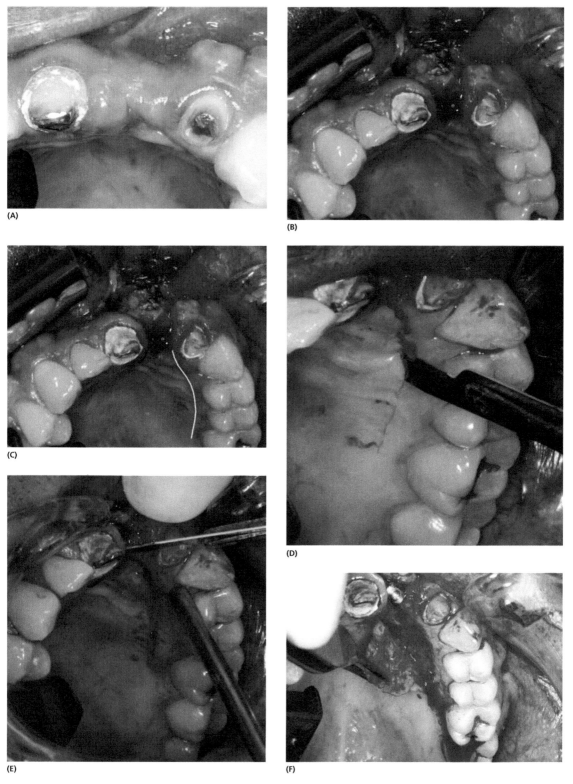

Figure 10.18 (A) Occlusal view of the edentulous space of tooth #9. (B) A papilla-sparing incision; also note that the incision is extended palatally. (C) A full-thickness incision is extended from the distal papilla-sparing incision to mesial aspect of the first molar (white line). Another small 4-mm full-thickness incision is extended from the mesial papilla-sparing incision (black line). (D) A split-thickness incision is made on the palatal aspect, starting from the first molar area and extending anteriorly. (E) The split-thickness incision is extended anteriorly and medially. (F) Completed palatal split-thickness incision.

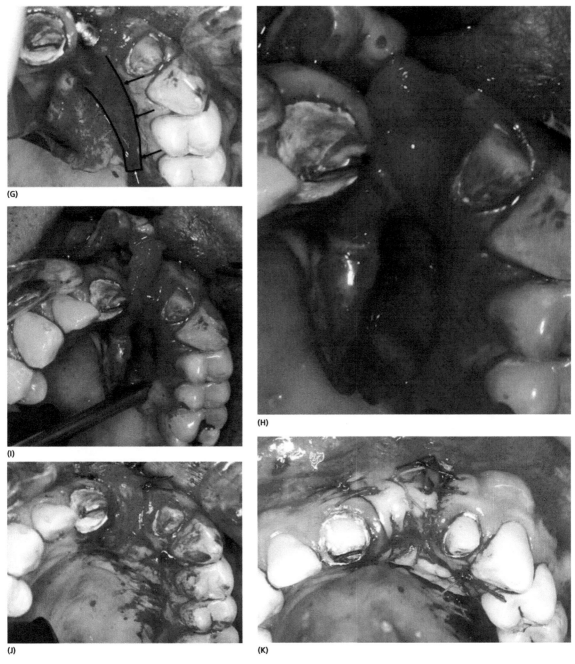

Figure 10.18 (*Continued*) (G) Outline of the planned finger flap; the initial full-thickness flap is around 3 mm from the CEJ of the teeth (black arrows), then a second full incision is made from the distal or second premolar (white arrow). Next, a third incision is made parallel to the initial incision and curved medially (gray arrows). (H) Pedicled finger flap reflected. (I) Pedicled finger flap reflected and rotated anteriorly. (J) Pedicled flap rotated and secured in place. (K) Final suturing of the buccal and palatal flaps.

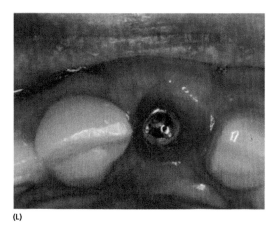

(L)

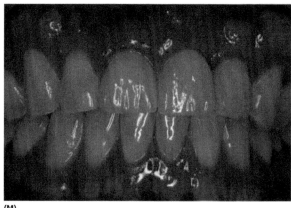

(M)

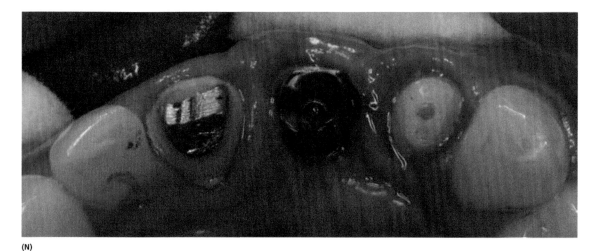

(N)

Figure 10.18 (*Continued*) (L) Final occlusal view showing increased tissue volume after exposure of the implant. (M) Final crown frontal view. (N) Final crown occlusal view.

soft-tissue thickness is needed, the flap can be rotated with the periosteum facing away from bone; this procedure allows for increased augmentation of the soft-tissue height. After securing the flap, a collagen or hemostatic dressing is placed in the area where the graft was harvested, and the area is closed with overlying resorbable sutures.

The buccal flap is then approximated to the palatal flap using standard suturing techniques (Figure 10.18K–N). On occasion, primary closure might not be achieved, and small areas of the pedicle may remain exposed; usually these areas will epithelialize over the pedicle without any loss of the graft. The use of a removable partial

denture (flipper) is not recommended as it may put pressure on the palatal pedicle, thereby compromising its inherent blood supply. Moreover, dentists will frequently encounter considerable difficulty with adjusting the denture to fit the space because of the volume of the grafted tissue on the palate. The author prefers the use of an Essex type of retainer as opposed to a conventional denture in these cases (Figures 10.19 and 10.20).

Free subepithelial connective tissue graft

Another variation of soft-tissue grafts around dental implants is the use of freestanding subepithelial connective tissue. Preparation of the recipient site depends

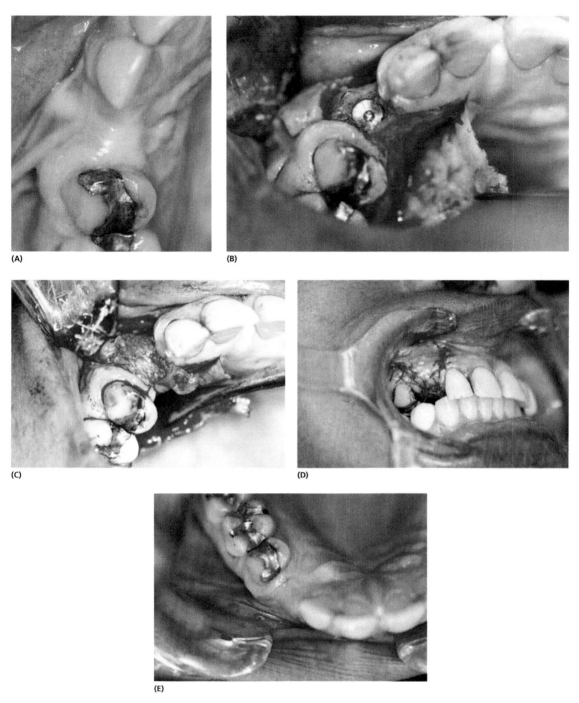

Figure 10.19 (A) Occlusal view before grafting. (B) Buccal and palatal flaps reflected. (C) Pedicled finger flap reflected. (D) Final suturing of the flaps. (E) View after healing of the graft.

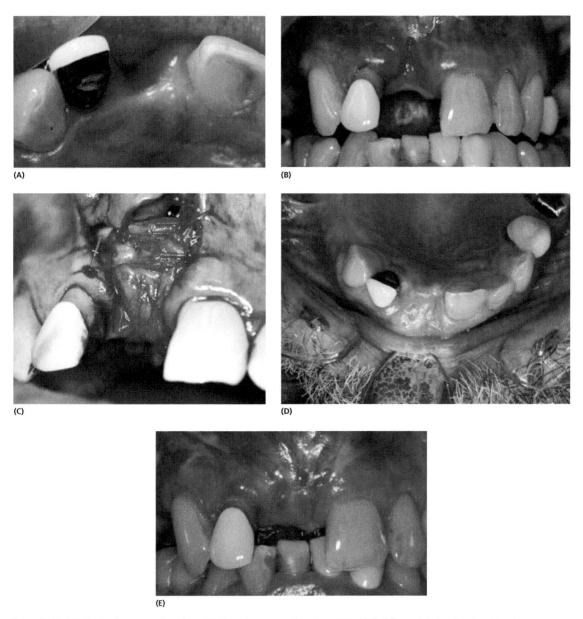

Figure 10.20 (A) Occlusal preoperative view. (B) Frontal preoperative view. (C) Pedicled flap rotated and sutured in place. (D) Occlusal postoperative view. (E) Frontal postoperative view.

on the timing of the soft-tissue graft. A split- or full-thickness flap is reflected, and a subepithelial connective tissue graft is harvested from the palate. The graft is trimmed and adapted to the buccal aspect of the flap. After the graft is appropriately sized, a resorbable suture such as 4–0 Vicryl is used to secure the graft to the buccal flap. The flap is sutured, and this closure will automatically secure the graft in place (Figure 10.21). An alternative option is to secure the graft to the recipient periosteal bed first and then suture the buccal flap over to completely cover the connective tissue graft[15] (Figure 10.22).

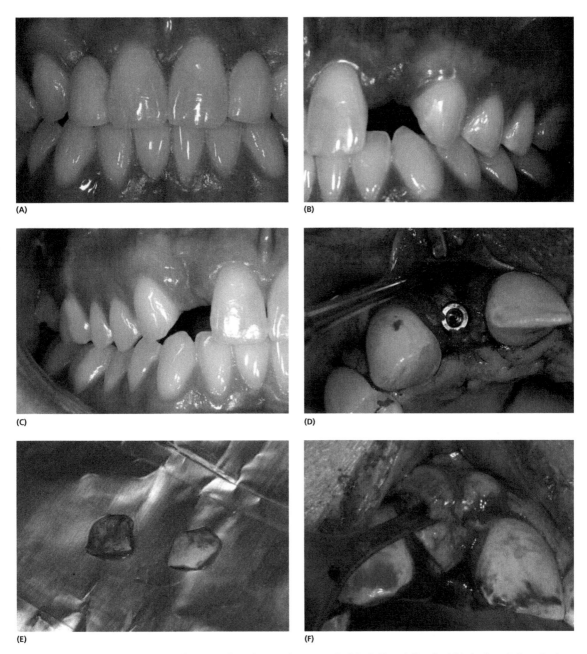

Figure 10.21 (A) Patient with congenitally missing laterals. (B) After removal of the bridge, clefting is visible in the soft tissue in the # 10 region. (C) After removal of the bridge, clefting is visible in the soft tissue in the # 7 region. (D) Implant in place. (E) Subepithelial connective tissue graft harvested from the palate. (F) Graft positioned in the desired position. Courtesy of Dr. David Cottrell.

Postoperative care

Pain management with over-the-counter medication or narcotics is recommended. Chlorhexidine 0.12% oral rinse bid for 10 days and warm normal saline oral rinses 3 to 5 times daily should be prescribed. Patients should be instructed not to use a water-pik or an electric tooth-brush around the graft area for 4 weeks. Cold packs to the face over the area for 10 minutes at a time, twice

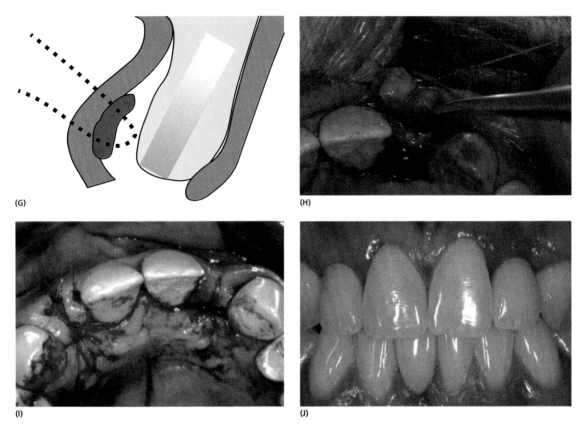

Figure 10.21 (*Continued*) (G) Graft secured to the buccal flap with a horizontal mattress suture. The dotted line is the suture, pink is the buccal flap, red is the subepithelial graft, and yellow is bone. (H) The suture is tied to secure the graft to the buccal flap. (I) Occlusal view with the graft in place on the right side and no graft on the left side. (J) Final crowns, teeth #7 and #10.

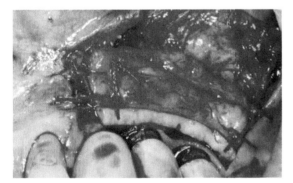

Figure 10.22 Subepithelial graft secured directly to the recipient site.

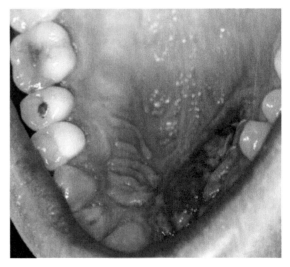

Figure 10.23 Dehiscence at the donor site.

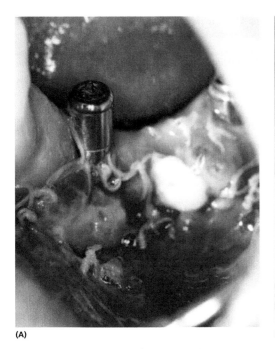
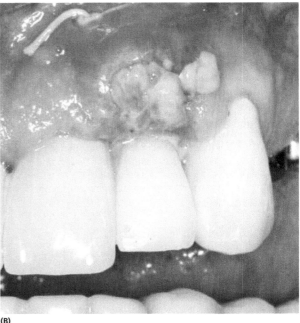

(A)   **(B)**

Figure 10.24 (A) Partial loss of epithelialized connective tissue graft. (B) Partial loss of subepithelial connective tissue graft.

an hour, for the first 6 hours and a soft diet for 1 week are encouraged. Smoking should be avoided for 4 to 6 weeks.

A follow-up appointment should be scheduled 7 to 14 days after surgery in order to examine the progress of healing. If a periodontal dressing is placed, it is usually discontinued at the same time as suture removal.

Management of complications
Bleeding

Bleeding could be encountered at the time of surgery or during the postoperative period. Bleeding is commonly managed with the application of pressure; this pressure will usually slow bleeding, and, if the source of the bleeding is identified, it can be cauterized or ligated. If no source is identified, several sutures can be placed along the course of the greater palatine artery to compress the artery; a local anesthetic with epinephrine can also be injected to slow the bleeding, and additional pressure can be applied.

Dehiscence at the donor site

Dehiscence at the donor site is one of the most common causes of postoperative discomfort (Figure 10.23). Conservative management is recommended; the area will granulate and completely heal within 3 to 4 weeks.

Partial or complete loss of the graft

Connective tissue grafts have a high success rate, but, in general, partial or complete loss of the graft is possible (Figure 10.24A, B). Usually management is conservative debridement of necrotic tissue. If any tissue appears fibrinous in nature, observation is recommended. One of the key factors in graft loss prevention is immobilization of the graft at the time of surgery.

References

1. Fürhauser R, Florescu D, Benesch T, Haas R, Mailath G, Watzek G. Evaluation of soft tissue around single-tooth implant crowns: the pink esthetic score. *Clinical Oral Implants Research.* 2005; 16(6): 639–44.

2. Olsson M, Lindhe J. Periodontal characteristics in individuals with varying form of the upper central incisors. *Journal of Clinical Periodontology.* 1991; 18(1): 78–82.

3. Olsson M, Lindhe J, Marinello CP. On the relationship between crown form and clinical features of the gingiva in adolescents. *Journal of Clinical Periodontology.* 1993; 20(8): 570–7.

4. Bhat V, Shetty S. Prevalence of different gingival biotypes in individuals with varying forms of maxillary central incisors: A survey. *Journal of Dental Implants.* 2013; 3(2): 116–21.

5. Sclar A. *Soft Tissue and Esthetic Considerations in Implant Therapy*. Quintessence Publishing, Chicago, 2003.

6. Sullivan HC, Atkins JH. Free autogenous gingival grafts. I. Principles of successful grafting. *Periodontics*. 1968; 6(3): 121–9.

7. Bjorn H. Free transplantation of gingival propria. *Svensk Tandlakare Tidskrift*. 1963; 22: 684–5.

8. Reiser GM, Bruno JF, Mahan PE, Larkin LH. The subepithelial connective tissue graft palatal donor site: anatomic considerations for surgeons. *International Journal of Periodontics and Restorative Dentistry*. 1996; 16(2): 130–7.

9. Rees TD, Brasher WJ. A technique for obtaining thin split-thickness grafts in periodontal surgery. *Oral Surgery, Oral Medicine, Oral Pathology*. 1970; 29(1): 148–54.

10. Dibart S, Karima M. *Practical Periodontal Plastic Surgery*. Blackwell, Oxford, 2006.

11. Langer B, Langer L. Subepithelial connective tissue graft technique for root coverage. *Journal of Periodontology*. 1985; 56(12): 715–20.

12. Zuhr O, Hurzeler M. *Plastic-Esthetic Periodontal and Implant Surgery a Microsurgical Approach*. Quintessence Publishing, Chicago, 2012.

13. Abrams L. Augmentation of the deformed residual edentulous ridge for fixed prosthesis. *Compendium of Continuing Education in General Dentistry*. 1980; 1(3): 205–13.

14. Scharf DR, Tarnow DP. Modified roll technique for localized alveolar ridge augmentation. *International Journal of Periodontics and Restorative Dentistry*. 1992; 12(5): 415–25.

15. Palacci P. *Esthetic Implant Dentistry, Soft and hard tissue management*. Quintessence Publishing, Chicago, 2001.

CHAPTER 11

Surgical Crown Lengthening

Serge Dibart

Department of Periodontology and Oral Biology, Boston University Henry M. Goldman School of Dental Medicine, Boston, MA, USA

History

There are two aspects to the crown lengthening procedure: esthetic and functional. In both cases, the goal of the surgical procedure is to re-establish the biological width apically while exposing more tooth structure. The biological width is defined as the sum of the junctional epithelium and the supracrestal connective tissue attachment.[1]

Gargiulo measured the dentogingival junction in humans and found that the average space occupied by the sum of the junctional epithelium and the supra-crestal connective tissue fibers was 2.04 mm.[2] Violation of that space by restorations impinging on the biological width has been associated with gingival inflammation, discomfort, gingival recession, alveolar bone loss, pocket formation, and other problems.[3,4]

In 1977, Ingber advocated a 3-mm distance of sound supracrestal tooth structure between the bone and prosthetic margins to ensure a harmonious and successful long-term restoration.[5] This allows for the reformation of the biological width plus sulcus depth. This can be achieved surgically (crown lengthening), orthodontically (forced eruption), or by a combination of both.[6–8]

The need for 3 mm of space between the bone and the gingival margin is a concept that has been around for a very long time. This concept, however, has been challenged because some authors found that there was considerable intra-individual and inter-individual variability to the supraosseous gingiva. Clinical variations in supra-osseous gingiva exist within and among patients for both similar and different tooth types and arches.[9]

Indeed, sometimes the 3 mm rule falls short, and inadequate bone recontouring results in inadequate gingival margins.[10] The latest literature advocates a pre-operative bone sounding at the surgical site to estimate the supracrestal dimension of the gingival tissue.[11] Perez *et al.*[12,13] did a human study involving clinical evaluation of the supraosseous gingivae before and after crown lengthening. They found that, when subjected to crown lengthening surgery, the postoperative supraosseous gingival dimension of a particular tooth could be estimated accurately (within 0.50 mm) by knowledge of its preoperative measurement. They also found an overall reduction in the supraosseous gingival dimension, ranging from 0.51 to 0.61 mm, 6 months postsurgically compared to the presurgical measurements. Hence, they concluded that the average 3-mm measurement used to estimate the amount of sound tooth structure needed after crown lengthening should be pre-empted by the supraosseous gingival dimensions of the particular tooth.[12,13] This is especially critical when operating in the esthetic zone.

Indications

- To improve a gummy smile in a patient with a high smile line.
- To rehabilitate a dentition that is compromised by the presence of extensive caries, short clinical crowns, traumatic injuries, or severe parafunctional habits.
- To restore gingival health when the biological width has been violated by a prosthetic restoration that is too close to the alveolar bone crest.

Manual of Minor Oral Surgery for the General Dentist, Second Edition. Edited by Pushkar Mehra and Richard D'Innocenzo.

Crown lengthening can be limited to the soft tissues when there is enough gingiva coronal to the alveolar bone allowing for surgical modification of the gingival margins without the need for osseous recontouring (i.e., pseudo pockets in cases of gingival hyperplasia). An external or internal bevel gingivectomy (gingivoplasty) is the procedure of choice for these cases.

The biological width has not been compromised, and, as a result, the soft tissue pocket is eliminated and the teeth exposed without the need for osseous resection. Unfortunately, the majority of cases will involve bone recontouring as well as gingival resection to accommodate esthetics and function. This is a more delicate procedure, which will require exposing the root surface, positioning gingival margins at the desired height, and apically re-establishing the individual biological width of the tooth or teeth that was premeasured.

The crown lengthening procedure will allow the restorative dentist to develop an adequate zone for crown retention without extending the crown margins deep into periodontal tissues. After the procedure is performed, it is customary to wait 6 to 8 weeks before cementing the final restoration. In the esthetic zone, a waiting period of at least 6 months is recommended before final impression.[14] This period will reduce the chances of gingival recession following prosthetic crown insertion, especially if the patient has the thin biotype.

Armamentarium

The armamentarium includes the basic surgical kit, plus the following:
- crown lengthening burrs and bone chisels or
- a piezoelectric knife and crown lengthening inserts.

Soft-tissue crown-lengthening technique

Soft-tissue crown lengthening is best accomplished with an external or internal bevel gingivectomy. The alveolar bone is left intact, the depth of the soft-tissue pocket is marked with a probe (bleeding points), and a gingivectomy knife (Kirkland or Orban [in the case of external bevel gingivectomy]) or a #15 blade (internal bevel gingivectomy) is used to eliminate the gingival excess.

Hard-tissue crown-lengthening technique

The optimal gingival line (margins) is determined after careful evaluation of the diagnostic wax-up. A surgical guide, prepared from the wax-up model, will help the surgeon re-create the ideal gingival line in the mouth (Figures 11.1 and 11.2). Using a #15 blade as a pencil, the surgeon outlines the incision and, following the surgical guide, keeps the blade at an angle to have a coronal internal bevel (Figure 11.3).

The full-thickness flap is then reflected, the secondary flap discarded, and the bone exposed. Using burrs, bone chisels, or the piezoelectric knife, the alveolar bone is recontoured to re-create the prerecorded space between the bone and the anticipated new margins (Figure 11.4). The flaps are sutured back in place (Figure 11.5) and the area left to heal for about 3 weeks before repreparing the teeth (supragingivally) and relining the temporaries. A waiting period of about 6 months, in temporaries, is recommended in the esthetic zone before final preparation and restoration (Figures 11.6 and 11.7).

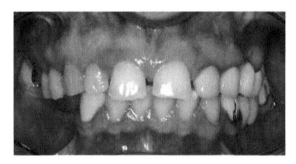

Figure 11.1 Frontal view. The patient, a 45-year-old woman, is unhappy with her smile and needs a major dental rehabilitation.

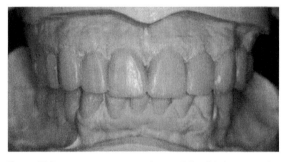

Figure 11.2 Diagnostic wax-up. This model will help create the surgical guide that will direct the surgeon's gingival incisions.

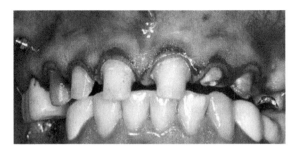

Figure 11.3 The submarginal incisions have been done with a #15 blade. This will be the new gingival margin line according the diagnostic wax-up. A temporary anchorage device (TAD) has been placed to intrude the right upper molars orthodontically.

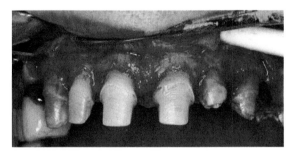

Figure 11.4 Full-thickness flap elevated and osseous recontouring done to re-establish the supraosseous gingival dimension.

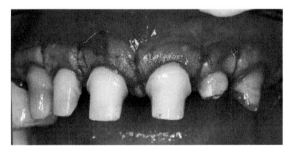

Figure 11.5 Flaps sutured back using 5-0 chromic gut single interrupted sutures.

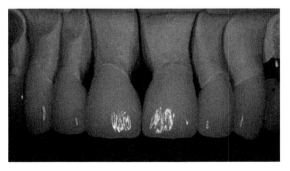

Figure 11.6 Final ceramic crowns before cementation.

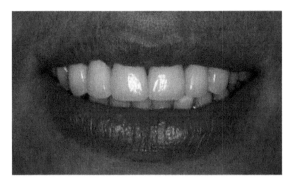

Figure 11.7 Patient's smile after cementation of the final prosthesis.

Acknowledgments

The author would like to thank Dr. Haneen Bokhadoor and Dr. Nawaf Al Dousari for contributing the clinical pictures to this chapter.

References

1. Cohen DW. Periodontal preparation of the mouth for restorative dentistry. Presented at the Walter Reed Army Medical Center, Washington, DC, June 3, 1962.
2. Gargiulo AW, Wentz FM, Orban B. Dimensions and relations of the dentogingival junction in humans. *Journal of Periodontology.* 1961; 32: 261–7.
3. Tarnow D, Sthal SS, Magner A, Zamzok J. Human gingival attachment responses to subgingival crown placement–marginal remodeling. *Journal of Clinical Periodontology.* 1986; 13: 563–9.
4. Parma-Benfenati S, Fugazzotto PA, Ruben MP. The effect of restorative margins on the post surgical development and nature of the periodontium. Part I. *The International Journal of Periodontics and Restorative Dentistry.* 1985; 5(6): 30–51.
5. Ingber FJS, Rose LF, Coslet JG. The biologic width. A concept in periodontics and restorative dentistry. *Alpha Omegan.* 1977; 10: 62–5.
6. Ingber JS. Forced eruption II. A method of treating nonrestorable teeth—periodontal and restorative considerations. *Journal of Periodontology.* 1976; 47: 203–13.
7. Pontoriero R, Celenza F Jr, Ricci G, Carnevale M. Rapid extrusion with fiber resection: A combined orthodontic-periodontic treatment modality. *International Journal of Periodontics and Restorative Dentistry.* 1987; 5: 30–43.
8. De Waal H, Castellucci G. The importance of restorative margin placement to the biologic width and periodontal health. Part II. *The International Journal of Periodontics and Restorative Dentistry.* 1994; 14(1): 70–83.

9. Becker W, Ochsenbein C, Tibbetts L, Becker BE. Alveolar bone anatomic profiles as measured from dry skulls. Clinical ramifications. *Journal of Clinical Periodontology.* 1997; 24(10): 727–31.

10. Brägger U, Lauchenauer D, Lang NP. Surgical lengthening of the clinical crown. *Journal of Clinical Periodontology.* 1992; 19(1): 58–63.

11. Scutella F, Landi L, Stellino G, Morgano SM. Surgical template for crown lengthening: a clinical report. *Journal of Prosthetic Dentistry.* 1999; 82(3): 253–6.

12. Perez JR, Smukler H, Nunn ME. Clinical evaluation of the supraosseous gingivae before and after crown lengthening. *Journal of Periodontology.* 2007; 78(6): 1023–30.

13. Perez JR, Smukler H, Nunn ME. Clinical dimensions of the supraosseous gingivae in the healthy periodontium. *Journal of Periodontology.* 2008; 79(12): 2267–72.

14. Pontoriero R, Carnevale G. Surgical crown lengthening: A 12-month clinical wound healing study. *Journal of Periodontology.* 2001; 72: 841–8.

CHAPTER 12

Endodontic Periradicular Microsurgery

Louay Abrass

Department of Endodontics, Boston University Henry M. Goldman School of Dental Medicine, Boston, MA, USA

Introduction

In the past decade, the field of endodontics has seen numerous advances, the scope of which have reached all facets of endodontic treatment in both conventional and surgical aspects. These technological advances have introduced new instruments and materials that did not exist before and revolutionized the way endodontic treatment is performed. This change could not be more evident than in the field of surgical endodontics, where both theoretical and practical aspects have completely transformed. The purpose of this chapter is to present to the surgical-minded general dentist the current standards and techniques in performing apical surgery with evidence-based rationales.

Problems with traditional endodontic surgery

Traditional apical surgery is viewed as an invasive, difficult, and less successful procedure than conventional endodontic treatment. Many reasons contribute to this belief, examples of which include working on a conscious patient in an area with restricted access, limitations in visibility, and operating on minuscule microstructures that are often obscured by bleeding. To manage these challenges, operators had to prepare large osteotomies to gain sufficient access that would accommodate the large surgical instruments that were traditionally used. This unnecessary removal of healthy buccal bone structure sometimes resulted in incomplete healing. The root apex was routinely resected with a 45-degree bevel angle with no biological or clinical imperative. Such a practice was performed merely to allow visualization of root canal anatomy and to facilitate retropreparation and retrofilling. This steep-bevel angle root resection created more problems than solutions. It exposed more dentinal tubules, which translated into an increase in apical leakage.[1,2] In addition, this method sacrificed more periodontal support of the buccal root surface, shortening the distance between the base of the gingival sulcus and the osteotomy site. This further predisposed the tooth for an endodontic–periodontal communication. This resection technique also frequently resulted in an incomplete root resection in which the root apex was merely beveled rather than excised and in which the lingual aspect of the root was never resected. Surgeons thus neglected to eliminate apical ramifications and lateral canals and failed to identify more lingually situated additional canals.[3,4] Finally, it produced a distorted and elongated view of the internal root canal anatomy that makes it harder to clearly and accurately identify and treat the apical anatomy. Figure 12.1 illustrates most of the common problems associated with conventional apical surgery and how microsurgical techniques can address and correct these deficiencies.

Comparison of traditional surgery to microsurgery

Introduction of the surgical operating microscope and ultrasonics paved the way in changing how endodontic surgery is performed (Figures 12.2 and 12.3). The

---

Manual of Minor Oral Surgery for the General Dentist, Second Edition. Edited by Pushkar Mehra and Richard D'Innocenzo.

microscope provides illumination and magnification of the surgical site where it is most needed. The ultrasonic tips allow a coaxial preparation of the root canal system to a depth of 3 mm that provides an optimum apical seal.[1] These two advances led to the miniaturization of surgical instruments. The net result was that all the previously mentioned developments revolutionized the traditional technique into a more precise method—an apical surgery with minimal healthy bone removal and a conservative shallow-bevel angle root resection. This transformation allows periradicular surgery to be performed on a solid biological and clinical basis.

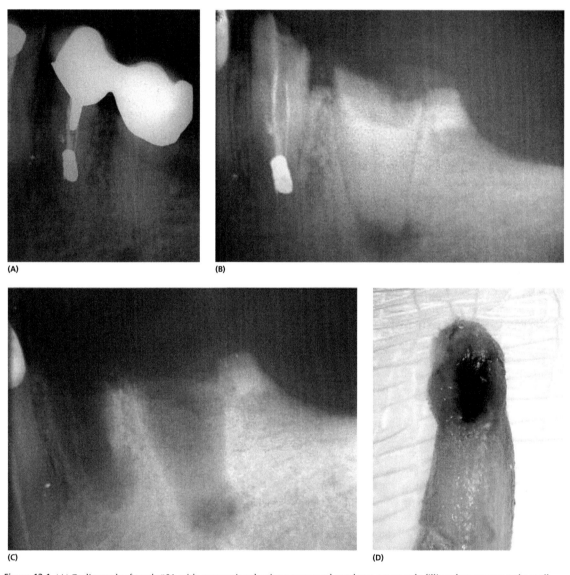

(A)　　(B)　　(C)　　(D)

Figure 12.1 (A) Radiograph of tooth #21 with conventional apicoectomy and amalgam retrograde filling that appears to be well centered within the root parameter. (All images in Figure 12.1 are of tooth #21.) (B) Due to failure of previous treatment and restorability issues, extraction was recommended. (C) Socket after extraction. (D) Buccal view of extracted tooth. Amalgam retrograde is visible.

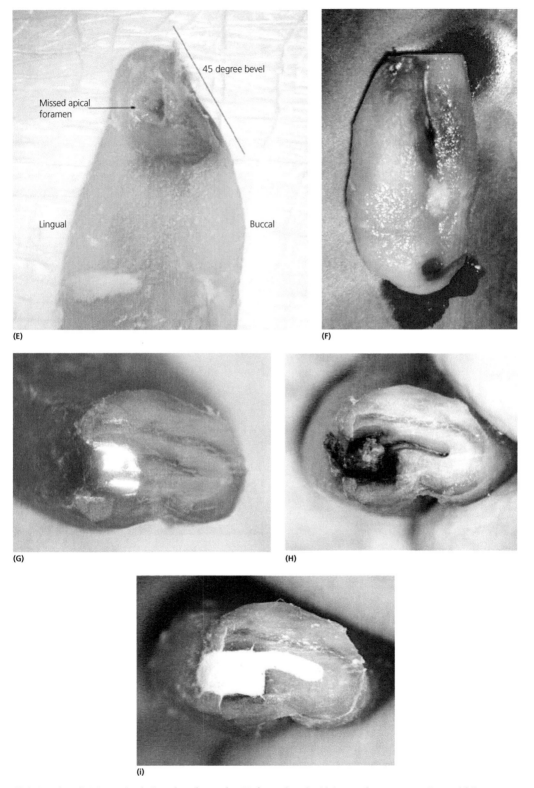

Figure 12.1 (*Continued*) (E) Proximal view that shows the 45-degree bevel with incomplete root resection and failure to eliminate apical ramifications. (F) This image shows 0-degree bevel root resection that eliminates the apical 3 mm of the root. (G) Microscopic inspection of the resected root surface reveals the buccally situated amalgam, the untreated lingual canal, and the missed isthmus. (H) Ultrasonic retropreparation of 3 mm depth that includes the buccal and lingual canals and the connecting isthmus. (I) Super EBA retrograde filling.

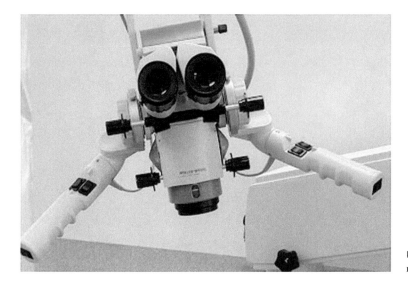

Figure 12.2 The surgical operating microscope.

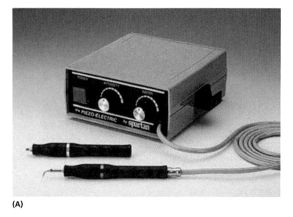

(A)

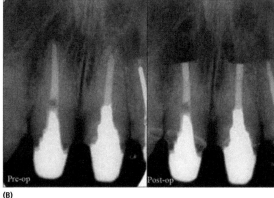

(B)

Figure 12.3 (A) The ultrasonic unit by Spartan. (B) An ideal case of periradicular microsurgery; note the 0-degree bevel angle root resection and the coaxial retropreparation.

The need for endodontic surgery

The success rate of endodontic treatment varies and has been reported to be as high as 94.8% or as low as 53% (Figure 12.4). This variability stems from many factors, such as the type of study, sample size, pulpal and periapical status, follow-up period, and number of treatment visits. Conventional retreatment has a lower success rate that ranges between 48 and 84% (Figure 12.5). One important fact remains: A certain percentage of failures will be encountered even when the root canal treatment has been carried out to the highest quality. The following etiological factors explain why some conventional endodontic treatments fail and eventually necessitate surgical intervention.

Anatomical factors

Careful examination of the root canal system reveals enormous complexities such as accessory canals, C-shaped canals, fins, and isthmuses (Figure 12.6). These microstructures are more abundant in the apical one-third of the root[5,6] and are farthest away from the operator's control. By providing a safe haven for bacteria from biomechanical instrumentation, these anatomical complexities can impair the treatment outcome in

Conventional endodontic success rate			
Author/year	# of cases	Follow-up (yr)	Success %
Strindberg 1956	529	4	87
Seltzer et al 1963	2921	0.5	80
Bender et al 1964	706	2	82
Grossman et al 1964	432	1–5	90
Ingle 1965	1229	2	91.5
Jokinen et al 1978	1304	2–7	53
Pekruhn 1986	925	1	94.8
Ray et al 1995	1010	1 and up	61.1

Figure 12.4 This table presents a summary and a comparison of multiple studies of conventional endodontic success rates. It clearly demonstrates that a 100% success rate is not achievable.

Conventional retreatment success rate		
Study	Follow-up (yr)	Success rate (%)
Strindberg (1956)	4	66
	7	84
Molven & Halse (1988)	10–17	71
Bergenholtz et al (1979)	2	48
Allen et al (1989)	0.5–1	73
Sjogren et al (1990)	8–10	62
Sundqvist et al (1998)	5	74

Figure 12.5 This figure summarizes the results of different studies in regard to conventional endodontic retreatment success rates. It clearly demonstrates the lower success rate associated with endodontic retreatment cases.

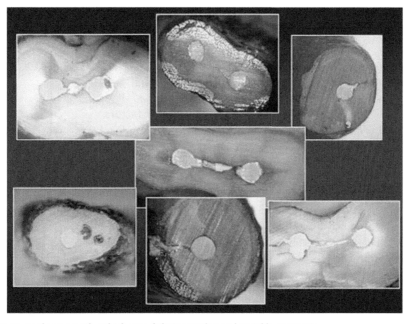

Figure 12.6 Cross sections of some teeth, which reveal their complex and variable anatomy.

cases in which the pulp space is infected. This contributes to the lower success rate of endodontic treatment in infected cases.

Bacteriological factors

Post-treatment apical periodontitis is caused by microbial infection that persists either in the intraradicular space or in the extraradicular area. Certain bacteria, such as *Enterococcus faecalis*, can withstand antibacterial measures, survive a restricted nutritional environment, and exist in the root canal as a single type of bacteria.[7] Although extraradicular infection has a lower prevalence than that of root canal infection, it could, nonetheless, be the etiological factor behind therapy-resistant apical periodontitis.[8] Additional studies have shown that bacteria such as *Actinomyces israelii*[9,10] and *Arachnia propionica*[11] can survive in the periapical tissue. Some can even invade periapical cementum.[12]

Histological factors

A non-microbial source of endodontic failure is the presence of periapical cysts, which represent up to 15% of all periapical lesions.[13,14] Periapical cysts exist in two structurally distinct classes: periapical true cysts and pocket cysts.[15] Pocket cysts contain epithelium-lined cavities that are open to the root canals. These can heal following non-surgical root canal therapy. On the other hand, true cysts are less likely to heal without surgical intervention.

Case selection

When an endodontic treatment fails, clinicians ought to carefully investigate to reveal the true etiology behind the failure. It is very important to reach a sound diagnosis, which leads to a treatment plan that addresses the disease rather than just the symptoms (Figure 12.7).

In assessing a previously root canal–treated tooth, the following three factors should be evaluated: (1) quality of previous endodontic treatment, (2) quality of coronal restoration, and (3) accessibility to the canals. Conventional retreatment should always be considered first. Surgical retreatment should be considered when access to canals is impossible or when the current endodontic treatment and coronal restoration seem to be of adequate quality (Figure 12.8).

Failures associated with silver points pose another challenging situation. Failing silver points usually present with gross leakage and corrosion byproducts. Surgical treatment can only marginally address these problems.

Because it is extremely difficult to adequately retroprepare and retrofill the canals to provide a good apical seal, every effort should be made to retreat these cases and to avoid surgery at any cost (Figure 12.9).

Indications

There are several reasons why this surgery should be performed. The operator should consider these indications and then either perform the surgery or refer the patient to someone who will perform the procedure according to current accepted standards.

Failure of previous endodontic therapy

When previous endodontic treatment seems to be of adequate quality and/or retreatment has already been attempted without further success, periradicular surgery becomes rightly indicated (Figure 12.10).

Failure of previous apical surgery

Clinicians should not hesitate to perform apical microsurgery on previously failed apicoectomies. This is especially true when it is evident that the previous surgery was inadequate or not performed according to the current standards of care (Figure 12.11). In these cases, it is common to discover an incompletely resected apex with malpositioned retrofilling material that is mostly placed outside the root canal perameter. Thorough presentation of such deficiencies was covered in a previous section of this chapter.

Iatrogenic factors

Procedural mishaps can occur during the course of endodontic treatment. Examples include canal transportation, perforation, ledge formation, blockage, or separated instruments (Figure 12.12). These complications are likely to result in incomplete biomechanical debridement and a compromised apical seal. Cases involving mishaps in the apical one-third of the canal are good candidates for apical surgery. However, if the error is located in the middle to coronal one-third of the root canal, then alternative approaches should be considered.

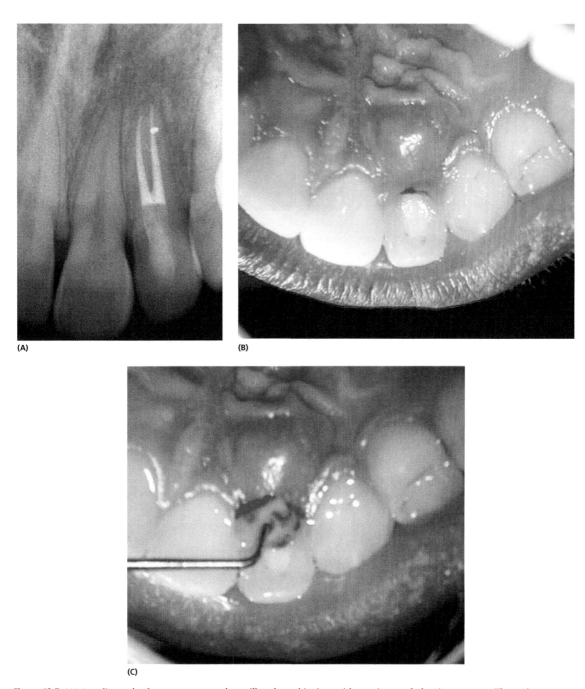

Figure 12.7 (A) A radiograph of a rare two-rooted maxillary lateral incisor with previous endodontic treatment. The patient presented with severe spontaneous pain and tenderness to percussion. (B) Clinical examination reveals localized palatal swelling. (C) Periodontal examination shows a 12-mm probing on the palatal surface associated with a purulent discharge; the diagnosis is periodontal abscess associated with a palatal developmental groove.

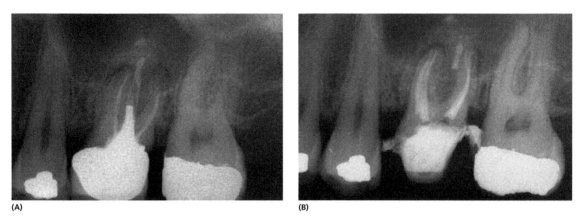

Figure 12.8 (A) A preoperative radiograph of tooth #14 that has a failing inadequate endodontic treatment. Close examination reveals the untreated second mesiobuccal (MB) root and an ill-fitting crown. (B) Crown removal and conventional retreatment are performed; the second mesiobuccal and second distiobuccal canals are localized and treated.

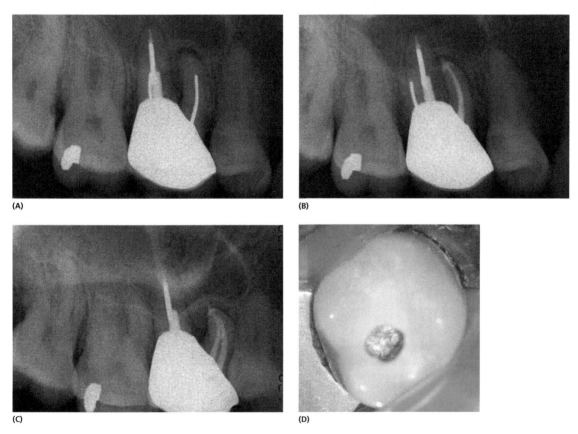

Figure 12.9 (A) Tooth #3, which has a previous endodontic treatment with silver points and a new crown of good quality. A symptomatic periapical lesion is limited to the MB root only. (B) Localized conventional retreatment of the MB root is performed to address the pathology without compromising the crown. (C) An angulated radiograph showing the two treated mesiobuccal canals. (D) The microscopic access needed to perform the retreatment.

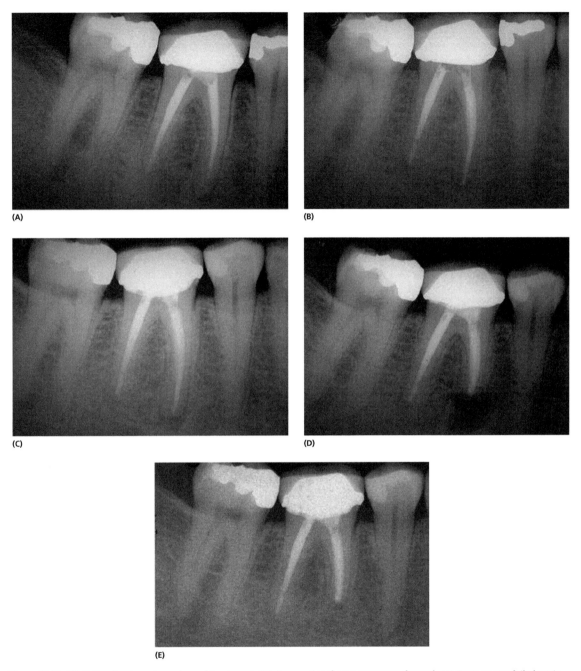

(A)

(B)

(C)

(D)

(E)

Figure 12.10 (A) Failing inadequate root canal treatment. (B) Conventional retreatment performed. (C) Retreatment failed again after 2 years. (D) Apical surgery performed. (E) Two-year recall demonstrates complete healing.

Anatomical deviations

Teeth can present with challenging root anatomy that complicates endodontic therapy and compromises complete debridement. Common examples include canal calcifications, blunderbuss apices, S- and C-shaped canals, and severe root curvatures. The case illustrated in Figure 12.13 shows a maxillary lateral incisor that presents with dens-in-dente, canal

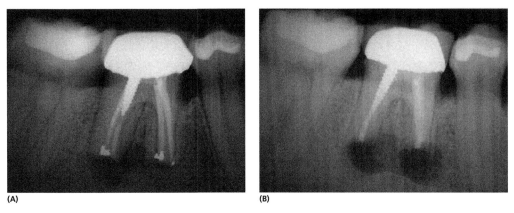

Figure 12.11 (A) Failed previous surgery where both mesiolingual (ML) and distolingual (DL) roots were not resected nor retroprepared. (B) Complete root resection with minimum bevel angle and 3 mm retrofilling.

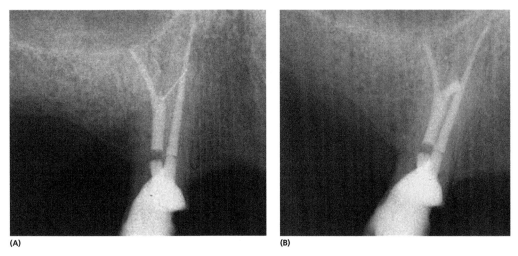

Figure 12.12 (A) Separated file in the MB root of tooth #12. (B) Instrument removed and canal retrofilled.

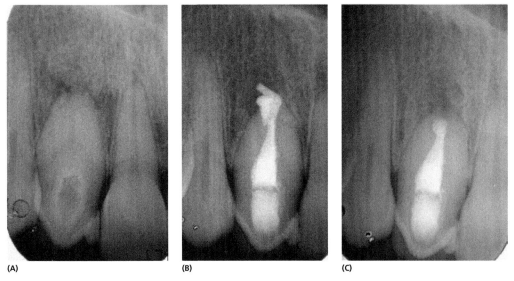

Figure 12.13 (A) Tooth #7 presented with dens-in-dente, canal calcification, and a blunderbuss apex. (B) A gross overfill of gutta-percha was difficult to avoid due to the large, irregular, and divergent walls of this blunderbuss apex. (C) Surgical correction of the overfill and the establishment of a precise apical seal using microsurgical techniques. The canal was retroprepared using a surgical ultrasonic tip and then retrofilled with Super EBA.

calcification, and a blunderbuss apex. Conventional endodontic therapy was initially performed. Despite the fact that the canal was localized and treated, it was still difficult to establish an apical seal due to the large, divergent, and irregular apical foramen. Microsurgery was performed to remove the gross overfill and establish a precise apical seal.

Contraindications

Of the few contraindications to endodontic surgery, only some are absolute. The majority of these conditions are only temporary and can either be corrected or managed by a knowledgeable surgeon. These contraindications can be categorized as dental, anatomical, and medical. The following sections will present each category in detail.

Tooth-specific factors

The restorability and the periodontal health of a tooth are important factors in planning treatment and determining a prognosis. Probing depth and mobility should be carefully assessed before surgery. Another concern is the clinical crown-root ratio the tooth exhibits. Apical surgery on a short-rooted tooth with significant attachment loss will further compromise the crown-root ratio (Figure 12.14). Moreover, such a course of treatment could result in an endodontic/periodontic communication, compromising the overall outcome of the surgery and leading to eventual tooth loss. In these situations, conventional retreatment should be considered if feasible. Otherwise, extraction may be the best solution.

Anatomical factors
The inferior alveolar nerve

The location of the mandibular canal and the mental foramen should be carefully assessed before surgery in the posterior mandible. The use of a microscope facilitates identification of the neurovascular bundle. The added magnification also assists in the preparation of the groove technique (a shallow horizontal groove in bone), a measure that prevents unintentional instrument slippage and avoids permanent nerve damage. However, in certain cases, the extreme proximity of the neurovascular bundle could render the procedure risky and, therefore, contraindicated (Figure 12.15).

The maxillary sinus

The apices of maxillary molar and premolar teeth can be in close proximity to the floor of the sinus (Figure 12.16). In some instances, the apices are located inside the sinus. A watchful examination of preoperative radiographs, coupled with careful surgical dissection under magnification, will minimize the chances of sinus membrane perforation. When the sinus membrane is inadvertently perforated, if meticulous surgical techniques and proper postoperative care were employed, the outcome of apical surgery will not be compromised and complications are usually minimal.[16]

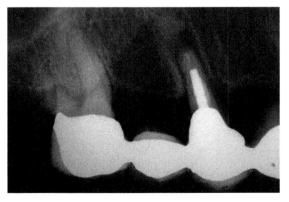

Figure 12.14 A radiograph of tooth #4, which has a poor crown–root ratio and a moderate attachment loss. Apical surgery is contraindicated.

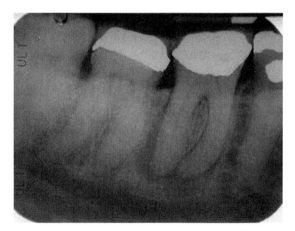

Figure 12.15 A radiograph that reveals the close proximity of the mandibular nerve and the mental foramen to the apices of teeth #29, 30, and 31. Apical surgery can be risky, and therefore, it might be contraindicated in certain cases to avoid permanent paresthesia.

Barrier placement is recommended to block the perforation area during the surgery and to ensure that foreign material or even a resected apex does not enter the sinus.[17] Telfa pads (Kendall Company, Mansfield, MA) are excellent materials to use as a sinus barrier (Figure 12.17). They can be cut to fit the perforation size, and they contain no cotton fibers that could contaminate the surgical field. To prevent the Telfa pad from getting dislodged into the sinus cavity, a suture is tied through its center, which will keep the barrier in place throughout the surgery and allow the operator to easily pull the barrier out at the end of the surgery. In addition, patients should be prescribed an antibiotic (1 g amoxicillin immediately following the perforation, continued with 500 mg tid for 24 hours) and a nasal decongestant for 5 days.

The second mandibular molar area

The mandibular second molar presents many difficult obstacles for apical surgery. Due to a thick buccal cortex of bone, lingually inclined roots, and close proximity of the apices to the mandibular canal, these teeth are usually poor candidates for surgery. In addition, as the far distal location in the dental arch impedes easy access, surgery becomes nearly impossible. For mandibular second molars, an alternative to surgery should be considered, such as retreatment or replantation.

Medical considerations

A thorough review of a patient's medical history is of paramount importance. All medical concerns should be answered before surgery. There are a few medical conditions that contraindicate endodontic surgery, such as clotting deficiencies, brittle diabetes, dialysis, and a compromised immune system. With certain other medical conditions, endodontic surgery should be postponed until the condition is treated or stabilized and no longer presents any risk to the patient. Good examples include recent myocardial infarction, radiation therapy, anticoagulant medications, and first and third trimesters of pregnancy. The decision for surgery should be evaluated on a case-by-case basis and in consultation with the patient's physician.

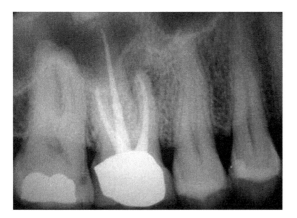

Figure 12.16 This radiograph demonstrates the close proximity of the maxillary sinus to the apices of the teeth in that quadrant.

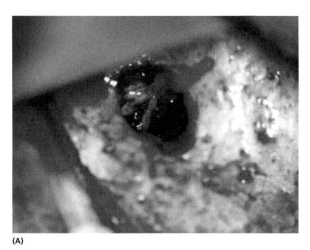

(A)

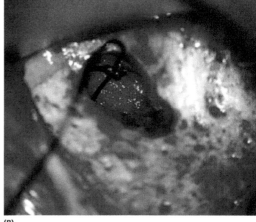

(B)

Figure 12.17 (A) Sinus perforation. (B) Barrier placement with suture.

The surgeon's skill and ability

One very important factor in case selection is the surgeon's level of knowledge and experience. Clinicians should carefully assess the difficulty of each case and decide who is best suited to perform the procedure. Challenging cases should be referred to endodontists or oral surgeons with microsurgical expertise.

Armamentarium

A basic endodontic surgery kit should contain the most commonly used instruments to perform periradicular surgical procedures. Key instruments and materials with their general use are listed in Table 12.1. The surgical kit should be supplemented with the following instruments and devices to perform apical microsurgery.

Surgical operating microscope

The microscope is defined as an instrument that gives an enlarged image of an object or substance that is minute or not visible with the naked eye. The incorporation of the operating microscope into apical surgery carries great benefits simply by providing illumination and magnification to a small surgical field. This will translate clinically into a more precise and conservative surgical procedure with minimal guesswork. It will also allow accurate assessment and excision of all pathological changes with very conservative removal of healthy structures. For the first time, the resected root surface can be clearly inspected for any anatomical complexities or microfractures.

Every microscope contains the following components: eyepieces, binoculars, objective lens, and the magnification changer (Figure 12.18). Magnification is determined by the power of the eyepieces (M_e), the focal length of the binoculars (f_t), the magnification changer factor (M_c), and the focal length of the objective length (f_0). Total magnification can be calculated using the following equation:

$$\text{Total magnification } M_t = f_t / f_0 \times M_e \times M_c$$

Recommended settings for a surgical operating microscope in endodontics are ×12.5 eyepieces, five-step magnification changer, 200 to 250 mm objective length, and 60 degrees or more inclinable binoculars.

Incorporating the microscope into general dentistry practice is costly and initially will slow the operator's speed due to the nature of the learning curve. However, it is the single most important element in performing apical surgery to the current standards. The use of magnifying

Table 12.1 Surgical kit

Examination instruments
Mirror, endodontic explorer, and periodontal probe

Soft-tissue incision, elevation, and reflection
#15C blade
Microblades
Periosteal elevators (Howard, #9 Molt, and #149)
Kim/Pecora retractors 1 through 4 (Hartzell & Sons, Inc.)
Tissue forceps

Osteotomy and root-resection instruments
Impact Air 45 handpiece
H 161 Lindemann bone cutting burr (Brasseler, Inc.)
Surgical-length round burrs

Curettage instruments
Small endodontic spoon curette
Periodontal curette (Columbia 13/14)
34/35 Jaquette and Mini-Jaquette scalers
#2/4 Molt curette

Inspection instruments
Micromirrors (5 mm round and modified rectangular)

Root-end preparation instruments
Ultrasonic unit (Spartan or Miniendo)
Surgical ultrasonic tips (KiS 1 through 6, BK3-R)

Root-end filling/finishing instruments
Retrofilling carrier (West carrier)
MTA pellet-forming block with KM-3/KM-4 placement instruments (Hartzell & Son, Inc.)
Micropluggers and ball burnishers
Polishing burrs

Suturing and soft-tissue closure
Castroviejo needle holder
Surgical scissors
Various suture types and sizes (5–0 and 6–0)
Sterile gauze for soft-tissue compression

Miscellaneous instruments and materials
Surgical aspirator
Irrigation syringes and needles
Stropko irrigator/drier with disposable microtip (Ultradent, Inc.)
Cut-Trol (50% ferric sulfate)
Super EBA (Bosworth, Inc.)
MTA (ProRoot by DENTSPLY/Tulsa, Inc.)
Racellet #3 epinephrine cotton pellet (Pascal Company, Inc.)
Methylene blue stain (Fisher Scientific, Inc.)
Microapplicator tips (Quick Tips by Worldwide Dental, Inc.)

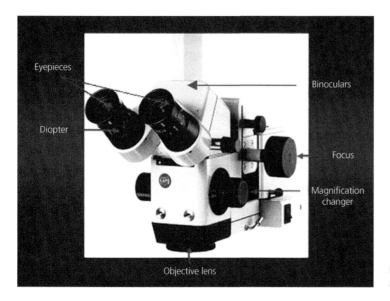

Figure 12.18 Components of the surgical operating microscope.

loupes with an added fiberoptic headlamp is helpful, but it is only the minimum requirement in performing apical surgery. Loupes can only provide a 2× to 6× range of magnification, which is marginally useful in anterior surgery. In surgeries involving posterior teeth, the microscope is absolutely essential due to restricted access, limited visibility, and far more complicated root anatomy.

The surgical microscope, in contrast to loupes, provides a wide range of magnification from ×3 to ×30. The lower range of magnification (×3 to ×8) provides a wider field of view and a high focal depth, which is practical for orientation. The middle range of magnification (×10 to ×16) is the working range, which provides adequate enlargement of the surgical field to perform most of the surgical steps. The highest range of magnification (×20 to ×30) is only used for fine inspection of the resected root surface. It has a shallow focal depth, and the focus can easily be affected by the slightest movement, such as the patient's breathing.

Microsurgical instruments

Many microsurgical instruments are miniaturized versions of traditional surgical instruments. Other instruments are specifically invented and designed to perform apical microsurgery.

The following is a list of microsurgical instruments and their general uses:

• **Microblades.** A #15C blade is the blade of choice in most surgical procedures. However, when the interproximal

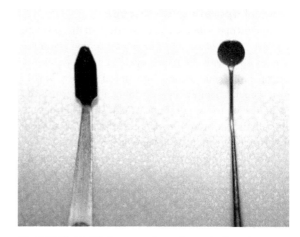

Figure 12.19 Modified rectangular and round micromirrors.

spaces are tight, such as in the anterior mandibular area, a microblade becomes more useful and will precisely incise the flap without any tissue damage.

• **Micromirrors.** A large variety of micromirrors is available on the market in different materials, shapes, and sizes. Only two micromirrors are needed, a round shape (5 mm in diameter) and a modified rectangular micromirror (Figure 12.19). Both can be purchased in stainless steel, sapphire, or diamond mirror surfaces. The sapphire and diamond micromirrors have scratch-free surfaces and are brighter than the stainless ones. They are also more costly.

• **Ultrasonic units and tips.** Ultrasonic units and tips have replaced the traditional micro handpieces. The two most widely used ultrasonic units are the Miniendo II (Analytic/SybronEndo) and the Spartan (Spartan/Obtura) (Figure 12.3). There are many different ultrasonic tips available on the market, but the three most popular are the KiS, CT, and BK3 (Figures 12.20, 12.21, and 12.22). All three types are very effective and precise; however, they vary in material, tip angulation, and design. The size of these tips is 1/10th the size of a conventional microhead handpiece. CT and BK3 tips are made of stainless steel, and they are also available with a diamond coating that improves their cutting efficiency. The BK3 tips

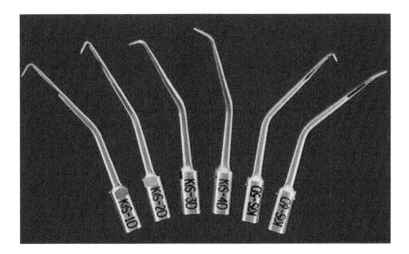

Figure 12.20 KiS ultrasonic tips.

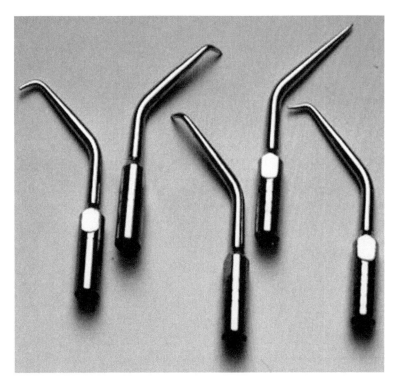

Figure 12.21 CT ultrasonic tips.

come in a set of two (BK3-R right, BK3-L left), and each tip has three bends that facilitate easy access to any preparation. BK3 right is designed for use in the upper right and lower left, and BK3 left is designed for use in the upper left and lower right. The KiS ultrasonic tips come in a set of six different tips, all of which are coated with zirconium nitride for smoother and more efficient cutting. The irrigation port is located

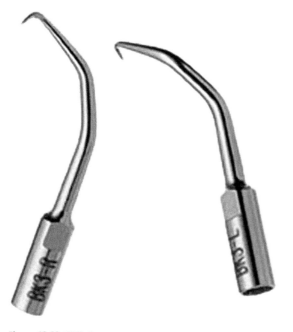

Figure 12.22 BK3 tips.

close to the 3-mm cutting tip. The KiS 1 tip has an 80-degree angled tip and is 0.24 mm in diameter. This thin-diameter tip is ideal for apical preparation on mandibular anteriors and premolars. The KiS 2 tip has a wider diameter and is ideal for wider preparation such as with maxillary anteriors. The KiS 3 tip has a double bend and a 70-degree angled tip. It is helpful in reaching the maxillary left and mandibular right posteriors. The KiS 4 tip is similar to the KiS 3 tip except that the tip angle is 110 degrees, which is designed to reach the lingual apex of molar. The KiS 5 tip is the counterpart of the KiS 3 tip. The Kis 6 tip is the counterpart of the KiS 4 tip.

- **Stropko irrigator/drier.** This device fits on a standard air/water syringe and uses a microtip needle (Ultradent, Inc.) to effectively irrigate and dry retropreparations. However, it should be used cautiously and only inside the retropreparation to reduce the chance of emphysema. It is recommended to change the pre-existing obtuse angle bend on the microtip needle to a 90-degree bend that is 3 mm in length (Figure 12.23). This manipulation will facilitate direct insertion of the tip into the retropreparation for a thorough drying with minimal disturbance of the delicate hemostasis of the crypt (Figure 12.24).
- **Retrofilling instruments.** Micropluggers, retrofilling carriers, and ball burnishers (Figure 12.25) are retrofilling instruments. Micropluggers come in ball ends ranging from 0.25 to 0.75 mm. They can be either straight-handled or double-angled. The straight-handled micropluggers come in two different

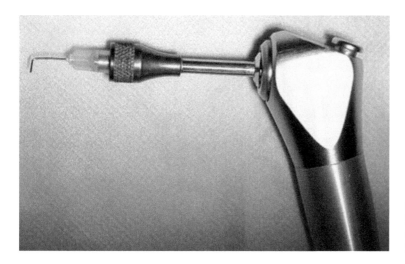

Figure 12.23 Stropko irrigator/drier. Note the microtip needle with the correct 90-degree bend that is 3 mm in length.

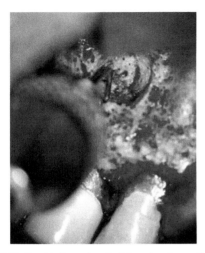

Figure 12.24 The 90-degree bend of the microtip needle will facilitate direct insertion of the needle tip into the retropreparation for a thorough drying with minimal disturbance of the delicate hemostasis of the crypt.

angles: a 90-degree tip for universal use and a 65-degree tip helpful for the lingual apex (Figure 12.26). The double-angled microplugger tips are offset by 65 degrees—one left and one right for left and right molar surgeries. The Super EBA retrofilling carrier has a flat surface that is designed to carry the retrofilling material into the retropreparation. Figure 12.27 shows the West carriers with straight and offset angles. Burnishers are ball shaped and are available in different sizes. They are used immediately following retrofilling material placement to adapt the retrofilling material into the retropreparation and to seal all the margins. If mineral trioxide aggregate (MTA) is to be used as the retrofilling material, then a carrier system is needed to transport this delicate material

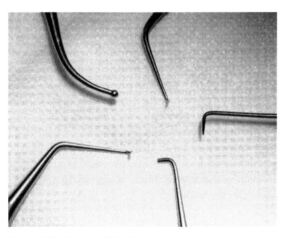

Figure 12.25 The retrofilling instruments.

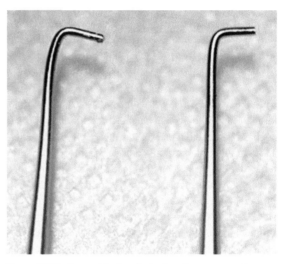

Figure 12.26 The straight-handled micropluggers come in two different angles: a 90-degree tip that is for universal use and a 65-degree tip that is helpful for the lingual apex.

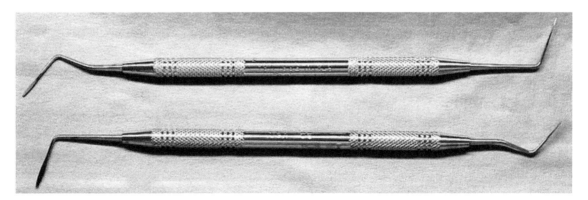

Figure 12.27 The West carriers.

into the retropreparation. A variety of Messing gun systems are available and can be used for this purpose. More recently, an MTA pellet-forming block has become available (Hartzell & Son, Concord, CA) and has proven to be more effective and less complicated than other systems. Directions for using this block will be provided later in the retrofilling section of this chapter.

Preoperative assessment

The prognosis following surgery depends on thorough preoperative medical, intraoral, periodontic, and radiographic evaluations as well as with good surgical technique and proper postoperative instruction.

Medical evaluation

A routine review of the patient's medical history and current medications should be performed, and, when necessary, additional medical consultations should be requested. As a general rule, no special precautions need to be taken when surgery is planned other than those that normally apply to routine dental procedures.[18] Special emphasis should be placed, however, on noting any blood-thinning medications, especially aspirin. They are so commonly prescribed that patients often forget to include it in their medical history. Aspirin should be discontinued at least 7 days before surgery, after discussion with the patient's primary care physician. Another consideration is the need to prescribe prophylactic premedication as is seen with patients with certain cardiac

conditions[19] and joint replacement. This will be covered elsewhere in the text.

Intraoral evaluation

A thorough oral examination should comprise all of the following:
- Patient's chief complaint
- Chronological history of the problem tooth
- Presence of swelling
- Tracing of existing sinus tract with a gutta-percha point (Figure 12.28)

Periodontal evaluation

The periodontal examination should include mobility, probing depth, and requests for preoperative scaling and/or root planing if needed. Probing depth measurements are an essential part of the consultation that aides in the diagnosis of vertical root fracture (Figure 12.29) or combined perioendo lesions. Detections of such periodontal involvements could drastically alter the treatment plan and save patients from undergoing unnecessary surgical procedures. If patient sensitivity prevents accurate probing, administration of a local anesthetic is recommended.

Radiographic evaluation

A radiological examination is essential and should include prior radiographs if available. Two radiographs taken from two different angles (straight on and mesially angulated) can uncover concealed anatomical structures by adding a third dimension to an otherwise two-dimensional image. Preoperative radiographs should be assessed in a systemic manner for the following:

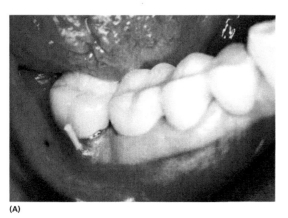

(A)

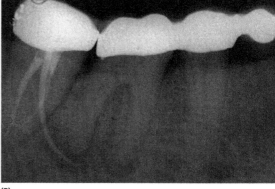

(B)

Figure 12.28 (A) Sinus tract opening buccal to tooth #31. (B) Radiograph of gutta-percha (GP) point traced to apex of tooth #30.

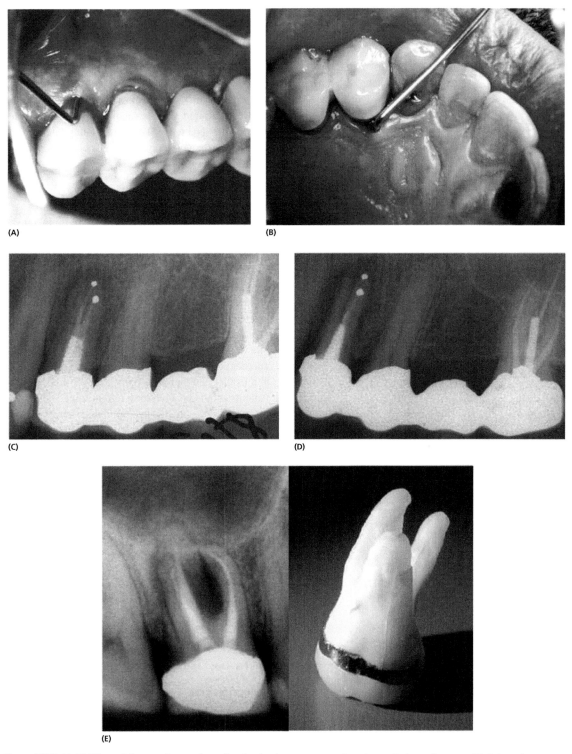

Figure 12.29 (A–B) Bilateral deep pockets on buccal and palatal areas—suggestive of a vertical root fracture. (C) J-shaped radiolucency commonly associated with root fracture. (D) Radiograph taken at slightly different angulation clearly shows the fracture. (E) Radiographic and clinical views of a vertical root fracture case.

- Approximate root length
- Number of roots and their configuration
- Degree of root curvature (Figure 12.30)
- Proximity of adjacent root tips, especially in anterior teeth (Figure 12.31)

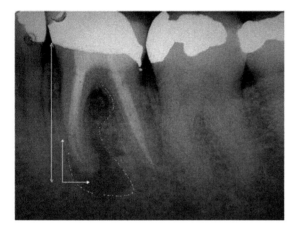

Figure 12.30 Preoperative radiographs provide valuable information such as the approximate root length, the number of roots and their configuration, and the degree of root curvature. The approximate size, location, and type of lesion can also be assessed.

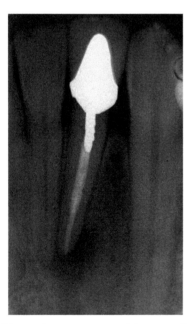

Figure 12.31 Note the close proximity of the apices of these two mandibular incisors. Patient should be made aware of the possible loss of vitality of the adjacent tooth after apical surgery.

- Proximity of anatomical structures including mandibular canal, mental foramen, external oblique ridge, zygomatic process, and the maxillary sinus
- Approximate size, location, and type of lesion
- Vertical root fracture or radiographic signs most commonly associated with it such as thickening of the periodontal ligament (PDL) surrounding lateral root surfaces, J-shaped lesions, or possible endodontic/periodontal lesions.

Preoperative medications

The following preoperative regimens are recommended:

- 0.12% chlorhexidine mouth rinse starting the day before surgery and continuing for up to a week after surgery to reduce the oral microflora.
- Ibuprofen 800 mg 1 hour before surgery, which is effective in reducing the inflammatory response and postoperative pain.[20]
- Tranquilizers for anxious patients such as valium (5 mg) one hour before the surgery. If a tranquilizer is used, another person must accompany the patient on the trip to the office and then back home after the procedure.
- Patients should be advised to refrain from smoking.
- As discussed previously, antibiotic prophylactic premedication should be prescribed when indicated.

Surgical technique

Anesthesia and hemostasis

The ability to achieve profound anesthesia and hemostasis in the surgical site is crucial in microsurgery. Profound anesthesia will eliminate patient discomfort and anxiety during, and for a significant time following, the procedure. Excellent hemostasis will improve visibility of the surgical site, allow microscopic inspection of the resected root surface, and minimize the surgery time.

Hemostatic control can be divided into preoperative, intraoperative, and postoperative phases. These phases are interrelated and dependent on each other.

Preoperative phase

An anesthetic solution containing a vasoconstrictor is indicated to achieve anesthesia and hemostasis.[21] While 2% lidocaine with a 1:100,000 concentration of epinephrine is recognized as an excellent anesthetic agent, clinical evidence suggests that a 1:50,000 concentration offers better hemostasis.[22,23]

The amount of the anesthetic solution containing 1:50,000 epinephrine that is necessary to achieve anesthesia and hemostasis depends on the size of the surgical site; however, 2.0 to 4.0 ml is usually sufficient. This amount of local anesthetic should be slowly infiltrated using multiple injections. Solution should be deposited throughout the entire submucosa superficial to the periosteum at the level of the root apices in the surgical site. It is worth mentioning that there is a narrow margin of error in delivering local infiltration. Skeletal muscles respond to epinephrine with vasodilation instead of vasoconstriction as they contain blood vessels that are mostly innervated with β2 adrenergic receptors. Thus, great care should be taken to avoid infiltrating into deeper skeletal tissue beyond the root apices and over basal bone instead of alveolar bone.

In the maxilla, anesthesia and hemostasis are usually accomplished simultaneously by local infiltration in the mucobuccal fold over the apices of the tooth in question and two adjacent teeth both mesial and distal to that tooth (five teeth total). This should be supplemented with a nerve block near the incisive foramen to block the nasopalatine nerve for surgery on maxillary anterior teeth, or near the greater palatine foramen to block the greater palatine nerve for surgery on the maxillary posterior teeth (Figures 12.32 and 12.33).

In the mandible, anesthesia and hemostasis are usually achieved separately. Anesthesia is established by a regional nerve block of the inferior alveolar nerve, using 1.5 cartridges of 2% lidocaine with 1:100,000 epinephrine. Hemostasis is established with two cartridges of 2% lidocaine with 1:50,000 epinephrine at the surgical site via multiple supraperiosteal injections into the mucobuccal fold. An additional supplement of a 0.5 cartridge is also injected into the lingual aspect of the tooth. The rate of injection will relate to the degree of hemostasis and anesthesia obtained. A rate of 1 to 2 ml/min is recommended.[24]

Injecting at a faster rate results in localized pooling of the solution, delayed and limited diffusion, and less than optimal anesthesia and hemostasis. It is essential to allow the deposited solution sufficient time to diffuse and reach the targeted area to produce the desired effects before any incision is made. The recommended wait time is usually 7 to10 minutes, until the soft tissue throughout the surgical site has blanched (Figures 12.34 and 12.35).

Intraoperative phase

The most important measure in achieving hemostasis is effective local vasoconstriction. Following osteotomy, curettage, and root resection, hemostasis needs to be established *again* as newly ruptured blood vessels immerse the bone crypt and the buccal plate with blood. The use of a topical hemostatic agent is frequently needed at this point during surgery to control bleeding. Such an agent maintains a dry surgical field that will allow microscopic inspection of the resected root surface, adequate

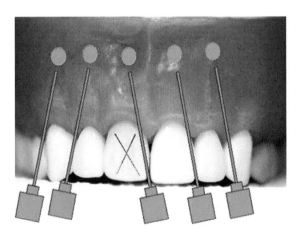

Figure 12.32 Local infiltration for surgery on tooth #8 should extend from tooth #6 to tooth #10 at the level of the root apices.

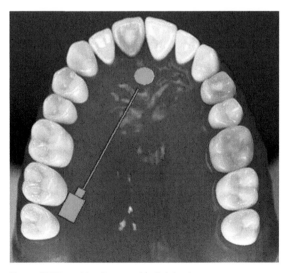

Figure 12.33 Incisive foramen block injection.

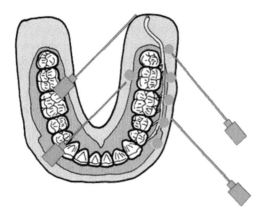

Figure 12.34 In the mandible, anesthesia is established by a regional nerve block of the inferior alveolar nerve, using 1.5 cartridges of 2% lidocaine with 1:100,000 epinephrine. Hemostasis is established with 2 cartridges of 2% lidocaine with 1:50,000 epinephrine at the surgical site via multiple supraperiosteal injections into the mucobuccal fold. An additional supplement of a 0.5 cartridge (also mainly for hemostasis) can be injected at the lingual aspect of the root.

visibility during ultrasonic retropreparation, and good isolation during retrofilling material placement.

Many topical hemostatic agents are available. The two most widely used by endodontists are epinephrine cotton pellets and ferric sulfate solution. The following is a presentation of the properties of these two chemical agents and their mechanisms of action.

Epinephrine pellets. Racellets are cotton pellets containing racemic epinephrine HCl (Pascal Company, Inc., Bellvue, WA). The amount of epinephrine in each varies depending on the number on the label (Figure 12.36). A Racellet #3 pellet contains an average of 0.55 mg of racemic epinephrine and is usually recommended for apical surgery. The Racellet pellets are inexpensive and highly effective in achieving hemostasis in the bone crypt via the vasoconstriction effects of epinephrine coupled with the pressure applied to these pellets.[25] It has been shown that one to seven pellets of Racellet #3 can be applied directly to the bone crypt and left for 2 to 4 minutes with no evident cardiovascular changes.[26]

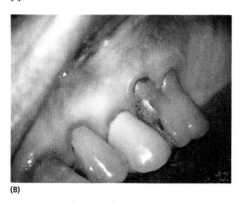

(A)

(B)

Figure 12.35 (A) Before anesthesia. (B) 10 minutes after local infiltration.

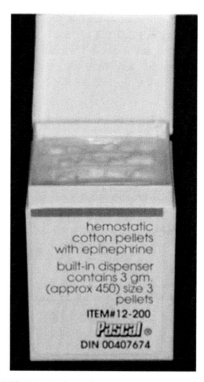

Figure 12.36 Epinephrine pellets.

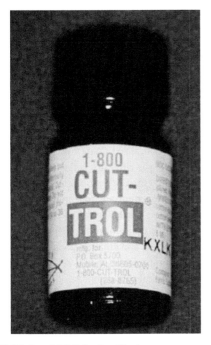

Figure 12.37 Cutrol (50% ferric sulfate).

Ferric sulfate. Ferric sulfate is another chemical hemostatic agent that has been used for a long time in restorative dentistry. Its mechanism of action is not completely clear, but it is believed to be due to agglutination of blood proteins when in contact with this very acidic solution (pH 0.21). The agglutinated proteins form plugs that occlude the capillary orifices to achieve hemostasis.

Ferric sulfate is commercially available in different solutions with different concentrations. The recommended solution for endodontic surgery is Cutrol, which contains 50% ferric sulfate (Figure 12.37). Cutrol is an excellent surface hemostatic agent on the buccal plate of bone and inside the bone crypt. It should be applied directly to the bleeding point with a microapplicator tip or a cotton pellet (Figure 12.38A). On contact with blood, this yellowish solution immediately turns dark brown. This color change is helpful in identifying any remaining bleeders that need to be addressed (Figure 12.38B).

Ferric sulfate is a very effective hemostatic agent that works instantly, but it is also cytotoxic and causes tissue necrosis. For this reason, it should not come in contact

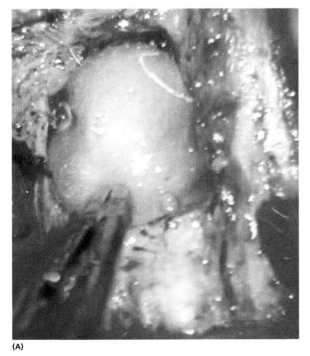

(A)

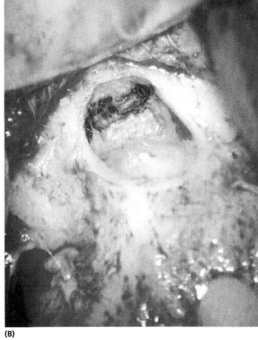

(B)

Figure 12.38 (A) Cutrol application to bone. (B) Bone color change.

with the flap tissue. This agent should be used as an adjunct to other hemostatic measures, and its use should be limited. For example, use ferric sulfate only if bleeding persists after using the epinephrine cotton pellet technique. When used correctly, as described in the previous paragraph, systemic absorption is unlikely since the coagulum stops the solution from reaching the blood stream.

Ferric sulfate also has been proved to damage bone and delay healing when used in large amounts and left in situ after surgery. It should therefore only be used in small amounts and should be immediately and gently irrigated with saline after application. If the coagulum is thoroughly removed and irrigated before closure, there is no adverse reaction.[27]

The following steps outline the most effective method to achieve local hemostasis quickly during apical surgery:

1. Complete all the cutting necessary (osteotomy and root resection) and then thoroughly remove all granulation tissue from the bone crypt.
2. Place a small Racellet #3 cotton pellet in the bone crypt and firmly pack it against the lingual wall (Figure 12.39A).
3. In quick succession, pack in additional Racellet pellets against the first pellet, until the entire crypt is filled with pellets (Figure 12.39B). Depending on the size of the crypt, this can take a variable number of pellets. A study by Vickers[26] has shown that up to seven Racellet #3 pellets can be safely used to fill the crypt. If more are needed due to the large size of the crypt, then some sterile cotton pellets should be added until the crypt is completely filled.
4. Apply pressure to these pellets with a blunt instrument (for example, back of a micromirror handle) for 2 to 4 minutes, until no further bleeding is observed (Figure 12.39C).
5. Remove all pellets one by one, except the last epinephrine pellet, which is left inside the crypt to avoid reopening the ruptured vessels (Figure 12.39D). This pellet should only be removed at the end of the surgical procedure before final irrigation and flap closure.

If small bleeders are still present on the buccal plate or inside the crypt, then Cutrol should be applied directly to the bleeding areas. Without disrupting the coagulum, the solution is quickly rinsed with saline to remove any excess. The coagulum formed should be left intact during the surgical procedure but must be thoroughly curetted and the corresponding area rinsed before closure.

Postoperative phase

Periradicular surgery should be performed within a reasonable amount of time so that complicated and hemostasis-dependent steps are completed before reactive hyperemia occurs. As the restricted blood flow returns to normal, it rapidly increases to a rate well beyond normal to compensate for localized tissue hypoxia and acidosis. Reactive hyperemia is clinically variable and unpredictable. It can be prevented or reduced by compressing the flap tissue for three minutes and applying firm finger pressure with saline-soaked gauze pads placed over the surgical site. This is done to induce hemostasis, prevent hematoma formation, and enhance good tissue reapproximation.[28] Flap compressions should be followed immediately with postsurgical cold compressions to the cheek.

Flap designs

The semilunar flap used to be the flap of choice for apical surgery (Figure 12.40). It is not advocated today for a number of reasons. The semilunar flap provides restricted surgical access and has limited potential for further extension if deemed necessary. It also carries the danger of postsurgical defects by incising through tissues that are not supported by underlying bone.[29] Furthermore, this type of incision results in maximum severing of periosteal blood vessels. This compromises the blood supply, which could lead to shrinkage, gapping, and secondary healing. Another disadvantage to the semilunar flap is the close proximity of the incision to the osteotomy site, which makes hemostatic control more challenging.

The following flap designs are recommended for periradicular surgery.

Full mucoperiosteal tissue flap

There are strong biological reasons to use this kind of flap whenever possible.[18,30] It maintains intact vertical blood supply and minimizes hemorrhage while providing adequate access. It allows a survey of bone and root structures, which facilitates excellent surgical orientation. However, as this flap involves the gingival papilla and exposes the crestal bone, it can carry a few potential risks including loss of tissue attachment, loss of crestal bone height, and possible loss of interdental papilla integrity.

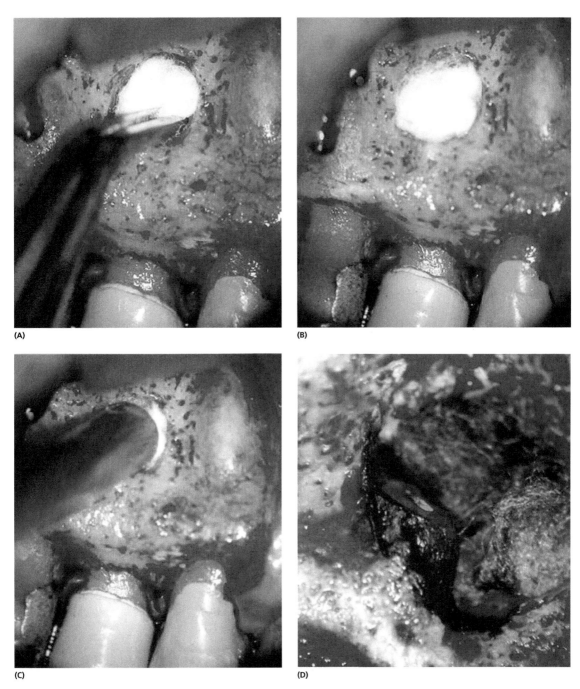

Figure 12.39 (A) Initial Racellet pellet placed inside the crypt. (B) Bone crypt filled with pellets. (C) Pressure applied on top of the pellets. (D) Racellet pellets removed until resected root is exposed, leaving at least one pellet against the crypt wall.

The two recommended designs for full mucoperiosteal tissue flaps for periradicular surgery are the triangular and rectangular (trapezoidal) designs.

The **triangular** flap design is the most widely used flap design in periradicular surgery, and it is indicated in the anterior and posterior regions of both the mandible and the maxilla. It requires a horizontal intrasulcular incision and a single vertical releasing incision (Figure 12.41).

The horizontal incision is made with the scalpel held near a vertical position, extending through the gingival sulcus and the gingival fibers down to the level of the crestal bone. When passing through the interdental region, care should be taken to ensure that the incision separates the buccal and lingual papillae in the midcol area. A microblade will ease this separation if the embrasure space is narrow (for example, mandibular anterior area). A clean incision located exactly midcol is vital to prevent sloughing of the papillae due to a compromised blood supply and to prevent the unesthetic look of double papillae.[18]

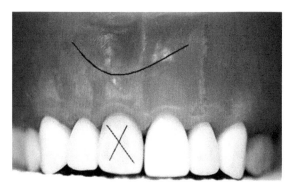

Figure 12.40 Semilunar flap design.

The vertical releasing incision is prepared between the root eminences parallel to the long access of the roots. In anterior surgery, the vertical incision is prepared in the flap perimeter closest to the surgeon. In posterior surgery, it always constitutes the mesial perimeter of the flap. It is important to keep the base of the flap as wide as the top so that the vertical incision is kept parallel to the vertically positioned supraperiosteal microvasculature and tissue-supportive collagen fibers.[31] In this manner, the least number of vessels and fibers are severed, which will translate into faster healing without scarring (Figure 12.42). Vertical incisions should terminate at the mesial or distal line angles of the teeth and never in the papillae or the mid-root area. A vertical incision also should meet the tooth at the free gingival margin at a 90-degree angle (Figures 12.41 and 12.43).

The advantages of the triangular flap design are simplicity, rapid wound healing, ease of flap reapproximation, and ease of suturing. A disadvantage, on the other hand, is the limited surgical access. In situations where more access is warranted, either the horizontal or the vertical incisions can be extended to allow some additional mobilization of the flap.

Alternatively, a rectangular flap design should be considered if maximum access is required.

The **rectangular** flap design is very similar to the triangular design except for the addition of a second vertical releasing incision (Figure 12.44). The rectangular flap design is indicated for anterior surgery when more access is needed. It is also used when multiple teeth will be operated on or when the roots are long (for example, cuspid).

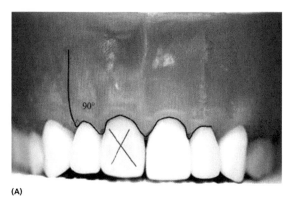

(A)

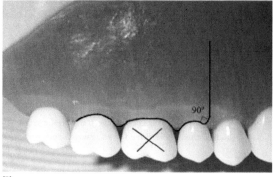

(B)

Figure 12.41 (A) Anterior triangular flap design. (B) Posterior triangular flap design.

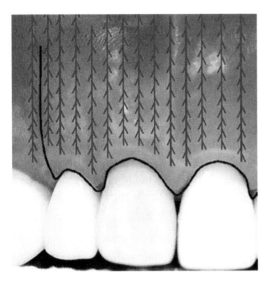

Figure 12.42 Vertical releasing incision is parallel to microvasculature.

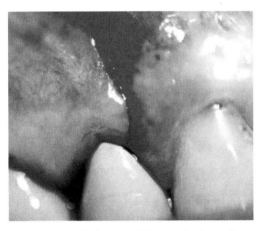

Figure 12.43 Vertical releasing incision terminating at the tooth line angle. It is perpendicular to the free gingival margin.

Potential disadvantages associated with this flap design include technique-sensitive wound closure and a greater chance for flap dislodgment.

Limited mucoperiosteal tissue flap (scalloped flap)

This limited tissue flap does not include the marginal and interdental gingiva within its perimeter. It is indicated in teeth with existing fixed restorations and in cases where esthetics are a major concern. The limited tissue flap can be used in both the maxillary anterior or posterior regions but only when sufficient width of the attached gingiva is available. It is usually contraindicated in the mandible because the attached gingiva is narrow in that region and esthetics are not a major concern.

An absolute minimum of 2 mm of attached gingiva from the depth of the gingival sulcus must be present before this flap design can be selected (Figure 12.45).[32] This submarginal flap design is formed by a scalloped horizontal incision and one or two vertical releasing incisions, depending on the surgical access needed (Figure 12.46). The scalloped incision reflects the contours of the marginal gingiva and provides an adequate distance from the depth of the gingival sulci.[18] It also serves as a guide for correctly repositioning the elevated flap for suturing.[25]

All the flap corners, either at the scalloping or at the junction of the horizontal and vertical incisions, should be rounded to promote smoother healing and minimize scar formation. The angle of the incision in relation to the cortical plate is 45 degrees to allow the widest cut surface as well as better adaptation when the flap is repositioned (Figure 12.47). This 45-degree bevel at the scalloped horizontal incision is made with the tip of

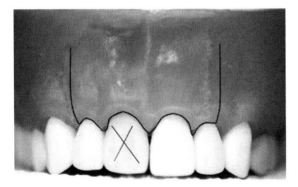

Figure 12.44 Rectangular flap design.

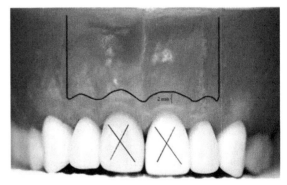

Figure 12.45 Rectangular submarginal flap design.

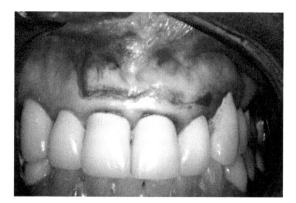

Figure 12.46 Triangular submarginal flap design.

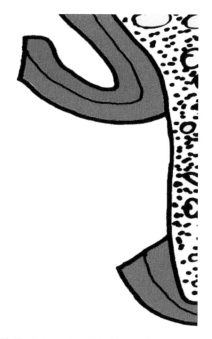

Figure 12.47 45-degree bevel incision angle.

the scalpel pointing away from the gingival sulcus. This adds an additional safety measure to protect the minimum 2 mm of attached gingiva.

The submarginal flap has the advantage of leaving the marginal and interdental gingiva intact in addition to leaving the crestal bone unexposed. The major disadvantage is the severing of supraperiosteal vessels, which could leave the unreflected tissue without a blood supply. This can be prevented by preserving an adequate width of unreflected gingival tissue, which will derive secondary blood supplies from the PDL and

intraosseous blood vessels. The healing of this flap seems to be quite similar to that of the full mucoperiosteal flap.[30]

Elevation and retraction

Tissue elevation always starts in the attached gingiva of the vertical incision (Figure 12.48A, B). This allows the periosteal elevator to apply reflective forces against the cortical bone and not the root surface while elevating the tougher fibrous tissue of the gingiva. Special attention should be paid to ensure that the periosteum is entirely lifted from the cortical plate with the elevated flap (Figure 12.49). The elevator should then be moved more coronally to elevate the marginal and interdental papilla atraumatically using the undermining elevation technique.[18] In this technique, all reflective forces should be applied to the bone and periosteum, with minimal forces on the gingival tissue (Figure 12.50A, B). Subsequently, the elevation continues in a more apical direction into the submucosa to expose the root tip area and to render the flap more flexible and movable.

At this point a retractor should be used to provide access to the periradicular tissue. The retractor tip should rest on bone with light but firm pressure and without any trauma to the flap soft tissue. The surgeon must ensure that minimal tension exists at all perimeters of the flap before the osteotomy. If tension exists, then one or both of the releasing incisions should be extended, or the reflected tissue should be elevated further. It is important to evaluate the cortical plate bone topography (flat, convex, or concave) to choose the right retractor tip—a shape that will fit the anatomy to maximize stable anchorage (Figure 12.51A, B). For example, if the cortical bone anatomy is convex, such as the area of the canine eminence or the zygoma, then a retractor with a concave or V-shaped tip will best fit this anatomy (Figure 12.52). An appropriate retractor tip will allow maximum surface contact between the retractor and bone to prevent unintentional retractor slippage and possible flap impingement.

For posterior mandibular surgery, the groove technique should be used to provide a stable anchor for the retractor. In this technique, a 15-mm shallow horizontal groove is prepared using the Lindemann burr. This groove is prepared beyond the apex for

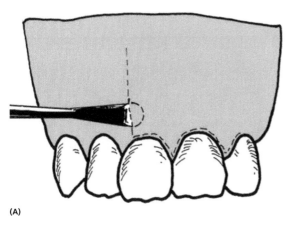

(A)

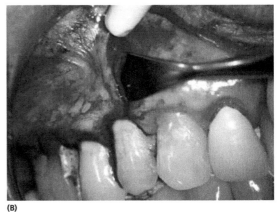

(B)

Figure 12.48 (A–B) Elevation starts at the middle portion of the vertical incision.

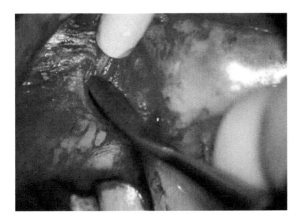

Figure 12.49 Visual inspection to ensure that the periosteum is included within the flap elevation and is completely lifted off the cortical plate.

molar surgery and above the mental foramen for premolar surgery. The use of a plastic cheek retractor underneath the surgical retractor provides better access and visibility to the surgical site while protecting the patient's lips at the same time (Figure 12.53). The amount of time that the tissue is retracted is an essential factor in the speed of healing. Although related literature does not give a specific recommendation, it seems logical to keep this time to a minimum. On the other hand, operators should take sufficient time to achieve the clinical goals of the surgical procedure.[29] By keeping the surgical site well hydrated with sterile saline, the time for the procedure can be extended seemingly indefinitely.

Osteotomy

The purpose of the osteotomy in endodontic surgery is to deliberately and precisely prepare a small window through the cortical plate of bone to gain direct visual and instrumental access to the periapical area. The osteotomy should allow identification of the root apex and thorough enucleation of the periapical lesion.

The osteotomy size should be as small as possible but as large as necessary.[33] However, a minimum diameter of 4 mm is absolutely essential. This is very important in order to allow a 3-mm root resection and to accommodate free manipulation of microsurgical instruments inside the bone crypt. An ultrasonic tip can be used to verify if the osteotomy is adequate. Ideally, the ultrasonic tip (which is 3 mm long) should fit freely inside the crypt without any contact with bone (Figure 12.54). When a larger lesion is encountered, the osteotomy might have to be further extended to ensure complete curettage of the lesion.

The osteotomy should be accurately prepared over the root apex to prevent any unnecessary overextension. This is an easy task when fenestration through the cortical plate is present. On the other hand, when the buccal cortical plate is intact and the lesion is limited to the medullary bone space, a careful assessment should precede any osteotomy preparation.

An important clinical clue in finding the apex is the estimated root length, which can be measured from a preoperative radiograph or obtained simply from the working length recorded in the patient's chart. The length measurement is then transferred to the buccal

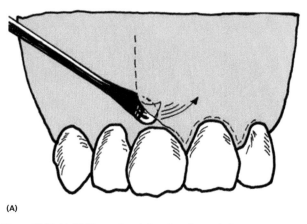

(A)

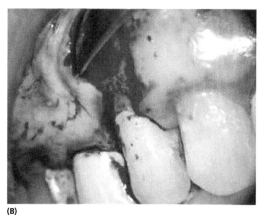

(B)

Figure 12.50 (A–B) The undermining elevation technique.

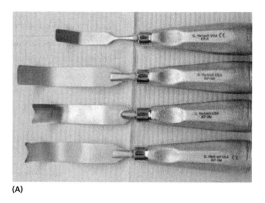

(A)

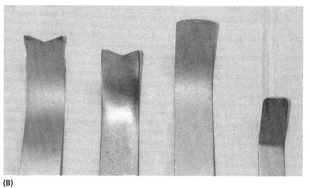

(B)

Figure 12.51 (A) The Kim/Pecora (KP) retractors 1 through 4 (Hartzell & Sons Co.). (B) A closer view of the different shapes of the KP retractor tips.

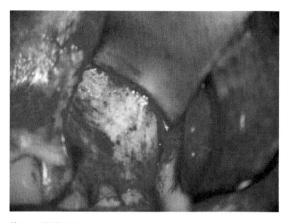

Figure 12.52 KP 2 retractor with a V-shape tip perfectly fits against the zygoma and provides maximum retention.

plate using a file or periodontal probe (Figure 12.55A, B). In addition to the length, the radiograph should be carefully examined for root curvature, position of the apex in relation to the cusp tip, and proximity of the apex to the adjacent apices or anatomical structures (mental foramen, mandibular nerve, and maxillary sinus). In most cases, a visual inspection of the buccal bone topography will reveal the root location and direct the surgeon to the root apex. In other cases, osseous palpation using an endodontic explorer is recommended to penetrate the thinned cortical plate into the lesion to confirm the exact location of the apex (Figure 12.56A, B).

If the operator is still unsure about the exact location of the apex, the following procedure can provide better

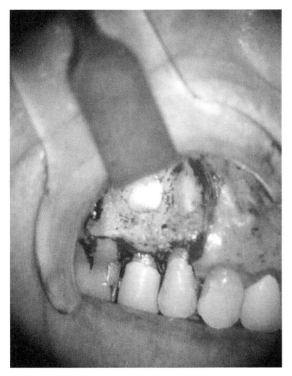

Figure 12.53 The use of the cheek retractor underneath the surgical retractor improves surgical access and provides added safety to patient's soft tissue.

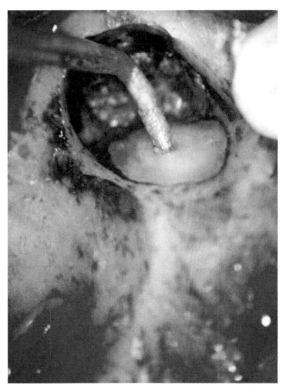

Figure 12.54 Ideal osteotomy size of 4 mm is confirmed with the use of an ultrasonic tip. It allows free manipulation of the microsurgical instruments inside the bone crypt.

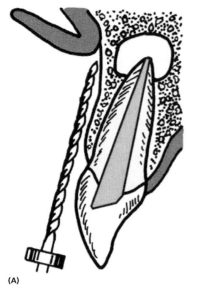

(A)

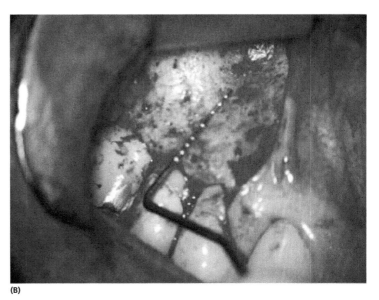

(B)

Figure 12.55 (A) Transferring the estimated root length measurement to the buccal plate using an endodontic file (adapted from *Practical Lessons in Endodontic Surgery* by DE Arens). (B) Measuring with a periodontal probe.

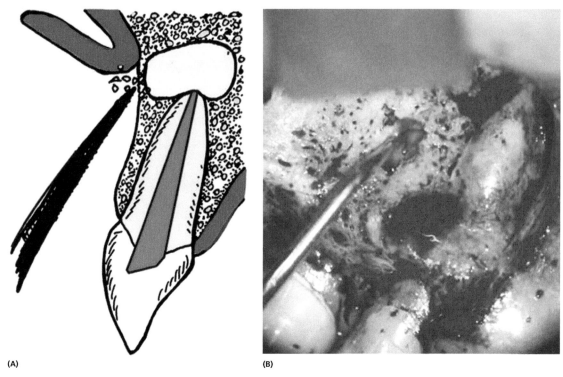

(A)   **(B)**

Figure 12.56 (A) Apical osseous palpation with endodontic explorer to locate exact location of the lesion (adapted from *Practical Lessons in Endodontic Surgery* by DE Arens). (B) Endodontic explorer breaking through the thin buccal plate and confirming the exact location of the lesion and the apex.

orientation. Using a surgical #1 round burr, an indentation is prepared on the cortical plate over the estimated location of the apex. The indentation is then filled with a radio-opaque material such as gutta-percha or tinfoil. A radiograph is taken with the marker in place to ascertain the location of the apex in relation to the marker (Figure 12.57A, B).

The osteotomy is usually accomplished with a Lindemann bonecutter burr mounted on a surgical high-speed handpiece, such as the Impact Air 45. It is used in a brushstroke fashion coupled with copious saline irrigation (Figure 12.58). The Lindemann burr has fewer flutes than conventional burrs, which results in less clogging and more efficient cutting with minimal amounts of frictional heat produced. The Lindemann burr also produces a smoother bone surface with divergent walls and fewer undercuts in comparison to a round burr. The advantage of the Impact Air 45 handpiece is that water is directed along the burr shaft while air is ejected out the back

of the handpiece, thus minimizing the chance of emphysema.

During the osteotomy preparation, it is essential to use the microscope at a lower magnification (4× to 8×) in order to make the distinction between bone and the root tip. The root structure can be identified by texture (smooth and hard), color (darker yellowish), lack of bleeding during probing, and the presence of an outline (PDL). When the root tip cannot be distinguished, the osteotomy site is stained with methylene blue dye, which preferentially stains the periodontal ligament (Figure 12.59) and identifies the root apex.[25,33,34]

Periradicular curettage

It is important to emphasize that periradicular curettage alone does not eliminate the origin of the lesion but, rather, temporarily relieves the symptoms. The purpose of the curettage is only to remove the reactive tissue, whether it is a periapical granuloma or cyst. It is usually performed before or in conjunction with root-end resection.

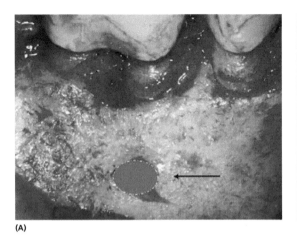

(A)

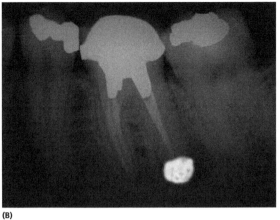

(B)

Figure 12.57 (A) Gutta-percha (arrow) placed into the indentation prepared over the estimated location of the apex. (B) The marker location is verified radiographically.

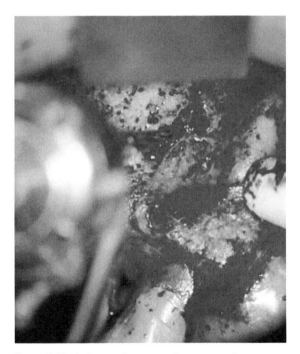

Figure 12.58 Lindemann bone cutter burr mounted on an Impact Air 45 handpiece.

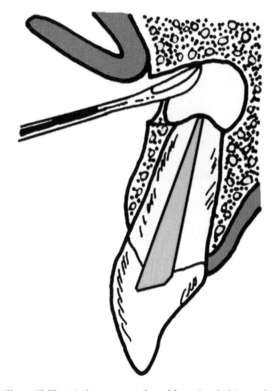

Figure 12.59 Apical curettage (adapted from *Practical Lessons in Endodontic Surgery* by DE Arens).

Curettage is accomplished with bone curettes (#2/4 Molt), with the concave surface of the instrument facing the bony wall first (Figure 12.59).[18] Pressure is applied only against the bony crypt until the tissue is freed along the lateral margins (Figure 12.60A–E). Then, the bone curette can be rotated around and used in a scraping motion. Once the tissue is loosened, tissue forceps are used to grasp the tissue and transfer it directly to the biopsy bottle. Periodontal curettes (Columbia 13/14, Jaquette 34/35, and mini-Jaquette)

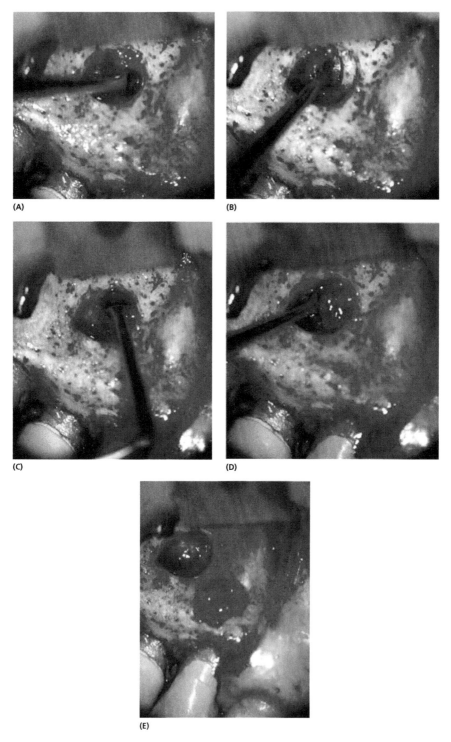

(A)

(B)

(C)

(D)

(E)

Figure 12.60 (A) Apical curettage using the back action of the spoon excavator. (B–D) The spoon is used circumferentially around the granulation tissue until the lesion is completely separated from the wall of the bone crypt. (E) The lesion is removed in one piece.

can be used to remove any remaining lesion tissue or tags, especially in the region lingual to the apex.

Apical root resection

This is also referred to as apicoectomy. Apical root resection is performed to ensure the removal of aberrant root entities and allow microscopic inspection of the resected root surface. Similar to the osteotomy, it is usually accomplished with the Lindemann burr in an Impact Air 45 handpiece using copious saline spray and under low magnification (4× to 8×) (Figure 12.61). The smooth resected root surface produced by the Lindemann burr facilitates microinspection (Figure 12.62).

There are two important factors to consider with this procedure: the extent of apical resection and the bevel angle.

Extent of apical resection

The amount of root resection depends on the incidence of lateral canals and apical ramifications. Apical resection of 3 mm at a 0-degree bevel has been shown to reduce lateral canals by 93% and apical ramifications of lateral canals, deltas, and isthmuses by 98% (Figure 12.63).[25] Additional resection does not reduce this percentage significantly.

The level of root resection may need to be modified due to the presence of the following factors:

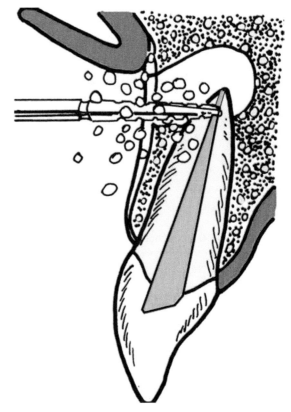

Figure 12.61 Apical root resection (adapted from *Practical Lessons in Endodontic Surgery* by DE Arens).

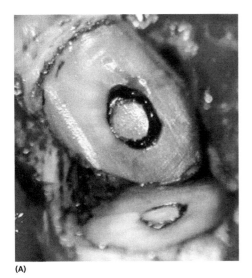

(A)

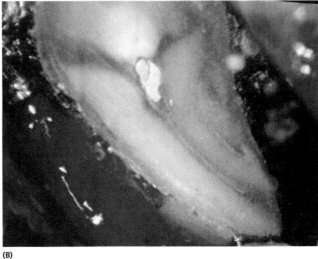

(B)

Figure 12.62 (A) The smooth and flat resected root surface produced with the Lindemann burr as viewed with the help of a micromirror following methylene blue staining. This picture shows gross apical leakage. (B) MB root of a maxillary molar, revealing a missed MB2 canal and an isthmus.

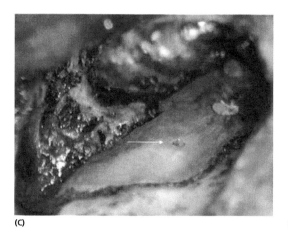

(C)

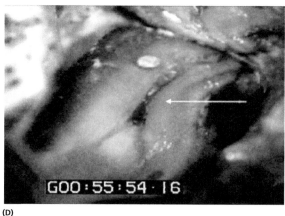

(D)

Figure 12.62 (*Continued*) (C) Untreated canal space (arrow). (D) Apical transportation. Note the off-center location of the GP fill compared to the original canals that are stained blue (arrow). Source: Syngcuk Kim. Reproduced with permission of Syngcuk Kim.

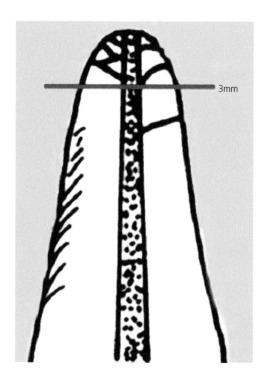

Figure 12.63 Three-millimeter apical root resection eliminates 93% of lateral canals.

- Presence and position of additional roots (for example, a mesiopalatal root of a maxillary molar that is shorter than the mesiobuccal root).
- Presence of a lateral canal at the root resection level (Figure 12.64).

- Presence of a long post and the need to place a root-end filling (Figure 12.65A, B).
- Presence and location of a perforation.
- Presence of an apical root fracture.
- Amount of remaining buccal crestal bone (a minimum of 2 mm should remain to prevent periodontic–endodontic communication).
- Presence of an apical root curvature (Figure 12.65C, D).

Bevel angle

Apical root resection should be performed perpendicular to the long axis of the root (Figure 12.66). This 0-degree bevel will ensure equal resection of the root apex on both buccal and lingual aspects.[35] In some situations, a 0-degree bevel might not be possible (for example, severe lingual inclination of an anterior tooth or wide roots in a buccolingual dimension). In these cases, the operator should use a small bevel angle (up to 10 degrees). This bevel should be kept to the smallest angle possible as the real bevel angle is almost always greater than what it appears to be depending on the angle at which the tooth is proclined in the alveolus. For example, mandibular and maxillary anterior teeth have lingual inclinations. Surgeons might resect the root at what seems to be a 10-degree bevel, but in reality the root is being resected at a bevel of 20 degrees or more. The surgeon should compensate for this distortion of perspective by minimizing the angle of the bevel, keeping it as close to 0 degrees as possible.[3,35]

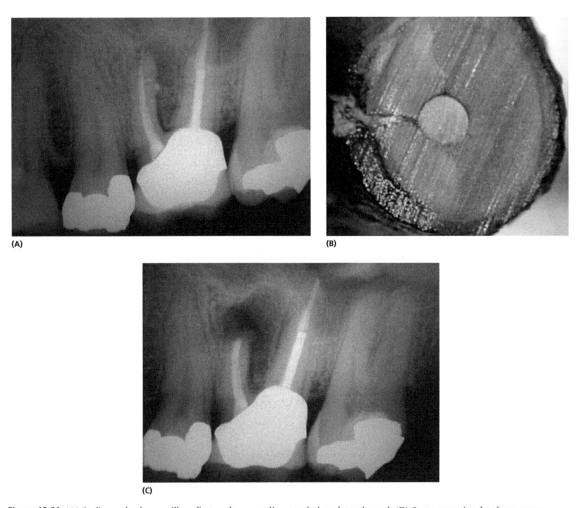

Figure 12.64 (A) Radiograph of a maxillary first molar, revealing an obvious lateral canal. (B) Some resection has been accomplished, but additional resection is necessary to eliminate the lateral canal as a possible avenue for leakage. (C) Radiograph of completed resection, retropreparation, and retrofill.

An important advantage of the perpendicular root resection is the minimal exposure of the dentinal tubules, which results in a reduction in apical leakage (Figure 12.67).[1] In addition, the root canal anatomy is no longer elongated in a buccolingual direction as it is by traditional wide-angled methods (Figure 12.68A, B), thus facilitating retropreparation and retrofilling procedures.

Figure 12.69 shows apical root resection being performed on tooth #4. An adequate osteotomy is prepared to expose the apical 3 mm of the root before resection (Figure 12.69A). Root resection is performed at a 0- to 10-degree bevel angle (Figure 12.69B). The root tip is completely separated and removed (Figure 12.69C, D).

Microscopic inspection of the resected root surface

The smooth surface of a perpendicular root resection will best prepare the root to reveal its hidden anatomy to microscopic inspection. This is usually accomplished under high magnification (16× to 25×) and after staining with methylene blue dye. Without the added clarity provided by the dye, magnification alone is insufficient for an accurate inspection. Like adding color to a black-and-white film, the dye adds borders and contrast to an otherwise monochromatic surgical field, revealing a surprising degree of additional detailed anatomy.

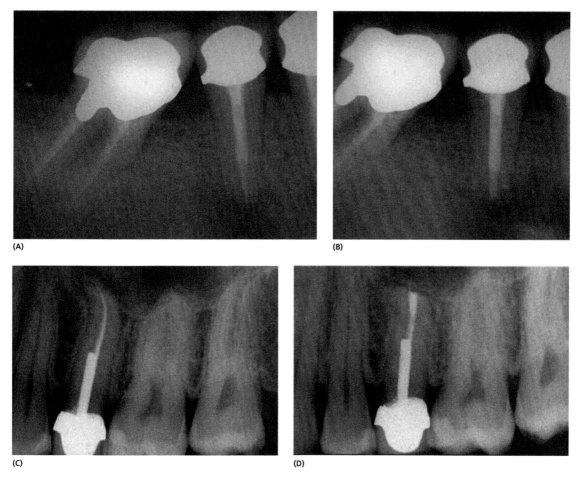

(A)

(B)

(C)

(D)

Figure 12.65 (A) A 3-mm root resection in this case will leave limited room for an adequate retropreparation and retrofilling. (B) Postoperative radiograph with a more conservative root resection. (C) Presence of apical curvature. (D) Root resection extended to eliminate the apical curvature so that retropreparation to a depth of 3 mm could be performed.

Methylene blue staining technique

The resected root surface has to be thoroughly dried using the Stropko drier before the application of the dye with a microapplicator tip (Figure 12.70A, B). After waiting a few seconds, the excess dye is rinsed with saline, and the root surface is dried again in final preparation for microinspection. At this time, the periodontal ligament and leaky areas are clearly defined by the blue stain. If the entire root tip has been resected, the PDL can be identified as a continuous line around the root surface (Figure 12.70B). A partial line indicates that only part of the root has been resected.

Microscopic inspection

Microinspection of the resected root surface is the single most important step in the entire surgical procedure. This novel method was not available during the period when traditional surgical techniques were employed. Only when it is performed accurately can a definite diagnosis be made to identify the true etiology of the disease.

An appropriately sized and shaped micromirror is used to reflect a clear and direct view of the resected root surface (Figure 12.71). Potentially leaky anatomy or suspicious microfractures can be confirmed by probing with the CX-1 microexplorer.

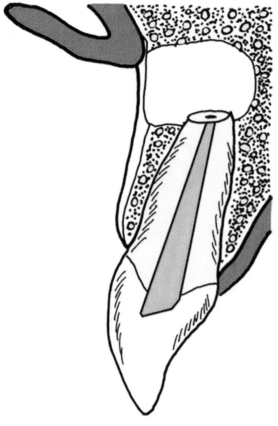

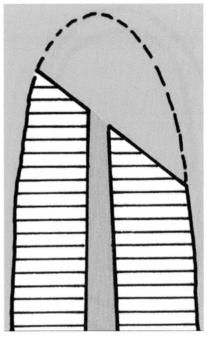

Figure 12.67 A 45-degree bevel angle will expose a large number of dentinal tubules and will barely resect the lingual aspect of the root.

Figure 12.66 A 0-degree bevel angle (adapted from *Practical Lessons in Endodontic Surgery* by DE Arens).

At this point, the resected root surface should be checked for the following anatomical and pathological details:

- Missed canals
- Isthmuses, fins, C-shaped canals, and accessory canals
- Leaky canals
- Microfractures
- Apical canal transportation
- Separated instruments.

After all of these structures and defects are identified, the operator can proceed with their treatments and corrections (Figure 12.72).

If an apical microfracture is discovered, further root resection and staining is performed until the fracture line is completely eliminated. If the fracture line persists, then either root amputation or extraction should be considered. All anatomical variations (such as isthmuses

and fins) should be included in the retropreparation to eliminate them as avenues for leakage. Separated instruments in the apical third of the canal can be effectively removed with the combination of the 3 mm root resection and retropreparation.

The majority of apical perforations and transportations can be simply corrected with root resection. When resection alone is inadequate to correct the problem, the transported canal will look off-center while the original untreated canal space will be more centered and stained in blue (as shown in Figure 12.62D). If further resection cannot be performed, then emphasis should be placed on treating the untreated canal rather than the deviated gutta-percha fill.

Ultrasonic retropreparation

The objective of retropreparation is to clean and shape the apical canal while providing at the same time a retentive cavity preparation to receive the root-end filling material and secure an apical seal.

An ideal retropreparation is best described as "a class one preparation that is at least three millimeters into root dentin with walls parallel to and coincident

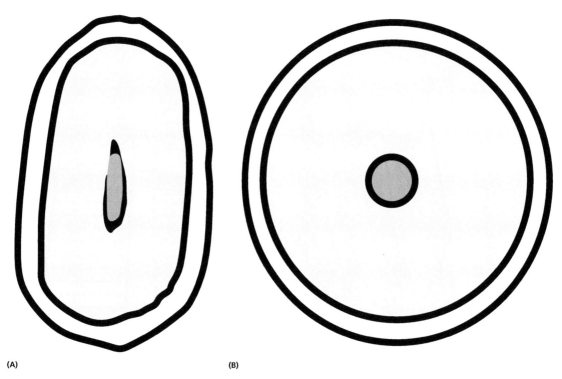

(A)   (B)

Figure 12.68 (A) A 45-degree bevel will produce a distorted elongated view of the canal in a buccolingual direction. (B) A 0-degree bevel will produce a more accurate and centered view of the canal shape.

with the anatomic outline of the pulpal space" (Figure 12.73).[4]

The outline of the preparation depends mainly on the anatomy of the exposed canal space in cross-section. For example, in the maxillary central incisor, the shape of the preparation will be round. In premolars and molars, the outline of the preparation will be more oval and narrow.

A preparation depth of 3 mm with a 0- to 10-degree root resection bevel angle is generally recommended (Figure 12.74).[1] This depth has been shown to significantly reduce apical dentin permeability and apical microleakage. Apical dentin permeability is directly related to the number of open dentinal tubules at the resected root end. Tidmarsh and Arrowsmith suggested that the angle of the bevel should be kept to a minimum to reduce the number of exposed dentinal tubules.[2] They also recommended that the canal to be retrofilled at least to the level of the coronal end of the beveled root to internally seal any exposed tubules (Figure 12.75).

Apical microleakage is the leakage along the interface between the filling material and the canal wall. Microleakage is dictated by two interconnected factors: the retrograde filling depth and the root resection bevel angle. Increasing the depth of the retrograde filling significantly decreases apical leakage.[1] If teeth are resected at 0 degrees to the long access, a retrograde filling with a depth of 1 mm is sufficient to prevent apical microleakage. But a steeper-beveled apex will require a deeper retrofilling. As the bevel angle increases to 30 and 45 degrees, the depth of the retrograde filling should be increased to 2.1 and 2.5 mm, respectively, to achieve a similar apical seal. This is due to the shorter buccal wall of the retroprepared canal space of a beveled resected apex (Figure 12.75).

Because a small bevel angle is sometimes necessary for good surgical access as opposed to the ideal 0-degree bevel angle and because it is difficult to accurately assess the extent of the bevel angle clinically, retrograde filling with a depth of 3 mm is recommended to minimize apical microleakage.

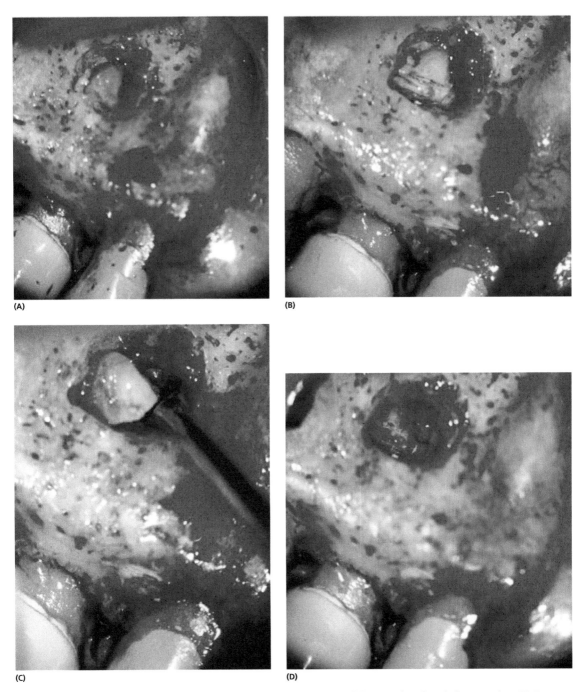

Figure 12.69 (A) An osteotomy has been prepared to expose the apical 3 mm of the root of tooth #4 before resection. (B) Root resection performed at a 0- to 10-degree bevel angle. (C) The root tip has been separated from the root. (D) Root tip removed.

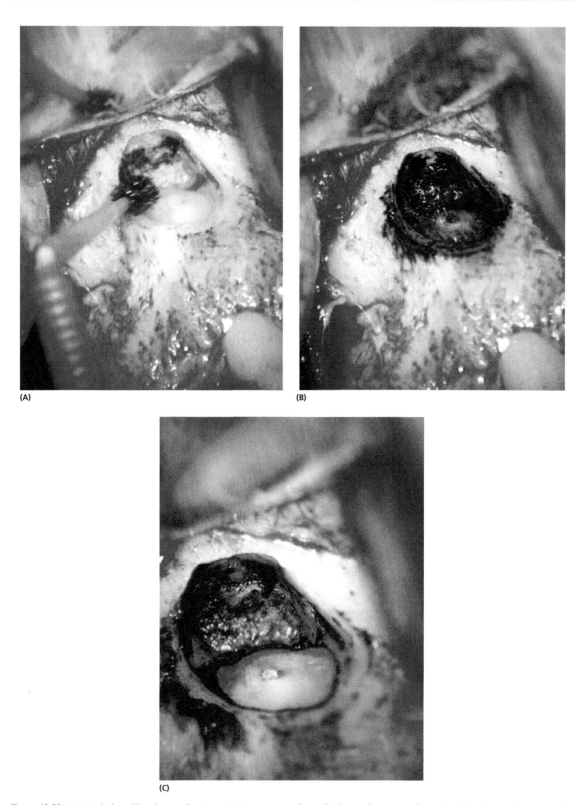

(A)

(B)

(C)

Figure 12.70 (A) Methylene blue dye application. (B) Dye generously applied over the root surface. (C) After rinsing the excess dye with saline, the PDL and any leakage around the GP are clearly stained in blue.

Using traditional endodontic surgery instruments and techniques, the objectives mentioned above are rarely achieved. Most traditional preparations are performed with a miniature contra-angle handpiece using small round or inverted-cone carbide burrs. These obsolete approaches often fail to execute retropreparation with

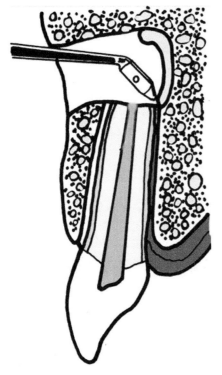

Figure 12.71 The micromirror is appropriately positioned to reflect a direct view of the resected root surface.

adequate depth that is parallel with the long axis of the root, and frequently result in unintentional lingual perforation. The net result is retrofilling that fails to achieve a hermetic seal due to its large size, shallow depth, and deviated location.

The use of ultrasonic tips in apical microsurgery eliminate most of the major inadequacies and complications associated with burr-type root-end preparations. The ultrasonic tips are 1/10th the size of a micro handpiece, and have diameters as small as 0.25 mm. When performed correctly and accurately, the ultrasonic technique provides the following advantages:

- Conservative preparations coaxial with the long axis of the root and of an adequate depth of 3 mm.
- Preparations that are confined to internal root canal anatomy.
- Precise isthmus preparations.
- Better access with unrestricted visibility.
- Thorough debridement of tissue debris.
- Smoother and more parallel walls.

The ultrasonic technique

After completing osteotomy preparation, apical root resection, crypt hemostasis, methylene blue staining, and microscopic root inspection, the ultrasonic retropreparation should be methodically performed using the following steps:

1. Selecting an ultrasonic tip with the appropriate tip angulations and/or diameter.
2. Thoroughly examining the stained resected root surface for all microanatomy at high magnification (16× to 25×).

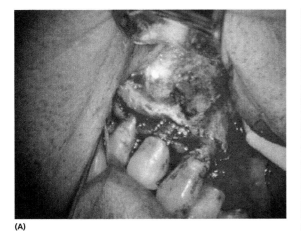
(A)

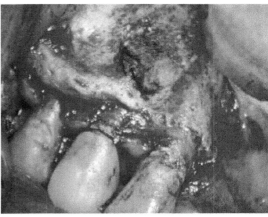
(B)

Figure 12.72 (A) Resected root viewed at 4× magnification. (B) 10× magnification.

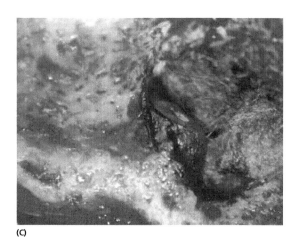

(C)

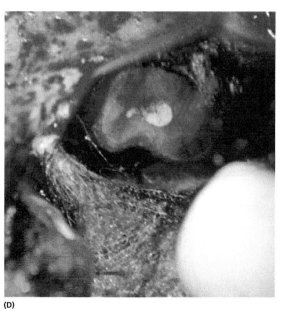

(D)

Figure 12.72 (*Continued*) (C) 16× magnification. (D) Microinspection of the resected root surface at 20× magnification with the use of the micromirror. The missed second canal and isthmus are clearly identified.

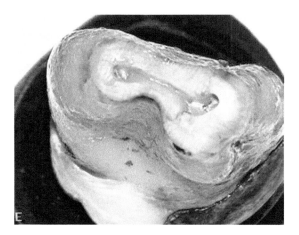

Figure 12.73 Ideal retropreparation outline that follows and includes the anatomic outline of the pulpal space. This is a case of a maxillary molar with fused roots and an isthmus that connects the buccal roots to the palatal root.

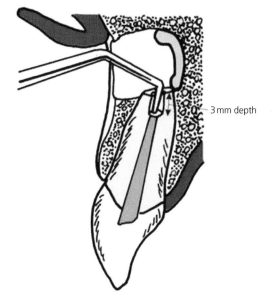

3 mm depth

Figure 12.74 Ultrasonic retropreparation depth of 3 mm with a 0- to 10-degree root resection bevel angle. Adapted from *Practical Lessons in Endodontic Surgery* by DE Arens.

3. Developing a mental image of the necessary retropreparation outline needed to include all anatomy (Figure 12.76).
4. Positioning the selected ultrasonic tip at the apex parallel with the long axis of the root (Figure 12.77). This can only be achieved at a lower magnification (4× to 6×), which has a wider field of view that allows the surgeon to observe the crown, the cervical root area, the root eminence, and the apical area all at the same time. This is important to prevent off-angle retropreparation and possible perforation.

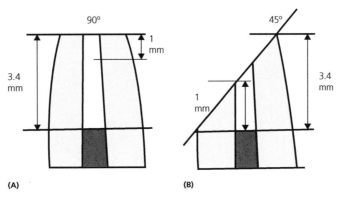

Figure 12.75 Increasing the depth of the retrograde filling significantly decreases apical leakage. (A) If teeth are resected at 0 degrees to the long access, a retrograde filling with a depth of 1 mm is sufficient to prevent apical microleakage. (B) A steeper-beveled apex will require a deeper retrofilling. As the bevel angle increases to 30 and 45 degrees, the depth of the retrograde filling should be increased to 2.1 and 2.5 mm, respectively, to achieve a similar apical seal. This is due to the shorter buccal wall of the retroprepared canal space of a beveled resected apex.

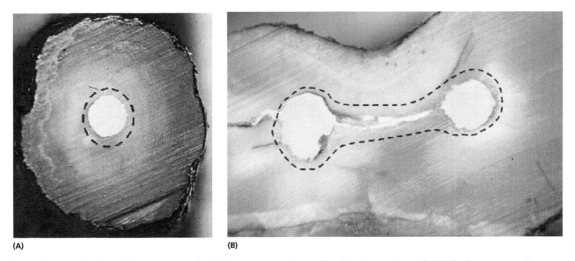

Figure 12.76 (A) The dotted line represents the ideal retropreparation outline for this round canal. (B) Ideal retropreparation outline of a mandibular molar mesial root. The outline includes both mesial canals and the connecting isthmus.

5. While maintaining the same orientation, activating the ultrasonic tip and retropreparing the apical canal with copious saline coolant to a 3 mm depth. This should be an easy task if the tip is parallel to the gutta-percha-filled canal (Figure 12.78). If resistance is encountered, then angulation of the tip should be slightly modified.
6. Using a microplugger to check the 3-mm depth of the preparation (Figure 12.79).

It is important to maneuver the ultrasonic tip in a gentle up-and-down brushing movement in order to cut effectively. Applying pressure too firmly will dampen its movement and render it ineffective.

If an isthmus is present between canals, the canals on the ends are prepared first without the connecting isthmus. The isthmus is then scored with the tip of a microexplorer (CX-1), producing a tracking groove.[35]

This groove will act as a guide for the ultrasonic tip and will help keep it centered during isthmus preparation. A narrow ultrasonic tip (such as KiS-1 or CT-1) is needed in this area because the isthmus is located in the thinner portion of the root, which can be perforated

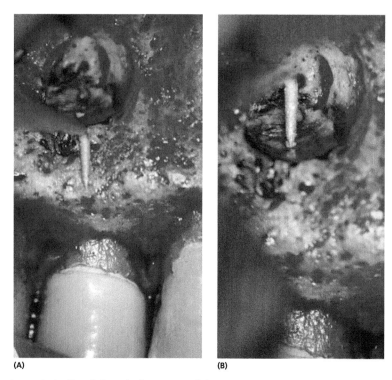

(A)   **(B)**

Figure 12.77 (A) An ultrasonic tip aligned along the long access of the root. (B) The tip transferred into the canal, keeping the exact orientation.

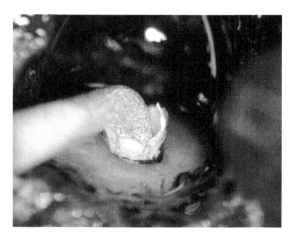

Figure 12.78 The tip is activated, and the canal is prepared to a depth of 3 mm (which is the length of the ultrasonic tip).

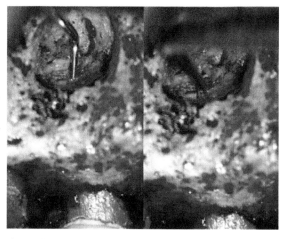

Figure 12.79 A microplugger is used to verify preparation depth and to condense down the GP.

easily. The isthmus is prepared using a light sweeping motion in a forward and backward direction connecting the two canals. The isthmus also has to be prepared to a 3-mm depth (Figure 12.80).

After the retropreparation is completed, the cavity is inspected with a micromirror at high magnification (16× to 25×). The surgeon should confirm that the walls are smooth and parallel and that the retroprepared

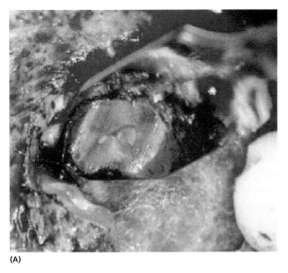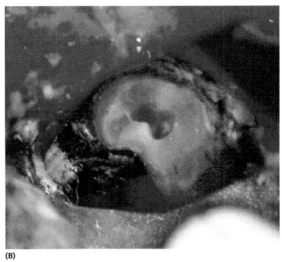

(A)   (B)

Figure 12.80 Isthmus retropreparation. (A) The resection of the root has been completed. (B) The two canals on each end of the isthmus are prepared first, followed by scoring of the isthmus with a tracking groove. Finally, the isthmus is prepared to the same depth as the two canals.

cavity outline has included all the microanatomy (Figure 12.81).

Any gutta-percha remaining on the walls needs to either be condensed with a microplugger or removed with a microexplorer. The use of an activated ultrasonic tip in chasing small pieces of gutta-percha is not only ineffective but can possibly result in widened preparation and unnecessary weakening of the walls.

Retrograde filling

The purpose of retrograde filling is to provide an adequate apical seal that will prevent the leakage of remaining bacteria and their by-products from the root canal system into the periradicular tissue. Ideal properties for a retrograde filling material as proposed by Grossman are summarized in Table 12.2.

Amalgam has previously been the most widely used root-end filling material. It is easily manipulated and readily available and seems to provide a good initial seal. However, amalgam use is no longer recommended due to its corrosion, leakage, staining of soft tissue, persistent apical inflammation, and lack of long-term success.[36,37]

The three retrograde filling materials currently recommended are Super EBA, mineral trioxide aggregate (MTA), and Endosequence Bioceramic.

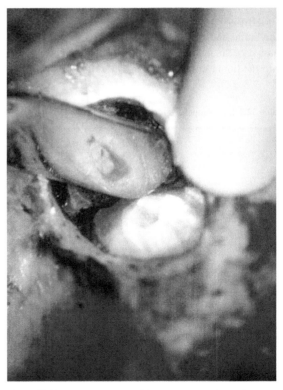

Figure 12.81 Microinspection of the retroprepared canal.

Super EBA

In 1978, Oynick and Oynick[38] suggested the use of Stailine (later marketed as Super EBA) as a retrograde filling material. They reported that Super EBA is unresorbable and radiopaque. Histological evaluation showed a chronic inflammatory reaction, which is considered normal in the presence of a foreign body, but it also showed the possibility of collagen fibers growing over the material.

Super EBA is a modified zinc oxide eugenol cement (Table 12.3). The eugenol is partially substituted with orthoethoxybenzoic acid to shorten the setting time. Alumina is added to the zinc oxide powder to make the cement stronger. Super EBA has a neutral pH, low solubility, and high tensile and compressive strength.[39] Several in vitro studies demonstrated that Super EBA has less leakage than amalgam and IRM.[39–41]

The advantages of Super EBA include fast setting time, dimensional stability, good adaptation to canal walls, and the ability to polish. However, it is a difficult material to manipulate because the setting time is greatly affected by temperature and humidity.

Preparation and placement of super EBA

The liquid and powder are mixed in a 1:4 ratio over a glass slab. Small increments of powder are incorporated into the liquid until the mixture loses its shine and the tip of the EBA does not droop when picked up with an EBA carrier.

When the right consistency is reached, the EBA mix is shaped into a thin roll over the glass slab. A 3-mm-long segment is picked up by the carrier and placed directly into the dried retroprepared cavity under midrange magnification (10× to 16×) (Figure 12.82). Using a microplugger of appropriate tip size and angulation, the EBA is gently condensed into the cavity (Figure 12.83). Placement and packing are repeated until the entire retroprepared cavity is filled. At this point, a microball burnisher is used to further condense the material and seal the margins while at the same time pushing aside any extra filling material (Figure 12.84). A periodontal curette can be used to carve away excess Super EBA (Figure 12.85). A dry field is maintained from the start of the retrofilling process until the Super EBA is completely set. Once the material sets, it can be polished with a composite finishing burr to a smooth finish (Figure 12.86).

Although polishing the Super EBA will remove extra filling material and produce an esthetically pleasing image of the retrofilled root-end, a recent study suggests that burnishing the EBA without polishing provides a better seal.[42]

Table 12.2 Ideal properties for retrograde filling materials

1. Readily available and easy to handle
2. Well-tolerated by periapical tissues
3. Adheres to tooth structure
4. Dimensionally stable
5. Bacteriocidal or bacteriostatic
6. Resistant to dissolution
7. Promotes cementogenesis
8. Non-corrosive
9. Does not stain tooth or periradicular tissue
10. Electrochemically inactive
11. Allows adequate working time, then sets quickly

Table 12.3 Bosworth's Super EBA retrofilling material composition

Powder
Zinc oxide 60%, alumina 37%, natural resin 3%, liquid eugenol 37.5%, orthoethoxybenzoic acid 62.5%

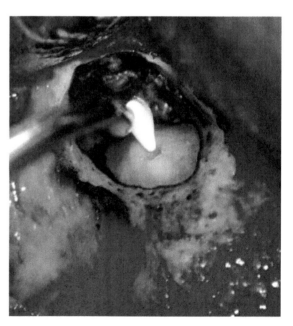

Figure 12.82 A 3-mm-long segment is picked up by the carrier and placed directly into the dried retroprepared cavity under midrange magnification.

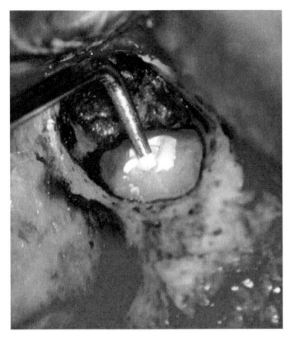

Figure 12.83 The Super EBA is condensed into the cavity.

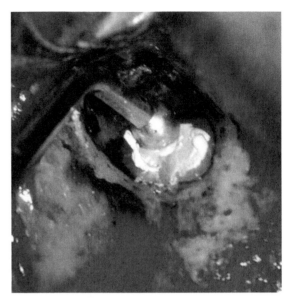

Figure 12.84 A microball burnisher is used to further condense the material and to seal the margins while pushing aside any extra filling material.

Mineral trioxide aggregate (MTA)

This relatively new material was developed by Torabinejad and coworkers in 1995,[43] and it has proven to be superior to other retrofilling materials. MTA is mainly composed of tricalcium silicate, tricalcium aluminate, and tricalcium oxide in addition to small amounts of other mineral oxides (Figure 12.87). Bismuth oxide is added to render the mix radiopaque.

MTA is biocompatible and hydrophilic and seems to provide excellent sealing properties that are not affected by contamination with blood.[43–45] MTA has a high pH, similar to calcium hydroxide. It is the only material with the ability to promote regeneration of the periodontal apparatus where new cementum is formed directly over MTA.

The two disadvantages of MTA are its long setting time (48 hours) and the difficulty in handling of the material. Due to the long setting time and solubility, the bone crypt area cannot be flushed with saline. Otherwise, the material would be washed out. The difficulty in handling MTA is due to its loose granular characteristics; it does not stick very well either to itself or to any instrument. Fortunately, the handling problem has been solved with the introduction of the MTA pellet-forming block.

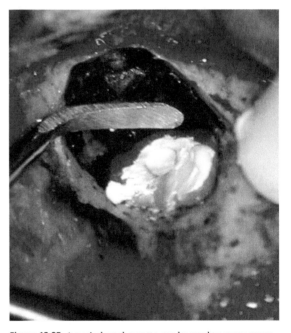

Figure 12.85 A periodontal curette can be used to carve away excess Super EBA.

To use the pellet-forming block, the MTA should be mixed to the proper consistency. If the MTA mix is too wet, the pellet will not form. If it is too dry, it will be crumbly and unmanageable. A proper mix should have

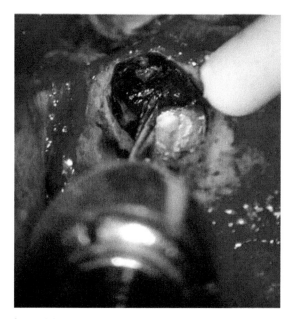
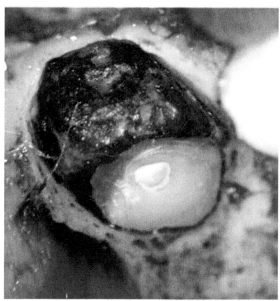

Figure 12.86 The material can be polished with a composite finishing burr to a smooth finish.

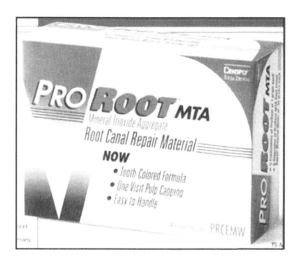

Figure 12.87 ProRoot MTA (by DENTSPLY/Tulsa Dental).

a matte finish and not a watery gloss. This system is simply composed of a block and a placement instrument (Figure 12.88). The block has precision grooves into which properly mixed MTA can be loaded using a spatula[46]; then any excess material outside the groove can be wiped off using a cotton swab (Figure 12.89). Finally, the placement instrument, which perfectly fits the groove, can be used to gently slide out the MTA (Figure 12.90). This forms a small pellet—shaped like

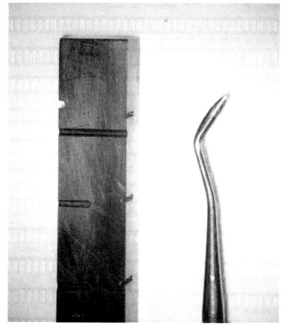

Figure 12.88 Pellet-forming block and placement instrument.

the groove—that should stick to the tip of the placement instrument (Figure 12.91). This MTA pellet can be precisely inserted into the root-end preparation and condensed with a microplugger and a ball burnisher.

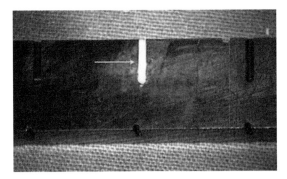

Figure 12.89 The groove filled with MTA.

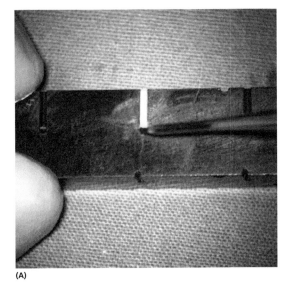

(A)

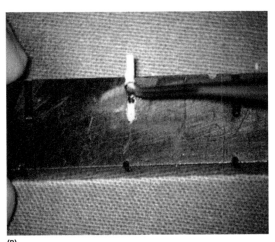

(B)

Figure 12.90 (A and B) The MTA pellet is carried out of the groove using the placement instrument.

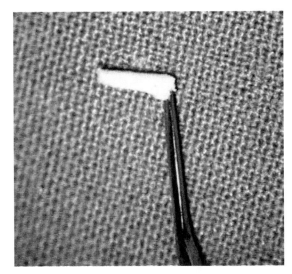

Figure 12.91 The MTA pellet on the placement instrument.

The excess material can be simply removed using a wet cotton swab (Figure 12.92A–E).

Endosequence bioceramic

Endosequence Bioceramic is a new material that was recently introduced by Brassler as a root-repair material and root-end filling material. It comes in putty or paste pre-mixed forms ready for immediate use. For the purpose of retrofilling, the putty form is the one recommended. It can be shaped into a thin roll over a glass slab and handled exactly like Super EBA.

This material seems to exhibit properties similar to MTA in terms of biocompatibility.[47] However, it is much easier to handle and has a shorter setting time.

Wound closure

Wound closure after the surgical procedure has three stages: reapproximation and compression, stabilization with sutures, and suture removal.

Reapproximation and compression

After surgery, the surgical site is thoroughly rinsed with copious saline to ensure the removal of any debris or blood clots. This should apply to the entire surgical field, including the surrounding buccal plate of bone, the periradicular bone cavity (except where MTA has been used), and the underside of the reflected flap.

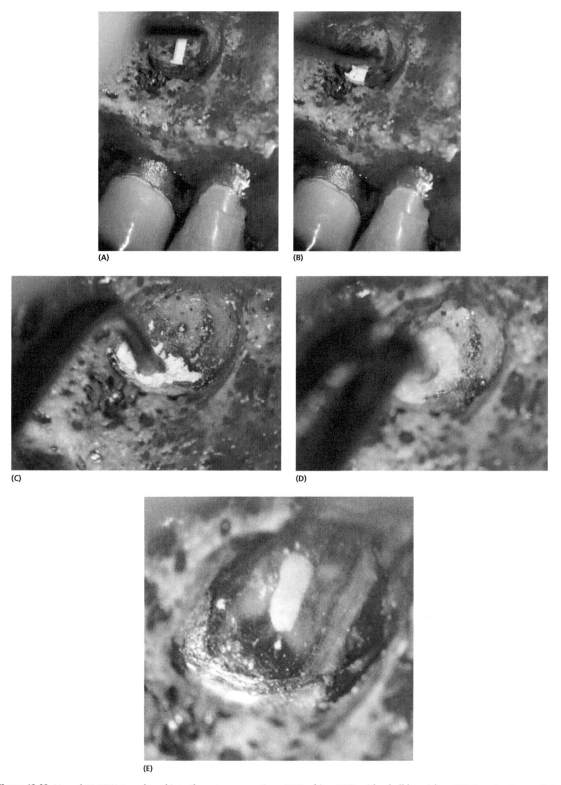

Figure 12.92 (A and B) MTA transferred into the retropreparation. (C) Packing MTA with a ball burnisher. (D) A wet cotton pellet is used to wipe off excess cement. (E) Microinspection of the MTA filling.

If ferric sulfate was used, it should be curetted and rinsed until fresh bleeding is observed. When epinephrine Racellet cotton pellets are used, they should be removed before final irrigation. Any loose cotton fibers should be removed from the bone crypt with the aid of microscopic inspection. Undetected cotton fibers left in situ will induce inflammation and retard healing.[35]

Accurate reapproximation of the tissue aids in the initiation of healing by primary intention. After the flap is repositioned, saline-soaked gauze is used to compress the wound site, using firm finger pressure for 3 to 5 minutes. This is essential for the creation of a thin fibrin clot between the flap and the bone and between the wound edges (Figure 12.93).[18,48]

Stabilization with sutures and suture removal

A variety of suture materials is available, each demonstrating advantages and disadvantages. Suture materials are divided into absorbable and nonabsorbable as well as monofilament or multifilament.

Silk sutures have been used for many years. They are easy to handle and inexpensive. Unfortunately, because silk sutures are braided, they exhibit a wicking effect in which they attract fluid and bacteria as early as 24 hours postoperatively, making them highly inflammatory to the wound.[49,50] However, with smaller suture sizes (5–0 or 6–0), proper suture placement, use of a chlorhexidine rinse, and timely suture removal in 48 to 72 hours, this problem can be minimized.[18]

Chromic gut sutures are resorbable. The treatment of these sutures with chromic acid prolongs their retention in tissues. Nevertheless, they are difficult to handle.

The use of synthetic monofilament sutures such as nylon is desirable. They are non-resorbable, available in small sizes, and cause minimal tissue reaction. They are the sutures of choice in areas with greater esthetic demand. The only disadvantage is their high cost.

Of the many suturing techniques available, the interrupted and sling suturing techniques seem to be the ones most commonly used because they are simple and effective. The interrupted suturing technique can be used for the vertical releasing incision, while the sling suture technique can be used for the sulcular incision.

Suture knots should always be placed away from the incision line to minimize microbial colonization in that area (Figure 12.94). The minimal number of sutures that provide adequate flap reapproximation should be used. All sutures should be removed in 48 to 72 hours.

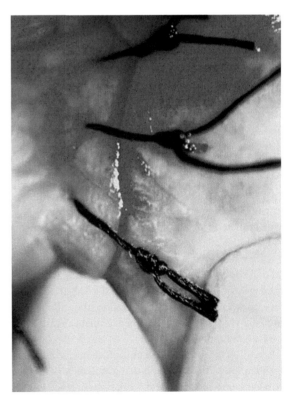

Figure 12.94 Interrupted suturing technique for the vertical incision; note the placement of the suture knots away from the incision line.

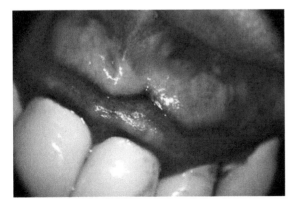

Figure 12.93 The flap is nicely reapproximated following saline wet gauze compression of 3 minutes.

Postsurgical care

Postoperative patient instructions should include the following:

1. Intermittent application of an ice pack to the surgical site (30 minutes on, 30 minutes off) starting immediately after the surgery and continuing for 6 to 8 hours.
2. Strenuous activity, smoking, and alcohol should be avoided.
3. Normal food is permitted, but hard, sticky, and chewy foods should be avoided.
4. Do not pull the lip or facial tissues.
5. Continue the use of analgesics given presurgically (600 mg ibuprofen every 6 hours as needed). Slight to moderate discomfort is expected for the first 24 to 48 hours. Narcotic analgesics are provided and should be used only as an adjunct to ibuprofen if needed.
6. Oozing of blood from the surgical site is normal for the first 24 hours. It can be managed with application of a wet gauze pack to the site, pressed in place with an ice pack.
7. The day following the surgery, chlorhexidine rinses should be used twice a day, continuing for 3 to 4 days. Warm salt water rinses can be used every 2 hours.
8. Brushing of the surgical site is not recommended until the sutures are removed. Cotton swabs can be used to clean the surgical site until then.

Surgical sequelae and complications

Oral and written postoperative instructions will minimize the occurrence and severity of surgical sequelae and will reduce patients' anxiety when and if problems develop.

Pain, swelling, and hemorrhage are the most common postsurgical complications. They can be easily managed with non-steroidal anti-inflammatory drugs, pressure, and ice application.

After 2 to 3 days, if signs of infection are present (for example, fever, pain, and progressive swelling with pus drainage), antibiotics should be considered. If patients develop a serious facial space infection, they should be immediately referred for emergency medical care and intravenous antibiotics.

Rarely, ecchymosis can develop. It is characterized by a discoloration of the facial and oral soft tissue due to the extravasation and subsequent breakdown of blood in the interstitial subcutaneous tissue. Usually, it occurs below the surgical site due to gravity. It can also develop in a higher site such as the infraorbital area (Figure 12.95).

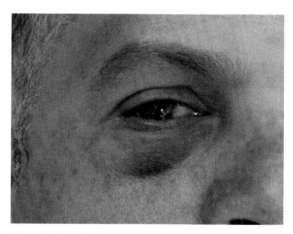

Figure 12.95 Ecchymosis in the infraorbital area following apical surgery in the maxilla.

Paresthesia can develop when surgery is performed near the mental foramen even when the surgical site is far from the nerve. It is usually transient in nature and is mainly caused by the inflammatory swelling of the surgical site, which impinges on the mandibular nerve. If the nerve has not been severed, normal sensation usually returns in few weeks, but it can take up to a few months. On rare occasions, paresthesia can be permanent.

Microsurgery success rate

Periradicular microsurgery is a predictable and successful treatment for endodontic failure when the previous root canal treatment and coronal restoration are of adequate quality. The reasons for an endodontic failure are not consistently obvious. Surgical treatment is, not always successful. Possible etiological factors for failure are as follows:

- Poor case selection
- Incomplete root canal space debridement
- Incomplete debridement of the canal isthmus
- Inadequate apical seal
- Missed canals
- Failure to manage the root-end or retrofilling material properly
- Vertical root fracture
- Endodontic–periodontic communication
- A recurrent cystic lesion.

Other uncertain factors, such as infected dentinal tubules, type of root canal filling, more coronally located lateral canals, and failure to use antibiotics, can also play a role.

When appropriate case selection criteria are used, endodontic microsurgery seems to have great success. One study showed a success rate of 96.8% after a 1-year follow-up.[51] With longer follow-up periods of up to 8 years of the same surgical cases, a success rate of 91.5% was achieved.[52] Similar results are reported for other long-term prospective studies.[53]

Conclusion

Periradicular surgery in the hands of operators who can perform the procedure accurately can be a great service for patients. With the presentation of this chapter, the author would like to bring a more thorough understanding of contemporary endodontic surgical techniques to general dentists who have an interest in incorporating this procedure into their practices. Needless to say, materials and methods in dentistry are changing constantly. It is the author's hope that readers will continuously enrich themselves with evidence-based literature relating to the study of endodontics for the purpose of providing better patient care.

Acknowledgments

I would like to express my deep appreciation for Dr. Alice P. Chen for her outstanding effort in editing and rewriting this chapter. I would also like to thank Dr. Syngcuk Kim for generously sharing some of his microsurgical slides. I am very grateful for the help I received from my assistants and staff in documenting and collecting clinical pictures and illustrations.

References

1. Gilheany PA. Apical dentin permeability and microleakage associated with root end resection and retrograde filling. *Journal of Endodontics*. 1994; 20(1): 22–6.
2. Tidmarsh BG. Dentinal tubules at the root ends of apicected teeth: a scanning electron micro-scopic study. *International Endodontics Journal*. 1989; 22: 184–9.
3. Carr GB. Common errors in periradicular surgery. *Endodontics Reports*. 1993; 8: 12.
4. Carr GB. Ultrasonic root-end preparation. *Dental Clinics of North America*. 1997; 41(3): 541–4.
5. Hess W. Formation of root canal in human teeth. *Journal of the National Dental Association*. 1921; 3: 704–34.
6. Hess W, Zurcher E. *The Anatomy of the Root Canals of the Permanent Dentition*. William Wood & Co., New York, 1925.
7. Sundqvist G. Microbiological analysis of teeth with failed endodontic treatment and the outcome of conservative re-treatment. *Oral Surgery, Oral Medicine, and Oral Pathology*. 1998; 85(1): 86–93.
8. Wayman BE. A bacteriological and histological evaluation of 58 periapical lesions. *Journal of Endodontics*. 1992; 18: 152–5.
9. Sundqvist G. Isolation of *Actinomyces israelii* from periapical lesion. *Journal of Endodontics*. 1980; 6: 602–6.
10. Nair PNR. Periapical actinomycosis. *Journal of Endodontics*. 1984; 10: 567–70.
11. Sjögren U. Survival of *Arachnia propionica* in periapical tissue. *International Endodontics Journal*. 1988; 21: 277–82.
12. Kiryu T. Bacteria invading periapical cementum. *Journal of Endodontics*. 1994; 20: 169–72.
13. Nair PNR. Types and incidence of human periapical lesions obtained with extracted teeth. *Oral Surgery, Oral Medicine, and Oral Pathology*. 1996; 81: 93–102.
14. Nair PNR. Non-microbial etiology: periapical cysts sustain post-treatment apical periodontitis. *Endodontics Topics*. 2003; 6: 96–113.
15. Simon JHS. Incidence of periapical cysts in relation to the root canal. *Journal of Endodontics*. 1980; 6: 845–8.
16. Freedman A. Complications after apicoectomy in maxillary premolar and molar teeth. *International Journal of Oral and Maxillofacial Surgery*. 1999; 28: 192–4.
17. Jerome CE. Preventing root tip loss in the maxillary sinus during endodontic surgery. *Journal of Endodontics*. 1995; 21: 422–4.
18. Gutmann JL, Harrison JW. *Surgical Endodontics*. Ishiyaku EuroAmerica, St Louis, MO, 1994.
19. Wilson W, Taubert KA, Gewitz M, Lockhart PB, Baddour LM, Levison M, *et al*. Prevention of infective endocarditis: Guidelines from the American Heart Association—A Guideline from the American Heart Association Rheumatic Fever, Endocarditis and Kawasaki Disease Committee, Council on Cardiovascular Disease in the Young, and the Council on Clinical Cardiology, Council on Cardiovascular Surgery and Anesthesia, and the Quality of Care and Outcomes Research Interdisciplinary Working Group. *Circulation*. 2007; 116: 1736–54.
20. Jackson D. Preoperative non-steroidal anti-inflammatory drugs for the prevention of postoperative pain. *Journal of the American Dental Association*. 1989; 119: 641–7.
21. Jastak JT. Vasoconstrictors and local anesthesia: a review and rationale for use. *Journal of the American Dental Association*. 1983; 107: 623–30.

22. Buckley JA. Efficacy of epinephrine concentration in local anesthesia during periodontal surgery. *Journal of Periodontology.* 1984; 55: 653–7.

23. Ciancio SG. *Clinical Pharmacology for Dental Professionals,* 3rd edn. Year Book Medical, Chicago, IL, 1989, pp. 146–148.

24. Roberts DH. *Local Analgesia in Dentistry,* 2nd edn. Wright, Bristol, UK, 1987, pp. 84–88.

25. Kim S, Pecora G, Rubinstein R. *Color Atlas of Microsurgery in Endodontics.* W.B. Saunders, Philadelphia, PA, 2001.

26. Vickers FJ. Hemostatic efficacy and cardiovascular effects of agents used during endodontic surgery. *Journal of Endodontics.* 2003; 28(4): 322–3.

27. Jeansonne BG. Ferric sulfate hemostasis: effect on osseous wound healing. II. With curettage and irrigation. *Journal of Endodontics.* 1993; 19(4): 174–6.

28. Gutmann JL. Posterior endodontic surgery: anatomical considerations and clinical techniques. *International Endodontics Journal.* 1985; 18: 8–34.

29. Peters LB. Soft tissue management in endodontic surgery. *Dental Clinics of North America.* 1997; 41(30): 513–28.

30. Harrison JW. Wound healing in the tissue of the periodontium following periradicular surgery. I. The incisional wound. *Journal of Endodontics.* 1991; 17(9): 425–35.

31. Cutright DE. Microcirculation of the perioral regions in the Macaca rhesus: part 1. *Oral Surgery.* 1970; 29: 776.

32. Lang NP. The relationship between the width of keratinized gingiva and gingival health. *Journal of Periodontogy.* 1972; 43: 623–7.

33. Kim S. Hemostasis in endodontic microsurgery. *Dental Clinics of North America.* 1997; 41(3): 499–512.

34. Cambruzzi JV. Molar endodontic surgery. *Journal of the Canadian Dental Association.* 1983; 49: 61–5.

35. Carr GB. Surgical endodontics. In: Cohen S, Burns RC, eds. *Pathways of the Pulp,* 7th edn. Mosby-Year Book, St Louis, MO, 1998, pp. 608–56.

36. Dorn SO. Retrograde filling materials: a retrospective success-failure study of amalgam, EBA, and IRM. *Journal of Endodontics.* 1990; 16: 391–3.

37. Frank AL. Long-term evaluation of surgically placed amalgam fillings. *Journal of Endodontics.* 1992; 18: 391–8.

38. Oynick J. A study for a new material for retrograde fillings. *Journal of Endodontics.* 1978; 4: 203–6.

39. O'Connor RP. Leakage of amalgam and super-EBA root-end fillings using two preparation techniques and surgical microscopy. *Journal of Endodontics.* 1995; 21: 74–8.

40. Bondra DL. Leakage in vitro with IRM, high copper amalgam, and EBA cement as retrofilling materials. *Journal of Endodontics.* 1989; 15: 157–60.

41. Briggs JT. Ten year in vitro assessment of the surface status of three retrofilling materials. *Journal of Endodontics.* 1995; 21: 521–5.

42. Forte SG. Microleakage of super-EBA with and without finishing as determined by the fluid filtration method. *Journal of Endodontics.* 1998; 24(12): 799.

43. Torabinejad M. Physical and chemical properties of a new root-end filling material. *Journal of Endodontics.* 1995; 21: 349–53.

44. Torabinejad M. Dye leakage of four root end filling materials: effects of blood contamination. *Journal of Endodontics.* 1994; 20: 159–63.

45. Torabinejad M. Histologic assessment of mineral trioxide aggregate as a root-end filling in monkeys. *Journal of Endodontics.* 1997; 23: 225–8.

46. Lee ES. A new mineral trioxide aggregate root-end filling technique. *Journal of Endodontics.* 2000; 26(12): 764–5.

47. Ma, J. Biocompatibility of two novel root repair materials. *Journal of Endodontics.* 2011; 37: 793–8.

48. Levine HL. Repair following periodontal flap surgery with the retention of the gingival fibers. *Journal of Periodontology.* 1972; 43: 99–103.

49. Lilly GE. Reaction of oral tissues to suture materials: Part III. *Oral Surgery.* 1969; 28: 432–8.

50. Lilly GE. Reaction of oral tissues to suture materials: Part IV. *Oral Surgery.* 1972; 33: 152–7.

51. Rubinstein RA. Short-term observation of the results of endodontic surgery with the use of the surgical operating microscope and Super-EBA as root-end filling material. *Journal of Endodontics.* 1999; 25: 43–8.

52. Rubinstein RA. Long-term follow-up of cases considered healed one year after apical microsurgery. *Journal of Endodontics.* 2002; 28: 378–83.

53. Zuolo ML. Prognosis in periradicular surgery: a clinical prospective study. *International Endodontics Journal.* 2000; 33: 91–8.

54. Arens DE, Torabinejad M, Chivian N, Rubinstein R. *Practical Lessons in Endodontic Surgery,* 1st edn. Quintessence, Chicago, IL, 1998.

CHAPTER 13

Dentoalveolar Trauma

Omar Abubaker[1] and Din Lam[2]

[1] Department of Oral and Maxillofacial Surgery, Medical College of Virginia School of Dentistry, Richmond, VA, USA
[2] Private Practice of Oral and Maxillofacial Surgery, Charlotte, NC, USA

Introduction

Dentoalveolar (DA) injuries are common in everyday dental practice. A DA injury can occur in different age groups, and depending on the age of the patient, his or her etiology can vary and thus alter how a general practitioner manages the case. The general practitioner plays an important role in preventing, triaging, and managing DA injuries. Contact sports and playground activities lead to most DA injuries in children and adolescents. The use of mouth guards and appropriate headgear during contact sports has helped decrease sport-related injuries.[1] Many of these sports-related injuries are isolated in the DA complex and can be managed easily in the office setting. In adults, DA injuries are caused by motor vehicle collisions, altercations, industrial accidents, and iatrogenic medical or dental accidents. Depending on the nature of the injury, the general practitioner may need to refer the patient to an emergency room for more comprehensive management.

History and examination

As in any office visit, the initial encounter with these patients begins with obtaining an accurate history. In addition to the standard medical and dental history, the following specific information should be obtained before managing these patients:

- **When:** Timing of the injury is paramount in the management of DA fractures. The prognosis of an avulsed tooth can dramatically decrease if management is delayed. Pulpal exposure greater than 48 hours is at risk for pulpal necrosis.
- **How:** Knowledge of the mechanism of the injury is important so the clinician can explore for other injuries. If one suspects an injury other than a DA complex, referral to either an emergency room or another specialist for comprehensive care is warranted.
- **Where:** The environment in which the injury occurred may have contaminated the injury site. Antibiotics may be needed to prevent infection of the wound.
- **What:** What treatment has been rendered so far? An avulsed tooth might be transported to the clinician in different media. Depending on the medium used, the clinician might provide different prognoses to the patient. A fractured dental alveolar complex might have been splinted together in the emergency room; it is prudent to know how long the fractured segment has been splinted together. Prolonged splinting might lead to ankylosis.

Clinical examination

A general survey of other body parts is warranted to detect any occult injury. The initial examination should begin with the patient's vital signs and mental status. Distressed patients who exhibit altered mental status and abnormal vital signs should be referred to the emergency room.

Extraoral soft tissue injuries are common in DA injury. Soft-tissue injuries must be cleaned and debrided

Manual of Minor Oral Surgery for the General Dentist, Second Edition. Edited by Pushkar Mehra and Richard D'Innocenzo.
© 2016 John Wiley & Sons, Inc. Published 2016 by John Wiley & Sons, Inc.

before determining the extent of the injury. Cleaning the wound can be easily achieved with surgical soap and copious use of normal saline solution. Debridement refers to removing devitalized tissue from the wound. Soft-tissue abrasion and contusion usually do not require surgical intervention. Conservative management with antibiotic ointment, a warm compress, and massage provides excellent clinical resolution. Lacerations should be evaluated for depth and injury to vital structures (i.e., the Stentson duct or facial nerve). Facial nerve paralysis and deep lacerations should alert the clinician to possible injury to vital structures. Hence, evaluation of facial animation and saliva flow should also be part of the clinical exam.

Intraoral examinations should focus on both soft and hard tissues. In many cases, an intraoral soft tissue injury can provide clues to the underlying injury. Ecchymosis in the vestibule and floor of the mouth can indicate maxillary and mandibular fractures, respectively. Clinicians should be alerted when these findings are noticed during the exam.

Like their extraoral counterparts, vital structures, such as salivary ducts, lingual nerve, and vascular structure, should be inspected. It is important to incorporate lip and tongue sensory evaluation as part of the examination. On detecting violation of ductal and neural structures, the patient should be referred to a specialist for repair. The floor of the mouth elevation can indicate lingual vein injury. This indication should cause concern about obstruction of the airway; the patient should be referred to the emergency room for possible impending airway embarrassment.

Hard-tissue evaluation can be broken down into the following three categories: dentition, dental–alveolar process, and underlying jawbone. Facial fractures in any of these categories can occur in multiple locations. Like many physical examinations, a systematic approach helps to avoid misdiagnosis. The first step in the diagnosis should be the patient's occlusion. A change in occlusion is a sign of a DA fracture. Other features seen in DA injuries include mobility of dental segments, step in occlusion, and soft-tissue ecchymosis in the vestibule and floor of the mouth. Teeth displacement is commonly seen in facial injuries. It is crucial to search for displaced segments of the teeth. If the avulsed segment was not found at the scene of the accident or during the examination, a dental X-ray may be taken to help locate avulsed segments embedded in the soft tissue. If the fragment remains missing, the patient should be referred to the emergency room for a chest radiograph to rule out aspiration.

Percussion tests can help to determine the involvement of periodontal ligaments, especially when no obvious tooth displacement (i.e., intrusion and contusion injury) is found during the examination. Painful simulation from percussion can suggest periodontal ligament injury. Traumatic intrusion can emit a metallic sound during percussion testing. Pulp testing is usually not performed after acute injuries. False-negative results are common during this time. Testing is usually delayed for several weeks until a follow-up appointment.

Radiographic examination

The radiographic examination is an important part of DA injury evaluation; however, the types of radiograph that are used are limited by their availability in the dental office. In many cases, multiple views are needed to evaluate the injury. The panoramic radiograph is an excellent form of screening, but it is not commonly available in all dental offices. Instead, by using a multiple periapical radiograph, possibly in combination with an occlusal radiograph, meaningful insight into the hard-tissue injury can be gained.

Radiographic findings can be subtle in many cases; they should be correlated with physical findings to make the final diagnosis. Typical radiographic findings are listed in Table 13.1. Radiography is also important in locating foreign bodies within soft tissue and determining the stage of root development. Because of recent advances in cone-beam computerized tomography (CT) scans, clinicians now have additional armamentarium to evaluate a DA injury. However, the clinician should always be mindful of exposing the patient to unnecessary radiation.

Table 13.1 Radiographic findings in common dental trauma injuries

Type of injury	Radiographic findings
Displacement	Widening PDL space
	Displacement of lamina dura
Root fracture	Irregular root surface/canal outline
Extrusion	Conical periapical radiolucency
Intrusion	Absence of PDL space

Classification

Dentoalveolar injury has been classified by many clinicians; the most commonly used classification was suggested by Sanders *et al.* (Table 13.2).[2] This classification is based on the description of the injury, the tooth structure involved, and the type and direction of displacement.

Treatment

Soft-tissue injury

Extraoral lacerations should be closed in layers using sterile technique and local anesthesia. Complex lacerations and injuries related to the esthetic unit or vital structure should be referred to an oral and maxillofacial surgeon for comprehensive care.

Unlike its extraoral counterpart, a soft-tissue injury in the oral cavity can be quite forgiving. Simple lacerations can be closed primarily using resorbable sutures; complex injuries can sometimes be restored by secondary healing without any major consequences.

Table 13.2 Classification of dentoalveolar injuries

Crown fracture
• Enamel
• Enamel + dentin
• Enamel + dentin + pulp involved
Root fracture
• Vertical fracture
• Horizontal fracture
○ Apical third
○ Middle third
○ Cervical third
Concussion
Injury to the tooth-supporting structures. Tooth will be sensitive to touch but no mobility or displacement.
Tooth displacement
• Intrusion
• Extrusion
• Labial
• Lingual
• Lateral
Avulsion
Displacement of tooth from its socket
Alveolar fracture
Fracture of alveolar bone in the presence or absence of a tooth

Adapted from Sanders 1979.[2]

Treatment of DA injuries should be based on the type of injury, patient cooperation, the time elapsed since the injury, and the patient's underlying dental and medical condition.

Crown fracture

Crown fractures can be easily repaired with minimal long-term sequelae. Figure 13.1 shows the algorithm used to treat this kind of injury. If only the enamel is involved, the tooth can be simply reshaped or restored with composite resin.

When a considerable amount of dentin is exposed, the dental pulp needs to be protected. Prolonged dentin exposure can lead to inflammatory hyperemia of the pulp, and it indirectly decreases the prognosis of the tooth. Dentin sealers, such as calcium hydroxide and glass ionomer cements, are commonly used in this situation. Although there is no difference in the clinical outcomes of these two materials, glass ionomer has been more popular because of its biomechanical properties in facilitating placement and crown restoration.

When the injury involves the pulpal tissue, it should be addressed as soon as possible. The management is determined by (1) root apex maturity, (2) amount of exposure, (3) pulpal exposure time, and (4) health of the pulp. Pulp capping or partial pulpotomy is used for small coronal exposure (<48 hours pulpal exposure time) in a healthy non-displaced tooth. When the exposure extends beyond the dentinocemental junction in an immature tooth, regenerative endodontic therapy should be performed (Figure 13.1). The regenerative endodontic procedure (REP) (Figure 13.2) promotes apexogenesis by removing necrotic tissue, sterilizing the infected canal, and recruiting stem cells for pulpal revascularization.[3] REP consists of two stages. In a mature tooth, pulpotomy can be done for small exposure (<48 hours pulpal exposure time); whereas conventional endodontic therapy is used for large exposure.

Root fracture

Management of root fractures depends on the location and direction of the fracture (Figure 13.3). Fractures involving the middle and apical one-third have a more favorable prognosis. In these cases, the fractured segment will be repositioned and immobilized for one month. Immobilization can be done with flexible wire and composite resin (Figure 13.4). There should be at least two adjacent teeth on either side of the injury to

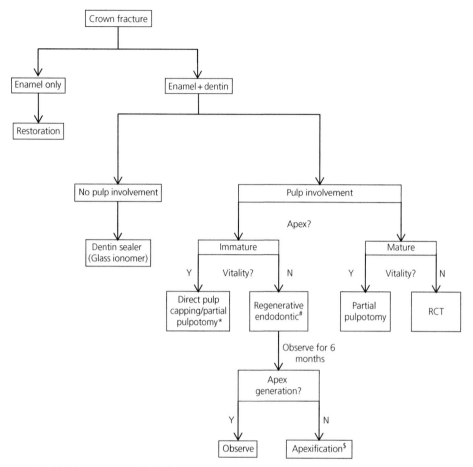

*Partial pulpotomy – removal of inflamed pulp tissue and the surrounding (1–3 mm) healthy pulp tissue.
#Regenerative Endodontic Procedure (REP) – technique allows apexogenesis. REP consists of removal of necrotic pulpal tissue, application of triple antibiotic paste, bleeding stimulation from minimal endodontic filing, and coronal seal with MTA.
$Apexification – apical seal with calcium hydroxide or MTA.

Figure 13.1 Algorithm for crown fracture.

provide proper stability. Definitive endodontic therapy may be needed to prevent internal or external resorption, but it should be delayed until 7 to 10 days after the injury. Fractures at the coronal one-third have poor clinical outcomes. In this type of injury, immobilization should last four months.

Concussion

Concussion is an injury to the tooth-supporting structure that does not cause mobility and displacement of the tooth. Teeth are usually sensitive to touch and

percussion. Fortunately, this type of injury carries a favorable outcome. Treatment consists of occlusal adjustment of the opposing dentition and follow-up examination to monitor pulpal health.

Tooth displacement

Tooth displacement can occur in multiple directions: labial, lingual, lateral, extrusion, and intrusion. Regardless of the direction of the displacement, most mobile teeth will stabilize over time with proper repositioning and immobilization. Repositioning can generally

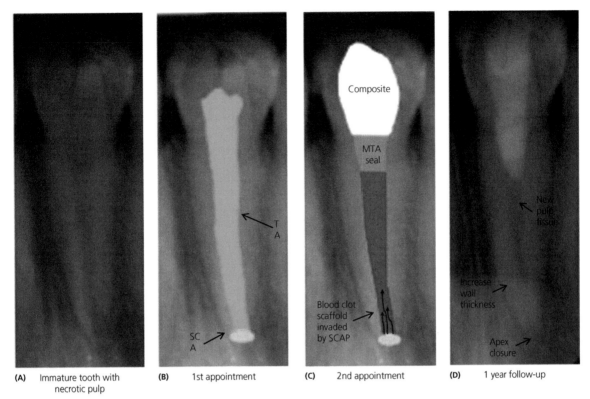

(A) Immature tooth with necrotic pulp   **(B)** 1st appointment   **(C)** 2nd appointment   **(D)** 1 year follow-up

Figure 13.2 Illustration of a regenerative endodontic procedure (REP).[3] (A) Immature tooth with necrotic pulp. (B) Removal of necrotic pulp and application of triple antibiotic paste (TAP) (ciprofloxacin, metronidazole, clindamycin; a 1:1:1 mixture). (C) After 3 to 4 weeks, minimal endodontic filing is done to stimulate bleeding from stem cell apical papilla (SCAP), and placement of an MTA coronal seal is also done. (D) Pulpal regeneration with apex closure. SCAP provides stem cells for pulpal regeneration.

be done using digital pressure. Local anesthesia should be administered before any manipulation. Once proper repositioning is done and the opposing occlusion is removed, the tooth is stabilized with composite resin and a flexible splint. The length of immobilization varies, depending on the type of displacement. Table 13.3 shows the duration of immobilization based on the type of injury.[4]

Compared to other displacement injuries, the traumatic intrusion of teeth has a less favorable outcome. Unlike other displacements, repositioning an intruded tooth is not always possible. Recent guidelines of the International Association of Dental Traumatology (IADT) recommend a new strategy that depends on the apical development of the intruded tooth.[5] Immature teeth with less than 7 mm intrusion should be allowed spontaneous eruption for 3 weeks. Orthodontic application should be used if no

movement is discerned at that time. Immature teeth with more than 7 mm intrusion should be repositioned orthodontically. Mature teeth follow a similar regime, but the cutoff measurement is 3 mm instead of 7 mm.

Orthodontic extrusion should be done slowly over a period of 3 to 4 weeks.[6] After the tooth is properly positioned, it should be splinted for 2 to 3 months. If the intruded tooth is a deciduous tooth, the tooth may be allowed to erupt for 4 to 6 weeks. If eruption does not occur during the given time, the tooth should be removed to prevent injury to the follicle of a succedaneous tooth and its proper eruption. Removal of this tooth should be done carefully to avoid injury to the adjacent tooth buds. Lastly, pulpal degeneration can occur in an intruded tooth; in this case, prophylactic pulpectomy with calcium hydroxide should be performed within 2 to 3 weeks.

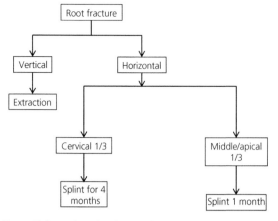

Figure 13.3 An algorithm for root fracture.

Table 13.3 Immobilization period for dentoalveolar injuries

Type of injuries	Duration
Tooth displacement	2 to 3 weeks
Root fracture (middle/apical)	1 month
Root fracture (coronal)	4 months
Intrusion	2 to 3 months
Extrusion	2 to 3 weeks
Replanted tooth (Dry time <60 min)	2 weeks
Replanted tooth (Dry time >60 min)	4 weeks
Alveolar fracture	4 weeks

Ellis 2008.[4] Reproduced with permission of Elsevier.

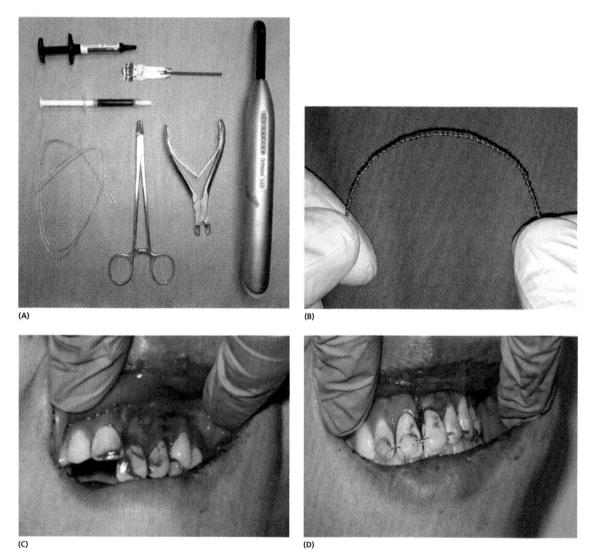

Figure 13.4 Flexible splint immobilization. (A) Splinting armamentarium: Dental composite, bonding agent, acid etch, 26-gauge wires, wire cutter, wire twister, and dental curing light. (B) Two 26-gauge wires are twisted together to serve as a splint. (C) A 20-year-old male with a dentoalveolar fracture. The fracture segment was repositioned back to its pre-injury form. (D) Wire and composite resin were used as a splint.

Avulsion

Commonly seen in dentists' offices, tooth avulsion carries a very poor prognosis if it is not handled properly. The prognosis is based on the following criteria:

1. Length of time the tooth has been out of the socket (dry time)
2. Baseline condition of the tooth and its periodontal health
3. Manner in which the tooth was preserved before replantation.

Figure 13.5 shows the algorithm used to manage this type of injury. Early involvement by the dentist is crucial for the survival of the avulsed tooth. At the scene of the injury, the patient or responsible person should be instructed to rinse the avulsed tooth with the patient's saliva and replant the tooth to the socket immediately. The tooth should be held by the crown without touching the root. If the tooth cannot be replanted at the scene, the avulsed tooth should be stored in a medium until a dentist can deliver care. Although Hank's Balanced Salt Solution (HBSS; Save-A-Tooth, Biologic Rescue Products, Conshohocken, PA) is the best medium, it is not always available at the time of injury. Alternative mediums, such as saliva and milk, are also acceptable.

The amount of time that the tooth has been out of the socket must be determined when the patient presents to the dental office. The prognosis of the tooth is best when it has been out of its socket for less than 60 minutes.[7] On the patient's arrival, if the tooth has already been replanted and seems to be in a good position, a dental radiograph should be obtained to confirm the tooth position and rule out other injuries. The tooth should then be splinted for the recommended period (Table 13.3). If the tooth position is less than ideal, manual adjustment without removing

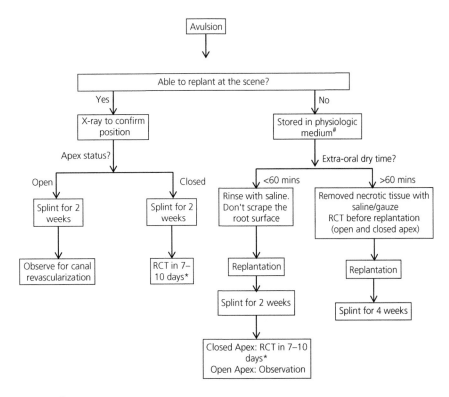

#Physiologic medium: Hanks solution, milk, and saliva.
*RCT – Calcium Hydroxide for 1 month followed by root canal filling with gutta percha.
Splint should not be removed while performing endodontic treatment.

Figure 13.5 An algorithm for tooth avulsion management.

the tooth from the socket should be done before splinting.

When the tooth has been out of the socket for less than 60 minutes, one should rinse the avulsed tooth with normal saline or Hank's Solution (HBSS) before replantation. The surface of the root should never be scraped or sterilized. Excessive manipulation of the root surface can destroy any viable periodontal tissue. When the dry time has been more than 60 minutes, the prognosis of the tooth is extremely poor. In addition to removing any non-vital tissue, endodontic therapy with calcium hydroxide should be performed before replantation.

An avulsed tooth with less than 60 minutes of dry time should be splinted for 2 weeks, whereas a tooth with more than 60 minutes of dry time should be splinted for 4 weeks. Root canal therapy is needed and can be performed safely at 7 to 10 days post-injury. The splint should not be removed during endodontic therapy. Initial endodontic therapy should include filling with calcium hydroxide or MTA. Definitive filling with gutta-percha can be performed 1 month later if no sign of resorption is appreciated.

Alveolar fracture

Alveolar fracture can present along with dental and soft-tissue injuries. Usually more than one tooth will be involved. Treatment options can vary based on the size of the fracture. If the fracture segment involves more than two teeth or extends above the pyriform rim or maxillary sinus in the maxilla or the basal bone of the mandible, these patients should be referred to an oral and maxillofacial surgeon for comprehensive care. This type of fracture may be better treated with an open surgical approach. Mild- to moderate-sized fractures can be managed in the dental office. The segment should be repositioned with digital pressure. Once the segment is correctly positioned, it should be immobilized with a wire splint for 4 weeks to allow osseous healing.

Pulpal management

Dental pulp is commonly involved in a DA injury. The goal of endodontic treatment is to eliminate any non-vital tissue that could lead to pulpal inflammation

and eventually to internal or external resorption. Vitality testing may yield false-negative results for up to 3 months. In this case, it is important to look for clinical and radiographical signs or symptoms of pulpal necrosis.

Figure 13.6 shows an algorithm that is useful in the management of pulpal tissue. Management of pulpal health is essential to tooth longevity. Timing and apex status are important factors in managing DA injuries. Endodontic therapy should not be performed until 7 to 10 days after the initial injury. Delaying endodontic treatment helps to prevent excessive manipulation of the injured tooth during its initial recovery phase, and it allows an immature tooth to revascularize its root canal system.

There are five treatment options available for pulpal management: (1) direct pulp capping/partial pulpotomy, (2) pulpotomy, (3) conventional endodontic therapy, (4) regenerative endodontic therapy, and (5) apexification.

Direct pulp capping/partial pulpotomy is indicated only for small exposures in both mature and immature teeth. Calcium hydroxide (CaOH) or MTA is used as a capping material to simulate calcific bridge formation. Pulpotomy is used for teeth with either large exposure or inflamed pulpal tissue limited to the pulpal chamber. When exposure extends beyond the dentoenamel junction (DEJ), conventional endodontic therapy should be performed in mature teeth, whereas regenerative endodontic therapy is indicated for immature teeth. Apexification is indicated when regenerative endodontic therapy fails to revascularize the necrotic pulpal tissue.

Unlike conventional endodontic therapy, initial endodontic therapy in a DA injury uses CaOH to prevent root resorption. If no resorption is observed for 1 month, conventional endodontic treatment with gutta-percha can be implemented.

Primary tooth injuries

Treatment of the injured primary tooth should focus on the well-being of the succedaneous tooth. Extraction of the primary tooth is indicated if the alternative treatment has the potential to damage the developing tooth bud. Another factor to consider is the amount of time remaining before the injured primary tooth undergoes exfoliation. If more

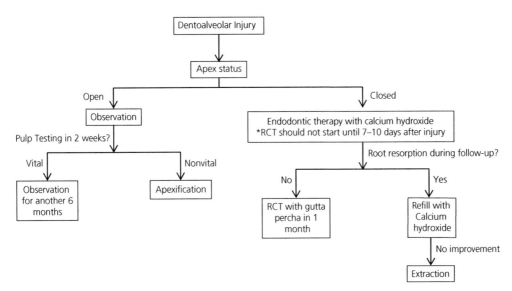

Figure 13.6 An algorithm for pulpal management in a DA injury.

than 1 year remains before exfoliation, appropriate treatment may be rendered; otherwise, the primary tooth should be extracted. Figure 13.7 illustrates an algorithm for the management of primary tooth injuries.

A primary tooth with lateral displacement may allow repositioning spontaneously. If manual repositioning is needed for proper occlusion, the tooth should be extracted to prevent injury of the underlying tooth bud. An intruded tooth that impedes the tooth buds or that fails to re-erupt spontaneously should be extracted. Minor extrusion can be repositioned and monitored; however, if the extrusion is too severe, the tooth should be extracted. An avulsed primary tooth should never be replanted into the socket. A crown fracture without pulp involvement can be managed using conventional restorative options. When pulpal tissue is involved, a primary tooth with an immature apex (<3 years old) can be treated via pulpotomy; however, in the mature apex (>3 years old), pulpectomy with zinc oxide and eugenol may be performed. Root fracture at the apical third can be splinted with wire and composite resin. Fracture at the middle or coronal thirds calls for extraction. If an apical fragment cannot be extracted easily, the fragment can be left behind for spontaneous resorption.

Postoperative instruction

Postoperative antibiotics should not be given routinely. Antibiotics should only be considered in noncompliant patients and those who have "through and through" lacerations. In such cases, a three-day course of penicillin or clindamycin is recommended.[8] The patient should stay on a soft diet for a week to prevent excessive occlusal trauma to the injured teeth. Strong emphasis should be placed on maintaining proper oral hygiene during recovery.

Follow-up appointments should be carried out bi-weekly during the first month, and then at 3 months, 6 months, and at 1-year intervals. Follow-up appointments may involve splint removal/adjustment, evaluation of pulpal tissue, occlusal adjustment, and radiography.

Conclusion

Dentoalveolar injuries can be a devastating experience for both patients and their caretakers. With appropriate management, both dentists and patients can experience rewarding clinical results.

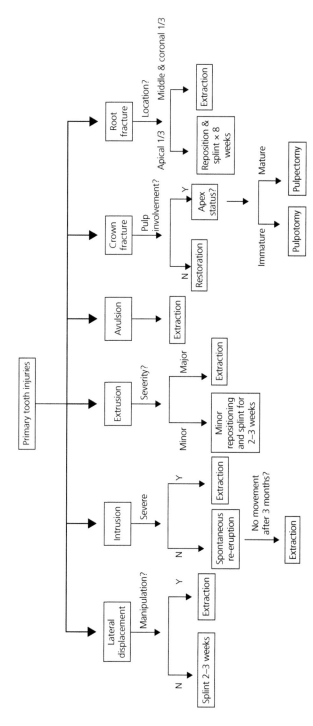

Figure 13.7 An algorithm for management of primary tooth injuries.

References

1. Abubaker AO, Papadopoulous H. Diagnosis and management of dentoalveolar injuries. In: Fonseca RA, *et al*. eds. *Oral and Maxillofacial Surgery, Vol. 2*, 2nd edn. Saunders, St Louis, 2009, p. 104.

2. Sanders B, Brady FA, Johnson R. Injuries. In: Sanders B, ed. *Pediatric Oral and Maxillofacial Surgery*. Mosby, St Louis, 1979.

3. Hargreaves KM, Law AS. Regenerative endodontics. Chapter 16. In: Hargreaves KM, Cohen S, eds. *Pathways of the Pulp*, 10th edn. Mosby Elsevier, St Louis, 2011, pp. 602–19.

4. Ellis E. Soft tissue and dentoalveolar injuries. In: Hupp JR, *et al*. eds. *Contemporary Oral and Maxillofacial Surgery*, 4th edn. Mosby, St Louis, 2008, p. 471.

5. Diangelis AJ, Andreasen JO, Ebeleseder KA, *et al*. International Association of Dental Traumatology guidelines for the management of traumatic dental injuries: 1. *Fractures and luxations of permanent teeth. Dental Traumatology.* 2012; 28(1): 2–12.

6. Turley PK, Joiner MW, Hellstrom S. The effect of orthodontic extrusion on traumatically intruded teeth. *American Journal of Orthodontics.* 1984; 85: 47.

7. Andreasen JO. The dental trauma guide. In: Andreasen JO, ed. *International Association of Dental Traumatology.* 2012. Available at <http://www.dentaltraumaguide.org>. Accessed 15 January 2015.

8. Abubaker AO. Use of prophylactic antibiotics in preventing infection of traumatic injuries. *Oral and Maxillofacial Surgery Clinics of North America.* 2009; 21(2): 259–64.

CHAPTER 14

Orofacial Infections

Thomas R. Flynn

Private Practice of Oral and Maxillofacial Surgery, Reno, NV, USA

Introduction

Correct management of a severe orofacial infection is one of the few ways in which a dentist can save a patient's life. The term *orofacial infection* is used here to describe an odontogenic infection that has spread beyond the alveolar process, causing swelling of the soft tissues of the oral cavity, face, or neck. The purpose of this chapter is to provide dentists with the knowledge that will enable them to safely manage their patients who present with orofacial infection.

The late Dr. Larry Peterson first articulated eight principles for the management of orofacial infections, which if followed in step-by-step, can guide dentists in their management of these infections. While these principles cannot guarantee an ideal result, they can help to ensure that the dental practitioner will meet the standard of care. These eight principles are the framework of this chapter. They are listed as steps next and form the major topic of each following section.

The use of prophylactic antibiotics in dentistry is also presented, based on the currently available scientific evidence.

Steps in the management of orofacial infections

1. Determine the severity of the infection
2. Evaluate host defenses
3. Decide: treat or refer
4. Treat surgically
5. Support medically
6. Choose an appropriate antibiotic
7. Administer the antibiotic appropriately
8. Re-evaluate frequently.

The first three of these steps can be accomplished within the first 5 minutes of the patient encounter. A focused clinical examination, guided by knowledge of head and neck anatomy, combined with a critical review of the patient's medical history and clinical response to the infection over the past few days, provide the basis for the all-important decision of step 3. If the dentist chooses the appropriate setting of care for the infected patient, a good outcome will most likely follow.

Step 1. Determine the severity of the infection

Severe orofacial infections are those that are likely to compromise the airway or threaten other vital structures, such as the brain and heart. We can identify severe orofacial infections by answering three questions:

1. Where is the infection?
2. How fast is the infection spreading?
3. Might this infection compromise the airway or vital structures?

Where is the infection?

Orofacial infections are caused by abscess-forming bacteria. To make matters worse, these bacteria are introduced deeply into the bone of the jaws, most commonly at the apex of a tooth or occasionally in a deep periodontal pocket. Bone, like teeth, is a calcified structure with a hard outer shell that encases the abscess-forming bacteria, blocking the drainage of pus to the external environment. Therefore, orofacial infections persist in the alveolar process until the cortical layer of

Manual of Minor Oral Surgery for the General Dentist, Second Edition. Edited by Pushkar Mehra and Richard D'Innocenzo.
© 2016 John Wiley & Sons, Inc. Published 2016 by John Wiley & Sons, Inc.

bone is resorbed. After the cortical plate is perforated, the infection can spread beyond the jaws into the soft tissues of the oral cavity and face, where it is deflected by anatomic barriers into potential spaces defined by bone, muscles, and fascial layers of dense connective tissue. Clinically, we see infection occupying these anatomic spaces as painful swellings of the face, mouth, or neck.

Perhaps the best way to remember the clinical anatomy of orofacial infections is to maintain a set of mental pictures of infections occupying the anatomic spaces of the head and neck. The series of clinical images in Figures 14.1, 14.2, 14.3, 14.4, 14.5, 14.6, 14.7, 14.8, 14.9, 14.10, 14.11, and 14.12 illustrate the appearance of patients with infections occupying each of these anatomic spaces, referred to as "deep fascial spaces" in the surgical literature. The anatomic spaces of the head and neck can also be grouped into the perioral spaces, the perimandibular spaces, the masticator spaces, and the deep neck spaces, as shown in Table 14.1. Anatomic details of these spaces, such as the borders, contents, relationships, and surgical approaches to each space are listed in Tables 14.2 and 14.3.

Infection in certain anatomic spaces is more dangerous than infection in others. We can grade the severity of infection in the various anatomic spaces based on the likelihood the infection will deviate, hinder therapeutic access to, or directly obstruct the airway or vital structures. The anatomic spaces of the head and neck are classified by their severity in Table 14.1.

Infections of the perioral spaces have low severity because these infections are not likely to interfere with endotracheal intubation (necessary to secure the airway for general anesthesia), and swellings there do not obstruct or deviate the airway. They can generally be approached via an intraoral incision.

Infection in the perimandibular spaces can cause trismus (difficulty opening the mouth widely) and elevation and swelling of the tongue, which can obstruct the airway and make endotracheal intubation difficult. Further, infection in either the submandibular space or the sublingual space can rapidly spread into the deeper neck spaces, where the airway is often deviated and compressed by swelling.

Infection in the masticator spaces causes severe trismus. This is due to inflammation and resulting pain in the muscles of mastication, perceived as stiffness when the patient attempts to open the mouth. Trismus interferes with visualization of the oropharynx, which is necessary not only for endotracheal intubation but also for evaluation of any swellings in the oropharynx.

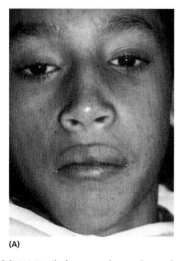 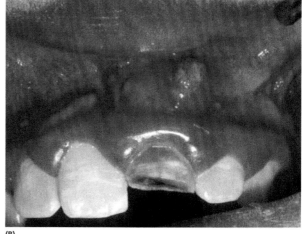

(A)   **(B)**

Figure 14.1 (A) Vestibular space abscess due to the upper left central incisor. Note the swelling of the lip, elevation of the ala of the nose, and effacement of the nasolabial fold on the affected side. (B) Intraoral view of the same patient. This early vestibular abscess is limited to the alveolar process, but, if left untreated, the vestibular fold may develop swelling. Source: Flynn TR. Anatomy of oral and maxillofacial infections. In: Topazian RG, Goldberg MH, Hupp JR, editors. *Oral and Maxillofacial Infections.* 4th edition. Philadelphia: WB Saunders Company; 2002. Reproduced with permission of Elsevier.

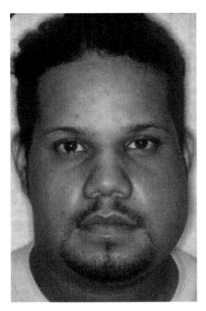

Figure 14.2 Buccal space abscess. Note the left facial swelling extending from the corner of the mouth posteriorly to the anterior border of the masseter (not seen). The swelling also extends from the zygomatic arch to the inferior border of the mandible. Source: Flynn TR. The swollen face. *Emergency Medicine Clinics of North America* 2000;15(Aug):481–519, used with permission.

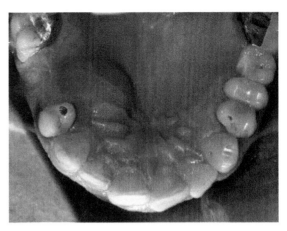

Figure 14.4 Palatal space abscess. This subperiosteal swelling was caused by periapical infection of the palatal root of the first bicuspid. Palatal abscesses are most often due to lateral incisors and the palatal roots of upper posterior teeth because their apices are close to the palatal cortical bone. Source: Flynn TR. Principles of management and prevention of odontogenic infections. In: Ellis E, Hupp JR, Tucker MR, editors. *Contemporary Oral and Maxillofacial Surgery.* 5th edition. St. Louis: Mosby; 2008, p. 291–315, p. 304, used with permission.

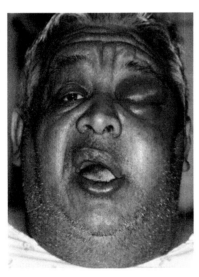

Figure 14.3 Infraorbital space abscess. In this patient, the central part of the infection extends from the upper lip to the infraorbital rim and from the nasal ala to the root of the zygomatic arch. The infection has spread from there into the periorbital space (eyelids), the buccal space, and the superficial temporal space, as seen by the convex swelling superior to the zygomatic arch. Source: Flynn TR. Surgical management of orofacial infections. *Atlas of the Oral and Maxillofacial Surgery Clinics of North America* 2000;8(Mar):77–100, p. 79, used with permission.

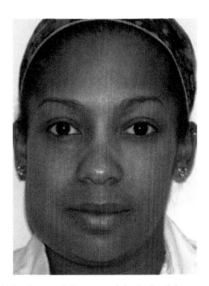

Figure 14.5 Abscess of the space of the body of the mandible. This mandibular subperiosteal abscess causes an enlargement in the same shape as the mandible. Therefore, it appears as if the right side of this patient's mandible is enlarged. The swelling stops at the inferior border of the mandible. Often the vestibular space in the region is infected as well. Source: Flynn TR. Complex odontogenic infections. In: Ellis E, Hupp JR, Tucker MR, editors. *Contemporary Oral and Maxillofacial Surgery.* 5th edition. St. Louis: Mosby; 2008, p. 317–336, p. 319, used with permission.

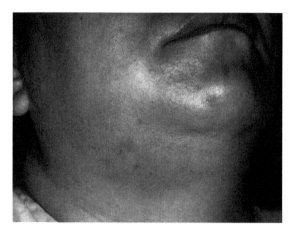

Figure 14.6 Submandibular abscess. This infection of the submandibular triangle is defined by the anterior and posterior bellies of the digastric muscles as they join inferiorly at the hyoid bone. The superior border of the infection is the inferior border of the mandible. Source: Flynn TR. Surgical management of orofacial infections. *Atlas of the Oral and Maxillofacial Surgery Clinics of North America* 2000;8(Mar):77–100, p. 79, used with permission.

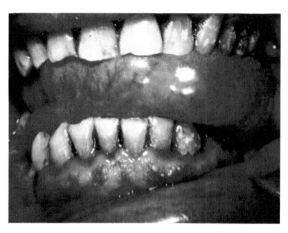

Figure 14.8 Sublingual space abscess. This severe sublingual space abscess has caused a large swelling of the floor of the mouth, which has elevated the tongue firmly into the palate. This swelling has thus made access for endotracheal intubation very difficult. Source: Flynn TR, Topazian RG. Infections of the oral cavity. In: Waite D, editor. *Textbook of Practical Oral and Maxillofacial Surgery.* Philadelphia: Lea & Febiger; 1987, p. 300, used with permission.

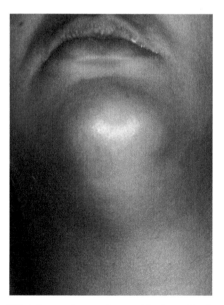

Figure 14.7 Submental space abscess. This abscess lies between the anterior bellies of the right and left digastric muscles. Its superior and inferior borders are the mandible and the hyoid bone, the same as in a submandibular abscess.

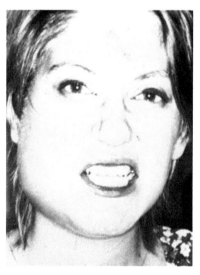

Figure 14.9 Submasseteric space abscess. There is pus between the masseter muscle and the ascending ramus of the mandible. Inflammation of the overlying masseter has caused severe trismus, seen as this patient's extremely limited interincisal opening. The swelling over the ramus blocks part of the view of the ear lobe, which is also characteristic of this infection. Source: Flynn TR. Anatomy of oral and maxillofacial infections. In: Topazian RG, Goldberg MH, Hupp JR, editors. *Oral and Maxillofacial Infections.* 4th edition. Philadelphia: WB Saunders Company; 2002. Reproduced with permission of Elsevier.

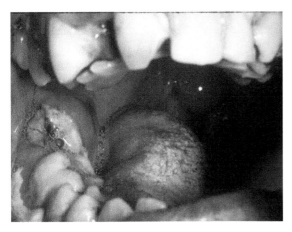

Figure 14.10 Pterygomandibular space abscess. This common orofacial infection lies between the medial pterygoid muscle and the ascending ramus of the mandible. Trismus is caused by inflammation of the medial pterygoid muscle, which makes it difficult to see beyond the teeth to the swelling of the anterior tonsillar pillar. Note also that the uvula is swollen and deviated to the opposite side by the mass effect of the swelling medial to the mandible. Source: Flynn TR, Topazian RG. Infections of the oral cavity. In: Waite D, editor. *Textbook of Practical Oral and Maxillofacial Surgery*. Philadelphia: Lea & Febiger; 1987, p. 300, used with permission.

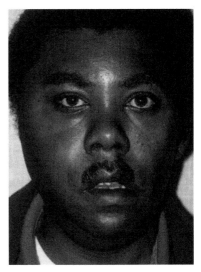

Figure 14.11 Masticator space abscess. This patient had a right facial swelling for 2 months before his presentation. Note the swelling of the entire right side of the face, extending from the attachment of the temporalis muscle on the cranium down to the inferior border of the mandible. Pus was encountered in the superficial and deep temporal spaces, the submasseteric, and the pterygomandibular space, which are all the components of the masticator space. Source: Flynn TR. The swollen face. *Emergency Medicine Clinics of North America* 2000;15(Aug):481–519, used with permission.

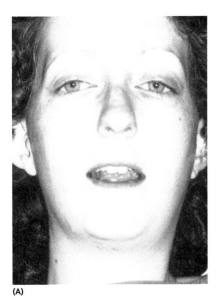

(A)

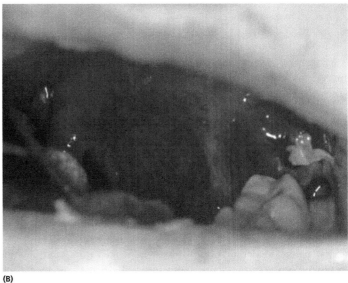

(B)

Figure 14.12 (A) Lateral pharyngeal space abscess, extraoral view. This patient has a postoperative infection that is causing some trismus, as seen by her limited interincisal opening. The swelling of the lateral pharyngeal space is seen as a tender fullness between the posterior belly of the digastric muscle and the anterior border of the sternocleidomastoid muscle. (B) Intraoral view of the same patient. Note that the anterior tonsillar pillar is swollen and is causing deviation of the uvula to the opposite side, plus blunting of the uvulopalatal fold on the left side. Source: Flynn TR. Anatomy of oral and maxillofacial infections. In: Topazian RG, Goldberg MH, Hupp JR, editors. *Oral and Maxillofacial Infections*. 4th edition. Philadelphia: WB Saunders Company; 2002. Reproduced with permission of Elsevier.

Table 14.1 Severity of anatomic space infections

Severity	Anatomic space
Low severity (Low risk to airway or vital structures)	The perioral spaces Vestibular Buccal Infraorbital Palatal Space of the body of the mandible
Moderate severity (Moderate risk to airway or vital structures)	The perimandibular spaces Submandibular Submental Sublingual The masticator spaces Pterygomandibular Submasseteric Superficial temporal Deep temporal (or infratemporal)
High severity (High risk to airway or vital structures)	The deep neck spaces Lateral pharyngeal Retropharyngeal Pretracheal
Extreme severity (extreme risk to airway or vital structures)	Danger space (space 4) Mediastinum Intracranial infection

Infection of the pterygomandibular space (between the medial pterygoid muscle and the mandible) is especially dangerous in this regard. Because the swelling is medial to the ascending ramus of the mandible, it is not visible externally. Trismus limits the ability to see beyond the teeth to the swelling of the anterior tonsillar pillar, which pushes the uvula to toward the unaffected side, as seen in Figure 14.10. Furthermore, pterygomandibular infections can rapidly pass around the medial pterygoid muscle and enter the lateral pharyngeal space, which is one of the high-severity deep spaces of the neck.

Trismus, therefore, is an ominous sign of infection that is of at least moderate severity. It hinders visualization of and access to the airway. In a study of severe odontogenic infections requiring hospitalization, trismus was present in 73% of cases. In the same study, dysphagia (difficulty swallowing) was found in 78% of these infections.[1,2,3,4] Infection found in the perimandibular or masticator spaces is of moderate severity, and these infections are often recognized by trismus or dysphagia.

Anatomically, the deep neck spaces occupy the loose connective tissue that surrounds the lateral and posterior sides of the oropharynx superiorly and the trachea and esophagus inferiorly. Thus, a swelling in any of these spaces can push the airway to one side, impinge on the airway and reduce its diameter, or even encircle the airway to literally strangle the patient. Loss of the airway is the most common cause of death in fatal odontogenic infections. In the preantibiotic era, the mortality of severe odontogenic infections was dramatically reduced from 54% to 10% due to immediate establishment of a secure airway by endotracheal intubation or tracheotomy, followed by aggressive surgical drainage of all infected anatomic spaces.[2] These findings not only point out the severity of infection in the deep neck spaces but also the primacy of airway security and surgical drainage over antibiotic therapy in the management of orofacial infections.

By the time an orofacial infection has progressed into the mediastinum (the space between the lungs, containing the heart) or the cranial cavity, the rate of morbidity and mortality is high. Even if the patient survives, organ damage, neurologic deficits, restrictive pulmonary disease, and painful scarring are likely. Because severe orofacial infections are accelerating in their anatomic and inflammatory potential, it is necessary for dentists to promptly detect and appropriately manage infections that are spreading beyond the low-severity anatomic spaces into the more threatening ones.

How fast is the infection spreading?

Based on the interaction of the virulence of the infecting bacteria and the host's systemic and immunologic resistance, some orofacial infections progress more rapidly than others. For example, the Group A beta-hemolytic streptococci that can cause strep throat are occasionally found in odontogenic infections. When these organisms become invasive, which fortunately is rare, they can cause necrotizing fasciitis (flesh-eating bacteria infection) or streptococcal toxic shock, resulting in hypotension and damage to multiple organ systems. Either of these infections can be fatal.

The rate of progress of a given infection is best assessed by a careful history. A patient with a large swelling that started only yesterday is in greater danger than one with a large swelling that has been present for a week or more. The patient shown in Figure 14.11 has a large swelling of all the masticator spaces (submasseteric,

Table 14.2 Borders of the deep spaces of the head and neck

Space	Borders					
	Anterior	**Posterior**	**Superior**	**Inferior**	**Superficial or medial§**	**Deep or lateral***
Buccal	Corner of mouth	Masseter m. Pterygomandibular space	Maxilla Infraorbital space	Mandible	Subcutaneous tissue and skin	Buccinator m.
Infraorbital	Nasal cartilages	Buccal space	Quadratus labii superioris m.	Oral mucosa	Quadratus labii superioris m.	Levator anguli oris m., Maxilla
Sub-mandibular	Ant. belly digastric m.	Post. belly digastric m. Stylohyoid m. Stylopharyngeus m.	Inf. & medial surfaces of mandible	Digastric tendon	Platysma m., Investing fascia	Mylohyoid, Hyoglossus, Sup. constrictor muscles
Submental	Inf. border of mandible	Hyoid bone	Mylohyoid m.	Investing fascia	Investing fascia	Ant. bellies digastric mm.*
Sublingual	Lingual surface of mandible	Submandibular space	Oral mucosa	Mylohyoid m.	Muscles of tongue§	Lingual surface of mandible*
Pterygomandibular	Buccal space	Parotid gland	Lateral pterygoid m.	Inf. border of mandible	Med. pterygoid muscle§	Ascending ramus of mandible*
Submasseteric	Buccal space	Parotid gland	Zygomatic arch	Inf. border of mandible	Ascending ramus of mandible§	Masseter m.*
Lateral pharyngeal	Sup. & mid. pharyngeal constrictor mm.	Carotid sheath and scalene fascia	Skull base	Hyoid bone	Pharyngeal constrictors & retropharyngeal space§	Medial pterygoid m.*
Retropharyngeal	Sup. & mid. pharyngeal constrictor mm.	Alar fascia	Skull base	Fusion of alar and prevertebral fasciae at C6–T4		Carotid sheath and lateral pharyngeal space*
Pretracheal	Sternothyroid-thyrohyoid fascia	Retropharyngeal space	Thyroid cartilage	Superior mediastinum	Sternothyroid-thyrohyoid fascia	Visceral fascia over trachea and thyroid gland

*Medial border.
§Lateral border.
m., muscle; Ant., anterior; Inf., inferior; Med., medial; Sp., Space; Post., posterior; Sup., superior; mid., middle; Lat., lateral.
Source: Flynn TR. Anatomy of oral and maxillofacial infections. In: Topazian RG, Goldberg MH, Hupp JR, editors. *Oral and Maxillofacial Infections.* 4th edition. Philadelphia: WB Saunders Company; 2002, p. 194, used with permission.

pterygomandibular, superficial and deep temporal), which has been present for 60 days. On the other hand, the two images seen in Figure 14.13 were taken only 4 hours apart. The first patient, with the slowly progressing infection, was infected by a mixed flora of alpha-hemolytic streptococci (*Streptococcus viridans*) and oral anaerobes; the second patient was infected by Group A beta-hemolytic streptococci. Clearly, a rapidly progressing infection is more severe than an indolent one.

Odontogenic infections generally pass through four stages of infection in their clinical course. In the first 3 days of symptoms, the inoculation stage occurs. This is

Table 14.3 Relations of anatomic spaces

Space	Likely causes	Contents	Neighboring spaces	Approach for I&D
Buccal	Upper bicuspids Upper molars Lower bicuspids	Parotid duct Ant. facial a. & v. Transverse facial artery & vein Buccal fat pad	Infraorbital Pterygomandibular Infratemporal	Intraoral (small) Extraoral (large)
Infraorbital	Upper cuspid	Angular a. & v. Infraorbital n.	Buccal	Intraoral
Submandibular	Lower molars	Submandibular gland Facial a. & v. Lymph nodes	Sublingual Submental Lateral pharyngeal Buccal	Extraoral
Submental	Lower anteriors Fracture of symphysis	Ant. jugular v. Lymph nodes	Submandibular (on either side)	Extraoral
Sublingual	Lower bicuspids Lower molars Direct trauma	Sublingual glands Wharton's ducts Lingual n. Sublingual a. & v.	Submandibular Lateral pharyngeal Visceral (trachea and esophagus)	Intraoral Intraoral–extraoral
Pterygomandibular	Lower third molars Fracture of angle of mandible	Mandibular div. of trigeminal n. Inf. alveolar a. & v.	Buccal Lateral pharyngeal Submasseteric Deep temporal Parotid Peritonsillar	Intraoral Intraoral–extraoral
Submasseteric	Lower third molars Fracture of angle of mandible	Masseteric a. & v.	Buccal Pterygomandibular Superficial temporal Parotid	Intraoral Intraoral–extraoral
Infratemporal & deep temporal	Upper molars	Pterygoid plexus Int. max. a. & v. Mand. div. of trigeminal n. Skull base foramina	Buccal Superf. temporal Inf. petrosal sinus	Intraoral Extraoral Intraoral-extraoral
Superficial temporal	Upper molars Lower molars	Temporal fat pad Temporal branch of facial n.	Buccal Deep temporal	Intraoral Extraoral Intraoral–extraoral
Lateral pharyngeal	Lower third molars Tonsils Infection in neighboring spaces	Carotid a. Internal jugular v. Vagus n. Cervical sympathetic chain	Pterygomandibular Submandibular Sublingual Peritonsillar Retropharyngeal	Intraoral Intraoral–extraoral

From: Flynn TR. Anatomy of oral and maxillofacial infections. In: Topazian RG, Goldberg MH, Hupp JR, editors. *Oral and Maxillofacial Infections*. 4th edition. Philadelphia: WB Saunders Company; 2002, p. 195, used with permission.

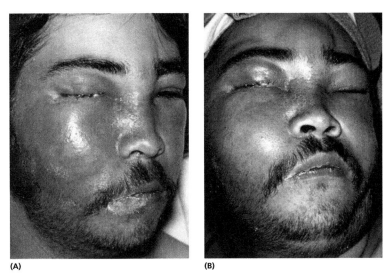

Figure 14.13 (A) Infraorbital, buccal, and periorbital abscess. This patient had a 3-day history of infection arising from the upper right first molar. Note that the swelling involves the cheek, infraorbit, and eyelids. It is even spreading across the bridge of the nose to the other eye. (B) The same patient four hours later. Note the rapid increase in this swelling, which was due to invasive Group A beta-hemolytic streptococci. At this point, early infection of the cavernous sinuses (right and left) was found. This case demonstrates how infections due to these streptococci can spread very rapidly. Source: Flynn TR, Topazian RG. Infections of the oral cavity. In: Waite D, editor. *Textbook of Practical Oral and Maxillofacial Surgery.* Philadelphia: Lea & Febiger; 1987, p. 301, used with permission.

due to the initial invasion of the soft tissues by bacteria, resulting in a mildly tender, soft, edematous swelling. At days 3 to 5, the cellulitis stage occurs, which is characterized by an exquisitely tender, indurated (hard), red, diffuse swelling. At days 5 to 7, an abscess begins to form, which is characterized by a central softening in the area of the cellulitis, a localizing of the infection, and often a decrease in tenderness. The skin overlying the forming abscess may become very soft and shiny due to undermining of the skin by the abscess beneath. The mucosa may undergo similar a similar process, with yellow pus visible through the intact mucous membrane. Finally, the resolution stage begins when either surgical or spontaneous drainage of the abscess is achieved.

Identification of the stage of infection is important because cellulitis occurs during the rapidly rising phase of the clinical course of the infection. By the time an abscess begins to form, the peak severity of the infection has generally been achieved. Therefore, cellulitis usually progresses more rapidly through the anatomic spaces than an abscess, giving rise to greater concern.

Might this infection compromise the airway or vital structures?

After determining the anatomic location of the infection and its rate of progress, the clinician should look for early signs of potential airway compromise. First, in the history, the dentist should ask if the patient has had to adopt measures that make it easier to breathe, such as sleeping sitting up in a chair overnight, or has had difficulty lying flat. In addition, the dentist should ask about the consistency of recent food intake. An inability to swallow solid food or even liquids indicates dysphagia, which may be due to an infection compressing the oropharynx and causing inflammation in the muscles of deglutition. Second, a careful examination for trismus may disclose an infection in the perimandibular or masticator spaces. Further, the patient's posture may reveal an adaptation to a deviated airway, such as the image in Figure 14.14, where a boy with a left lateral pharyngeal space infection deviates his head toward the opposite shoulder in order to position his upper airway over his deviated trachea.

Infections causing infraorbital, periorbital (eyelid), or orbital swelling can threaten the eye or the brain via the

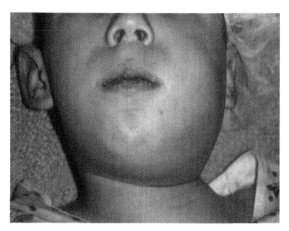

Figure 14.14 Buccal, submandibular, and lateral pharyngeal space abscess. A boy with a rapidly spreading infection that has pushed the trachea to the opposite side. In order to straighten his airway and make breathing easier, he has deviated his head toward his left shoulder, thus positioning his upper airway over his lower airway. Emergency surgery to secure the airway and drain the infection was necessary. Source: Flynn TR, Piecuch JF, Topazian RG. Infections of the oral cavity. In: Feigin RD, Cherry JD, editors. *Textbook of Pediatric Infectious Diseases*. 4th edition. Philadelphia: JB Lippincott; 1998, p. 142, used with permission.

cavernous sinus. Infections deep in the neck can threaten the heart via the mediastinum.

Step 2. Evaluate host defenses

A patient's resistance to infecting microorganisms depends not only on the immune response but also the systemic capacity to withstand the effects of the inflammatory response to infection. For example, an otherwise healthy, young athlete can better withstand the fever, dehydration, and interruption of nutrition that may accompany infection than a frail, elderly individual who suffers from cardiovascular disease.

Immune system compromise

Table 14.4 lists the most common diseases that compromise the immune system.

Diabetes is at the top of the list, as the most common immunocompromising disease. Diabetics suffer from a white blood cell defect that inhibits chemotaxis, the ability of the white blood cell to migrate to the site of infection. Elevated blood sugar is directly correlated with the degree of impairment of the immune system, so evaluation of the level of diabetes control is

Table 14.4 Immunocompromising diseases/conditions

Diabetes
Steroid therapy
Organ transplants
Malignancy
Chemotherapy
Alcoholism
Malnutrition
End-stage renal disease
End-stage AIDS

important in the infected individual. The dentist can inquire about the hemoglobin A1c (HbA1c, or glycosylated hemoglobin) test result, which corresponds to the average blood sugar level over the previous 3- to 4-month period. HbA1c levels under 7 are the therapeutic goal; levels over 8 represent increasingly poor control of diabetes. When a patient does not know his or her latest HbA1c result, the clinician may suspect poor compliance with the prescribed diabetes regimen. Fasting blood sugar levels over 225 mg/dl are correlated with increased infection rates.

Corticosteroids are used with increasing frequency in the management of respiratory diseases, such as asthma and chronic obstructive pulmonary disease (COPD). They suppress T-cells, which primarily attack intracellular pathogens, such as viruses and tuberculosis. Fortunately, the bacteria responsible for most orofacial infections are extracellular pathogens that are attacked by a combination of antibodies elaborated by B-cells and phagocytes that engulf and kill the bacteria. Nonetheless, current or recent steroid therapy warrants caution and may indicate the need for perioperative administration of steroid medication in order to prevent iatrogenic adrenal insufficiency.

Organ transplantation is increasingly common and is accompanied by chronic administration of immunosuppressive drugs to combat rejection. Such drugs include cyclosporine, azathioprine, tacrolimus (Prograf®), and sirolimus (Rapamune®). These drugs inhibit both T-cell and B-cell function. Therefore, host resistance to orofacial infection is more significantly reduced than in corticosteroid therapy.

Cancer chemotherapeutic agents inhibit the growth of rapidly dividing cells, such as malignant tumor cells. To varying degrees, however, chemotherapeutic drugs also inhibit the growth of white blood cells, which must divide rapidly in order to mount an anti-infective response. The effects of these agents may also remain for a prolonged period after the chemotherapeutic regimen has been completed. Therefore, patients are considered immunocompromised for 1 year after cessation of chemotherapy.

Ongoing malignancy, alcoholism, and malnutrition (including extreme diets) have also been associated with a poorly understood decreased immune response, perhaps by the common mechanism of malnutrition.

End-stage renal disease causes accumulation of urea in the blood, which directly suppresses white blood cells and other components of the immune system.

Until the final stages of acquired immune deficiency syndrome (AIDS), the human immunodeficiency virus (HIV) infection affects T-cells primarily, which makes the person living with HIV potentially more susceptible to intracellular infections, such as tuberculosis, viral infections such as oral herpes, and certain pneumonias. Resistance to yeast and fungal organisms is also decreased, as seen in oropharyngeal candidiasis, one of the clinical markers of AIDS. Fortunately, however, resistance to the common odontogenic infections caused by extracellular pathogens does not decline dramatically until AIDS is severe. Descriptive studies of orofacial infections in HIV-positive individuals have shown that their incidence is not increased, but the intensity of the infection and the therapeutic management is greater than in HIV-negative persons.

Systemic reserve

Host defenses are also assessed by the systemic response to the infection and by evaluation of the systemic reserve of the individual patient. Younger individuals mount the febrile response to inflammatory byproducts, which enhances immune function at core temperatures below 39.4°C (103°F). Above this level, fever becomes destructive, and it should be managed. However, people over 65 years of age do not develop fever to the same degree as younger people. Therefore, with aging, fever becomes a less reliable sign of the systemic response to infection.

Fever increases fluid loss by evaporation and sweating, which can cause dehydration. Severe dehydration can be recognized by parching of the lips and loss of skin turgor, but a more sensitive indicator of dehydration is the color of the urine, which increases in its amber-yellow coloration as dehydration progresses.

The local inflammatory response is classically described as the five cardinal signs of swelling, redness, increased temperature, pain, and loss of function. As the intensity of these signs increases, the severity of infection also increases.

As the inflammatory response progresses on the local and systemic levels, the physiologic demands on the human organism increase. Cardiac work increases in response to pain, dehydration, and fever, which also increase metabolic demands for energy and oxygen. Surgical trauma may add to the biologic stresses on the individual. Therefore, the dentist must evaluate the ability of the individual to tolerate the systemic demands of the infection, the inflammatory response to the infection, and the therapeutic management of the infection.

Step 3. Decide: treat or refer

Orofacial infections can be classified as low, moderate, or high anatomic severity primarily by their anatomic location but also by the other factors discussed above, such as rapid progression, immune system compromise, or decreased systemic reserve. In general, low-severity infections can be safely treated by a general dentist comfortable with the surgical and medical management of orofacial infections. Moderate-severity infections should be treated by an oral and maxillofacial surgeon, possibly on an outpatient basis. High-severity infections should be treated by an oral and maxillofacial surgeon in the hospital setting, possibly with the consultation of infectious disease specialists, intensivists, anesthesiologists, and other surgeons. Oral and maxillofacial surgeons are most familiar with orofacial infections and can manage the dental, oral, and surgical needs of the patient in the most conservative, yet effective manner.

In step 1, the dentist evaluates the possibility that the airway may be compromised. If it is clear that the airway is in immediate danger of being lost or obstructed, the patient should be transported immediately to the nearest hospital by the emergency medical system. If the patient is stable, however, the dentist must decide whether the given infection can be treated in the dental office or should be referred to an oral and maxillofacial surgeon.

The criteria for referral to an oral and maxillofacial surgeon are listed in Table 14.5. If impending airway compromise is likely, the oral and maxillofacial surgeon will take steps to secure the airway, including possible hospitalization, endotracheal intubation, emergency

Table 14.5 When to refer to an oral and maxillofacial surgeon

Impending airway compromise
Threat to vital structures (heart, brain)
Trismus (limited oral opening)
Dysphagia (difficulty swallowing)
Fever greater than 38.3°C (101°F)
Dehydration
Infection of moderate or high severity anatomic spaces
  Perimandibular spaces
  Masticator spaces
  Deep neck spaces
Need for general anesthesia
Need for inpatient control of systemic disease

surgery, culture and sensitivity testing, intravenous antibiotics, and intensive care. Trismus and dysphagia suggest infection in the perimandibular (submandibular, sublingual, submental) spaces or the masticator (submasseteric, pterygomandibular, superficial and deep temporal) spaces. Treatment of infection in these spaces will often involve hospitalization, securing the airway, tooth extraction, intraoral and possibly extraoral incision and drainage, and intravenous antibiotics. Infection in the deep neck spaces (lateral pharyngeal, retropharyngeal, pretracheal), the mediastinum, or the cranial cavity may require even more intensive therapy and consultation with medical specialists.

Sometimes, a relatively minor infection may require the care of an oral and maxillofacial surgeon, such as the patient with a systemic condition requiring concomitant medical management. Examples include the patient on coumadin anticoagulant therapy, insulin-dependent diabetics, or those requiring general anesthesia for patient management reasons.

Low-severity infections, such as those involving the perioral spaces (vestibular, infraorbital, buccal, subperiosteal, space of the body of the mandible), can be managed in the office setting by the general dentist. Fortunately, such infections are much more common than the moderate- and high-severity infections described above.

In doubtful cases, the wisest choice is to refer the infected patient to a higher level of care because the oral and maxillofacial surgeon will have access to all of the ancillary services provided by medical specialists and hospital facilities when needed. The rising rates of antibiotic resistance in oral pathogens, the increasing complexity of medical management of preexisting diseases,

and the variability of host responses to infection can make referral even more strategic now than in prior years.

Step 4. Treat surgically

Because the organisms that cause orofacial infections are abscess-formers that are introduced deeply into the bone of the jaws, surgical drainage is the most important treatment we can offer.

Another feature common in dental infections is biofilm formation. Antibiotics do not penetrate biofilms well. Furthermore, biofilm-bound bacteria are generally in a quiescent state in which they do not actively incorporate antibiotics. Physical removal appears to be the best strategy for eradicating biofilms, when possible.

Essentially, the treatment of almost all dental infection is surgical, ranging from the excavation of decay and gingival curettage to extraction and incision and drainage. Such is the nature of the diseases dentists treat; it has been so since before antibiotics were introduced.

The goals of the surgical management of orofacial infection are to remove the cause of the infection, provide drainage of abscess and cellulitis, and debride the infected wound. These are generally accomplished in one setting.

Remove the cause

Removing the cause of infection may require extraction, endodontic therapy, or periodontal debridement. The decision to remove or retain an infected tooth is based on the severity of the infection and the restorative needs of the patient. Extraction is more likely to be immediately successful in removing the source of infecting bacteria, but of course it may inhibit subsequent oral function. Enhanced oral function, however, must not take precedence over systemic priorities.

Drain the infection

Low-severity orofacial infections can generally be drained intraorally. As shown in Figure 14.15, an incision is made with a scalpel blade in the oral vestibule, often slightly toward the alveolar process from the depth of the vestibular fold, directly over the site of maximum swelling. The incision is usually 1.5 to 2 cm in length, commonly oriented parallel to the vestibular fold. The incision is carried through the mucosal epithelium and submucosa, which is recognized by slightly

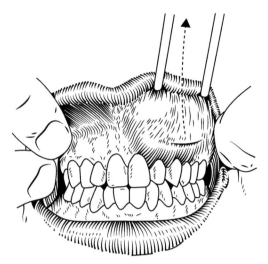

Figure 14.15 Intraoral incision and drainage. The horizontal incision over this vestibular abscess is shown at the solid line. The dotted arrow indicates the direction of blunt dissection into the vestibular space and the infraorbital space, as necessary. After thorough dissection, debridement, and irrigation of the infected space, a drain is sutured to one lip of the incision with a non-resorbable suture. Source: Modified from Flynn TR, Topazian RG. Infections of the oral cavity. In: Waite D, editor. *Textbook of Practical Oral and Maxillofacial Surgery.* Philadelphia: Lea & Febiger; 1987, p. 290, used with permission.

less resistance to the scalpel when the fibrous submucosa is penetrated. Often, the pus-containing abscess is encountered just below the submucosa, and drainage ensues. The pus can be cultured with aerobic and anaerobic swab culturettes immediately on entering the abscess cavity, before all the pus has been evacuated.

The next step in the incision and drainage procedure is to explore and debride the site of infection. A hemostat is introduced through the incision into the wound in the closed position. Within the depth of the wound, the hemostat beaks are opened, and then the hemostat is withdrawn in the open position. This procedure breaks up any septa within the abscess cavity, opening up any loculations to further drainage and debridement. A hemostat should never be closed within the tissues lest healthy tissue, especially a nerve or other structure, be crushed inadvertently. A key surgical principle is to bluntly explore the entire swelling by introducing the closed hemostat to the periphery of the swelling in all directions. The surgeon can verify that he or she has explored the entire infected site by counterpalpation for the tip of the hemostat with the non-dominant hand.

The hemostat can also be used to explore the facial cortical plate of the bone for a perforation, usually over the apex of the causative tooth. This provides a drainage pathway to the exterior (the oral cavity) for periapical infection.

Any grossly visible necrotic tissue is removed from the wound in order to minimize the bioburden of bacterial debris, inflammatory byproducts, and dead white blood cells that must be removed during healing. Microscopic debris and bacteria are further removed with copious irrigation of the wound using sterile saline solution.

Finally a drain, which may consist of a sterilized tubular Penrose drain (available in ¼-inch diameter size) or a strip of sterilized dental dam or surgical glove material, is sutured to one lip of the incision with a non-resorbable suture, such as 3–0 or 4–0 silk. Avoid using a latex drain in a latex-allergic patient. The purpose of the drain is to keep the wound open, allowing further drainage to occur over the next 1 to 3 days. When a drain is not used, the wound may close too early, allowing the abscess to reform.

Surgical pitfalls

As shown in Figure 14.16A, there are certain locations in the oral vestibule where an incision should be avoided. These include the sites of frenula, where an incision crossing a frenulum will heal slowly with significant scarring and considerable pain due to muscle pull across the incision. Instead, an incision oriented parallel to and just to either side of the frenulum will allow good access to the infection yet afford prompt, pain-free healing.

The incision for drainage of a palatal abscess is shown in Figure 14.16B. The incision is oriented parallel to the course of the greater palatine artery, and it is carried only through the mucosa and submucosa. The incision is not carried directly to the bony palate because the greater palatine artery and vein lie just superficial to the bone. Instead, blunt dissection with a hemostat allows exploration of the abscess cavity. During the dissection, the beaks of the hemostat are spread in the anteroposterior direction, parallel to the course of the vessels, which minimizes the risk of severe bleeding.

Another location in the oral vestibule to be managed with surgical caution is the region of the mental foramen and the mental nerve, in the mandibular bicuspid region.

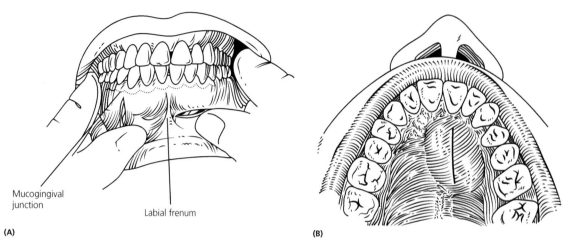

(A)

Mucogingival junction

Labial frenum

(B)

Figure 14.16 (A) Incision placement near a frenum and the mental foramen. The incision near the mental foramen and nerve should be oriented parallel to the nerve fibers and not carried deeply. Blunt dissection is used to minimize trauma to the nerve fibers. The incision at the labial frenum is placed to one side of the mandibular labial frenum, rather than across it. This minimizes the painful delayed healing caused by cutting across a frenum. (B) Incision placement for a palatal abscess. The incision is oriented parallel to the course of the greater palatine artery and vein. The incision is not carried directly to bone in order to avoid brisk hemorrhage from those vessels. Instead, blunt dissection with a hemostat is used to explore the abscess cavity, spreading the beaks of the hemostat parallel to the vessels. Source: Flynn TR. Surgical management of orofacial infections. *Atlas of the Oral and Maxillofacial Surgery Clinics of North America* 2000;8(Mar):77–100, p. 86, used with permission.

After the mental nerve exits from the mandible at the mental foramen, it rises superiorly toward the oral mucosa and runs in the submucosa in an obliquely anterior and medial direction into the lip. The mental nerve ramifies into at least three separate bundles soon after it leaves the mental foramen, branching into ever-finer filaments in its course to the lip and chin. An incision in this location should run parallel to the course of the mental nerve, which may sometimes be seen through the mucosa when the lip is firmly stretched anteriorly. The incision should be carried only partially through the submucosa, which is then bluntly dissected with a fine mosquito hemostat, spreading the beaks parallel to the nerve fibers. This stretches, rather than tears the nerve fibers in the region. If nerve fibers are unavoidably encountered, the direction of force application tends to cause only minor nerve injury that is likely to recover spontaneously. Alternatively, the dentist may wish to refer such cases to an oral and maxillofacial surgeon with more experience in the required careful dissection.

Incision and drainage of a cellulitis is to be encouraged rather than avoided. The old adage that surgical drainage before abscess formation may cause the infection to spread does not appear to be true. Experience has shown that when pus is not encountered during incision and drainage, the patient still gets better. In a series of severe odontogenic infections requiring hospitalization, complications such as an increased length of hospital stay, further spread of the infection, and the need for a second operation were not increased in the patients in whom no pus was encountered at surgery.[1,2] Good microbiologic samples were obtained from both the cellulitis wounds (no pus) and from the abscess wounds with pus. Draining a cellulitis aborted the spread of the infection into deeper anatomic spaces. Therefore, it is appropriate to use the same thorough exploration and debridement of the site of infection, whether or not pus is encountered at incision and drainage. The wound is kept open with a drain in order to allow infected fluid, including pus that may form later, to be evacuated.

Step 5. Support medically

Medical support for the infected patient includes hydration, nutrition, and control of systemic disease.

Hydration

Prolonged fever increases both sensible (e.g., perspiration, urination) fluid losses and insensible fluid losses, such as evaporation from the skin. Dehydration can precipitate cardiovascular instability and shock, especially in an elderly patient with a compromised cardiovascular system. The normal fluid requirement is about 2.1 liters per day, which increases by 800 ml per degree of fever per day. Therefore, a patient with a temperature of 37.7°C (100°F) would need to take in at least 3.7 liters per day (roughly 4 quarts of liquid). For an outpatient, the dentist must encourage the patient to force oral fluids. Temperatures over 38.3°C (101°F) may be managed best by intravenous hydration in a hospital setting.

Nutrition

Caloric requirements increase in the febrile adult by 3 to 5% per degree per day. Oral infection, however, can decrease appetite and the ability to ingest solid food. Therefore, liquid nutritional supplements consisting of commercially available protein-calorie shakes may aid in maintaining adequate caloric support of fever and the metabolic protein requirements of healing. The goal is to provide at least the normal daily protein and calorie requirement in the liquid supplement, with additional nutritional support coming from the diet as tolerated by the patient.

Control of systemic disease

Systemic diseases can increase the complexity and risk of an infection like an accelerant on a fire. The major organ systems that increase concern are the cardiac, respiratory, metabolic, hematologic, and immunologic systems.

The functional capacity of the heart and lungs, while not affecting resistance to infection directly, determines the ability of the individual to sustain the potentially damaging physiologic loads imposed by hypoxia, fever, dehydration, malnutrition, and the trauma of surgery. The patient with preexisting cardiac or respiratory disease, whether diagnosed or not, is at significantly greater risk when stressed by infection. Support of the patient with cardiac or respiratory disease includes minimizing stress with effective local anesthesia (while minimizing epinephrine in the cardiac patient), sedation as necessary, and monitoring oxygen saturation while using supplemental oxygen inhalation. Poorly compensated patients may require inpatient management.

Infection itself can raise the blood sugar of a diabetic patient. Counteracting this effect, however, is the likely decreased caloric intake of the patient with oral infection and recent surgical intervention. Therefore, blood glucose control may not readily be achieved by the patient's customary insulin or oral antihyperglycemic regimen. This problem is complicated further by the fact that inadequate control of blood sugar decreases host resistance to infection, necessitating fairly tight glucose control. Accordingly, the patient may need to use a sliding scale of regular (short-acting) insulin dosages based on frequent blood sugar measurements. The patient's physician may provide an individualized insulin dosage scale, based on that patient's historical responses to insulin.

In the perioperative period, the ability to achieve hemostasis is of prime concern to the surgeon. An increasing proportion of the population is using some type of anticoagulant drug, generally either an antiplatelet drug like aspirin or clopidogrel (Plavix®) or a warfarin class drug, such as coumadin, which inhibits clotting factor synthesis. Anticoagulants are used in chemoprevention of myocardial infarction and stroke, as well as to prevent thromboembolism, especially in elderly patients with atrial fibrillation. Because emergency surgery is the rule in infection, anticoagulated patients may require rapid reversal of their anticoagulation as well as emergency management of postoperative bleeding. Anticipation of the problem, especially by requesting medical management, is most effective. This is best achieved in the hospital setting.

Immune system compromise, discussed earlier, is also managed most commonly in the hospital, where isolation, advanced aseptic techniques, and co-management by physician colleagues are available. Further, high-dose intravenous broad-spectrum antibiotic therapy can be administered in the inpatient setting.

In summary, basic medical support is often available on an outpatient basis, but patients with complex medical needs may require inpatient medical support, even if their orofacial infection is otherwise minor.

Step 6. Choose an appropriate antibiotic

The usual pathogens of orofacial infections are the alpha-hemolytic streptococci also known as the *Streptococcus viridans* (Group A streptococcus) and the oral anaerobes of the genera *Prevotella*, *Porphyromonas*, *Parvimonas* (formerly *Peptostreptococcus*), and *Fusobacterium*. The anaerobes outnumber the aerobes by a factor of 10; they are found in 94% of orofacial infections. Therefore, when taking cultures of these infections, both aerobic and

Table 14.6 Most frequent pathogens isolated in orofacial infections

Microorganism	% of Cases
Streptococcus milleri group	65
Peptostreptococcus species	65
Other anaerobic streptococci	9
Prevotella species (*oralis, melaninogenica*, etc.)	74
Porphyromonas species (*gingivalis*, etc.)	17
Fusobacterium species	52

Data from: Sakamoto H, Kato H, Sato T, Sasaki J. Semiquantitative bacteriology of closed odontogenic abscesses. *The Bulletin of Tokyo Dental College*. 1998 May;39(2):103–7.

anaerobic culture and antibiotic sensitivity testing should be performed using appropriate culture swabs that support the transport of both types of bacteria. The most frequent pathogens of orofacial infections are listed in Table 14.6.

In the past, much consideration has been given to choosing among the antibiotics that are considered effective against the usual pathogens of orofacial infections. For example, when a new study indicated a slightly greater laboratory effectiveness of one antibiotic compared to another, clinicians have been swayed to change their antibiotic of choice based on the results of the new study. Ultimately, however, the best evidence of the effectiveness of antibiotics in orofacial infections are randomized, blind clinical studies that compare the cure rate of two or more antibiotics in direct comparison.

Recently, a systematic review of the available randomized, blind clinical trials comparing a penicillin-family antibiotic with at least one other antibiotic in the treatment of orofacial infections was performed. Because the results of all available high-quality studies were compared in this systematic review, its conclusions can be considered very reliable. The results of the systematic review are summarized in Table 14.7. There was no significant difference in clinical cure at 7 days between the control antibiotic (a penicillin) and the test antibiotic (a variety of newer antibiotics) in any of the eight studies. The conclusions of this review are that when the appropriate surgery (root canal therapy, periodontal debridement, extraction, and/or incision and drainage) is done, the choice of antibiotic among those commonly used for orofacial infection can be based on the patient's medical history, relative pharmacologic safety, and cost.[5]

Another important randomized clinical trial was performed that reinforces for clinicians the concept that the primary treatment of dental pain is the appropriate dental procedure, not a course of antibiotics. In this study, patients presenting to a hospital emergency room with toothache, in the absence of facial swelling, were treated with either an antibiotic plus an analgesic or an analgesic alone. Only 10% of the subjects developed a facial swelling, and they were evenly divided between the antibiotic and the non-antibiotic groups. The only factors that predicted the later development of orofacial infection were the presence of an amalgam restoration and a periapical radiolucency greater than 1.5 mm in diameter.[6] Thus, definitive dental care, not antibiotics, is the indicated treatment for toothache.

Antibiotic resistance is a mounting problem, even in orofacial infections. Table 14.8 shows the increasing rate of antibiotic resistance in orofacial infections during the 1990s.

The American Dental Association Council on Scientific Affairs has published a policy on the prevention of antibiotic resistance in dentistry.[7] The policy states that narrow-spectrum antibiotics (penicillin, clindamycin, and metronidazole) should be used for "simple" infections, and broad-spectrum antibiotics (amoxicillin, amoxicillin with clavulanic acid, tetracycline, and azithromycin) may be used for "complex" infections. However, the policy did not define the difference between simple and complex infections. A practical definition of simple and complex odontogenic infections can be proposed. Simple odontogenic infections are those in which the swelling is limited to the alveolar process or the vestibular space, the current antibiotic prescription is part of the first treatment course, and the patient is not immunocompromised. Conversely, a complex infection involves swelling extending beyond the vestibular space, previous treatment failure or recurrence of infection, or immune system compromise.

The costs of a 1-week prescription of various antibiotics commonly used in orofacial infections are compared in Table 14.9. It is interesting to note that amoxicillin has recently become less expensive than penicillin V. A further advantage of amoxicillin is the less frequent dosing, at three times per day, which improves patient compliance with the prescribed regimen. Clindamycin is more than three

Table 14.7 Clinical trials of antibiotics in orofacial infections

Reference	Year	N	Intervention group	Comparator group	Surgical control	Significant difference between groups?	Comment
Gilmore et al. 1988[18]	1988	49	PCN	CLI	N	N	Only surgery was I&D; EXT/RCT performed only after study completion.
von Konow and Nord 1983[19]	1983	60	ORN	PCN	N	N	Only surgery was I&D; 2 subjects in each group did not receive surgery. Fewer days of pain in ornidazole group (p<.05); more failures in PCN group (NSD).
Mangundjaja and Hardjawinata 1990[20]	1990	106	CLI	AMP	N	N	Only surgery was I&D; EXT/RCT performed only after study completion. Not all subjects were cured by 7d.
Lewis et al. 1993[21]	1993	78	AM/CL	PCN	N	N	Surgery was either I&D or EXT or RCT. Greater pain reduction at 1 to 2d & 2 to 3d in amoxicillin/clavulanate group; otherwise NSD in swelling, temperature, lymphadenopathy, or pain.
Davis and Balcom 3rd, 1969[22]	1969	49	LIN (im&po)	PCNG(im&po)	N	N	9 patients had trauma and fractures, including osteomyelitis.
Matijević et al., 2009[23]	2009	90	AMOX	CEPH	Y	N	Antibiotic groups had shorter treatment time than surgery alone (not statistically significant).
Ingham et al. 1977[24]	1977	37	MET	PCNG (im once daily)	N	N	Subjects received "appropriate surgery when necessary." At 24 to 48h, "marked clinical improvement" was noted in all subjects.
Al-Nawas et al. 2009.[25]	2009	19	MOXI	AM/CL	N	N	Only study of hospitalized patients, requiring extraoral and/or intraoral I&D. Cure = improving trismus, no pain on palpation, afebrile.

AM/CL = Amoxicillin/clavulanate; AMOX = amoxicillin; AMP = ampicillin; CEPH = cephalexin; CLI = clindamycin; EXT = extraction; I&D = incision and drainage; LIN = lincomycin; MET = metronidazole; MOXI = moxifloxacin; N = No; NSD = no statistically significant difference; ORN = ornidazole; PCN = penicillin V; PCNG = penicillin G; RCT = root canal therapy; Y = yes.
Adapted from: Flynn TR. What are the antibiotics of choice for odontogenic infections, and how long should the treatment course last? *Oral and Maxillofacial Surgery Clinics of North America* 2011;23(November):519–36.

Table 14.8 Increasing penicillin resistance rates among oral pathogens

Year	% of Cases PCN Resistant	Country
1991 (Brook et al.[26])	33	USA
1992 (von Konow et al.[27])	38	Sweden
1995 (Lewis et al.[28])	55	UK
1999 (Flynn et al.[1])	54	USA

times the cost of amoxicillin, and amoxicillin/clavulanate (Augmentin®) is more than four times the cost of amoxicillin. The American Dental Association's policy recommends amoxicillin/clavulanate only for sinus involvement in orofacial infections,[7] and the above-cited systematic review found no clinical advantage of this broad-spectrum antibiotic in dental infections.[5] Thus, there is no overriding reason to use amoxicillin/clavulanate as a first-line antibiotic in orofacial infections.

Table 14.9 Oral antibiotic costs

Usual antibiotic	Usual dose (mg)	Interval (h)	Retail cost/1 week 2012* ($)	Amoxicillin cost ratio
Penicillins				
Amoxicillin	500	8	11.99	1.00
Penicillin V	500	6	12.29	.03
Augmentin®	875	12	49.69	4.14
Augmentin XR®	2000	12	51.59	4.30
Dicloxacillin	500	6	24.29	2.03
Cephalosporins (generation)				
Cephalexin Caps (1st)	500	6	17.99	1.50
Cefadroxil (1st)	500	12	41.19	3.44
Cefuroxime (2nd)	500	8	82.99	6.92
Cefaclor ER (generic)	500	12	69.59	5.80
Cefdinir (3rd)	600	24	102.99	8.59
Erythromycins				
Erythromycin base	500	6	83.59	6.97
Clarithromycin (Biaxin XL®)	500	24	31.09	2.59
Azithromycin (Zithromax®)	250	12	82.59	6.89
Telithromycin (Ketek®)	800	24	240.99	20.10
Anti-anaerobic				
Clindamycin (generic)	150	6	28.99	2.42
Clindamycin (2 T generic)	300	6	57.98	4.84
Clindamycin (generic)	300	6	38.99	3.25
Metronidazole	500	6	29.99	2.50
Other				
Trimethoprim/sulfamethoxazole	160/800	2	11.99	1.00
Vancomycin	125	6	762.99	63.64
Ciprofloxacin	500	12	17.69	1.48
Moxifloxacin (Avelox®)	400	24	167.99	14.01
Doxycycline	100	12	11.99	1.00
Linezolid (Zyvox®)	600	12	1,776.99	148.21

Usual doses and intervals are for moderate infections and are not to be considered prescriptive.
Amoxicillin cost ratio = Retail cost of antibiotic for 1 week/retail cost of amoxicillin for 1 week.
*Retail cost/1 wk = Retail price charged for a 1-week prescription at a large national pharmacy chain. Courtesy of Joshua Avery, CPhT.

Based on the above considerations, plus overall pharmacologic safety and cost, the antibiotics of choice for orofacial infections are listed in Table 14.10. Perhaps due to recent overuse of clindamycin for antibiotic prophylaxis in patients not allergic to penicillin, the rate of resistance among the oral streptococci has risen to 17% of strains in a recent study.[1] Because of this resistance as well as cost considerations, amoxicillin should be considered the first antibiotic of choice in non-allergic patients with orofacial infections. Clindamycin is the first antibiotic of choice in penicillin-allergic patients.

Table 14.10 Empiric antibiotics* of choice for outpatient orofacial infections

	Antibiotic of choice
	Penicillin
	Clindamycin
	Azithromycin
Penicillin allergy	Clindamycin
	Metronidazole
	Moxifloxacin

*Empiric antibiotic therapy is used before culture and sensitivity reports are available. Culture samples should be taken in cases of complex infections.

Among the newer macrolide (erythromycin-family) antibiotics, azithromycin (Zithromax®) has a better safety profile than clarithromycin (Biaxin®). This is mainly due to the fact that azithromycin is metabolized by a slightly different enzymatic pathway than the other macrolides, which results in fewer interactions with other drugs, some of which can be life threatening. For patients with a penicillin allergy, clindamycin is the first antibiotic of choice, followed by metronidazole. Metronidazole has been used alone successfully in orofacial infections, when combined with appropriate surgery.

The fluoroquinolones (Cipro® family) are a family of synthetic antibiotics that have significant, potentially life-threatening drug interactions, and they are chondrotoxic. The fluoroquinolones have been shown to damage growing cartilage in young animals. They have also been associated with Achilles tendon rupture in adults. The fourth-generation fluoroquinolones have the best effectiveness against the oral pathogens, and moxifloxacin (Avelox®) is the best known antibiotic in this family. Because of their high cost as well as significant and frequent drug interactions and toxicities, the fluoroquinolones are not first-line antibiotics in dentistry. The fluoroquinolones should be avoided in pregnant women and children under 18; their use should be limited to complex cases managed by specialists.

Within these parameters, an individual patient's medical history must be considered when the clinician chooses an antibiotic. Table 14.11 lists the general pharmacologic characteristics of the commonly used antibiotics.

Step 7. Administer the antibiotic appropriately

Table 14.11 lists the usual dose and dosage interval for the antibiotics commonly used to treat orofacial infections. Pediatric dosages are listed by weight, which requires knowledge of the weight of the pediatric patient and calculation of the correct dose. Often, the clinician will have to choose the preparation of the given antibiotic that most closely matches the calculated dose.

Historically, the duration of the antibiotic regimen has been 7 to 10 days, based on a theoretical aim of minimizing the likelihood of development of antibiotic resistance and decreasing the likelihood of recurrence of the infection. However, two recent randomized clinical trials have shown that a 3- to 4-day course of an antibiotic, combined with the appropriate dental treatment, had equally good cure rates as a 7- to 10-day course of the antibiotic.[8,9] It has been postulated that a shorter antibiotic course will result in decreased antibiotic resistance, but this theory has not been scientifically demonstrated in orofacial infections. Because patient compliance with the prescribed antibiotic course declines as symptoms resolve, usually around 3 to 4 days, it makes practical clinical sense to prescribe antibiotics for only 3 to 4 days when the appropriate dental care is performed.

Certain antibiotics antagonize each other. This is true with the macrolides (erythromycin family) and the lincosamides (clindamycin family). Therefore, clindamycin and erythromycin are not combined.

Patient compliance with the prescribed regimen is better when the number of pills and the frequency of dosing is reduced. This fact may cause the clinician to favor the administration of an antibiotic that requires a three-times-per-day schedule, such as amoxicillin, versus a four-times-per-day antibiotic, such as penicillin.

When contemplating an antibiotic prescription, the clinician must be aware of the patient's past medical history and current medications. This requirement has become even more important recently because the aging population is being treated with an increasing array of new and old medications. Further, the newer antibiotics seem to have much more frequent drug interactions and untoward side effects than older antibiotics. The dentist may need to consult an up-to-date reference, some of which are online, in order to check for possible drug interactions between the contemplated antibiotic and the patient's current medications.

Step 8. Re-evaluate frequently

Increasing severity of infection warrants increasing the frequency of follow-up examinations. For outpatients, the most concerning cases of infection may need to be seen daily until definite improvement is noted. If incision and drainage has been performed, the drain is usually removed 2 to 3 days after placement. By this time, the patient will be able to report a definite change in the level of malaise (general feeling of being unwell) for the better or the worse. Changes in malaise often precede a visible increase or decrease in swelling, fever, trismus,

Table 14.11 Pharmacology of commonly used antibiotics in orofacial infection

Antibiotic	Spectrum	Dosage (po)	Mode of action	Side effects	Comments
Penicillin V	Oral streptococci Oral anaerobes *Actinomyces* *Eikenella* species **Resistant:** Staph Enteric flora *Bacteroides fragilis*	500 mg qid Children: 25–50 mg/kg/day	Bactericidal Interferes with cell wall synthesis of bacteria in their growth phase.	Allergy—may cause anaphylactic shock (~0.05%) Rare GI disturbances Superinfection by resistant bacteria may occur. Rash in 3% of patients, serum sickness in 4%.	Produces lower blood levels than IV Pen. G. Excreted by kidneys. Administer before meals.
Amoxicillin (Semisynthetic penicillin)	Oral streptococci Oral anaerobes *Actinomyces* **Resistant:** Staphylococci *Pseudomonas* spp.	500 mg tid OR 875 mg bid Children: 20–50 mg per /kg/day	Bactericidal Interferes with cell wall synthesis of bacteria in their growth phase.	Allergy – may cause anaphylactic shock. Most common cause of antibiotic- associated colitis Diarrhea in 10% of patients	Less effective against oral streps than penicillin V; has replaced ampicillin because of tid dosing.
Amoxicillin + clavulanic acid (Augmentin®)	Oral streptococci Oral anaerobes *Actinomyces* Staphylococci Enteric Gram-negative rods *H. influenzae*	500 mg tid children: 20–40 mg/kg/day	Bactericidal Interferes with cell wall synthesis of bacteria in their growth phase. Clavulanic acid inhibits penicillinase made by staphs and most Gram-negative rods.	Allergy may cause anaphylactic shock. Common cause of antibiotic-associated colitis. Diarrhea in 9% of patients; less frequent with bid dosing (less clavulanate).	Less effective against oral streps than penicillin V Not effective against methicillin-resistant *S. aureus*. Improved coverage for staph and enteric flora.
Azithromycin (Zithromax®)	Some oral streptococci Some staph Atypical pathogens in HIV+ patients **Resistant:** Most staph *Bacteroides fragilis*	500 mg on day 1, then 250 mg/day for days 2–5 Children: 10–12 mg/kg on day 1, then 5 mg/kg/day for days 2–5	Bactericidal or bacteriostatic. Interferes with protein synthesis during growth phase. Active uptake of the antibiotic by phagocytes may improve coverage over *in vitro* data.	GI upset: less common than with other macrolides.	Fewer drug interactions than with the other macrolides; concentrates in phagocytes at up to 15x concentration in serum.

Drug	Spectrum / Resistance	Dose	Mechanism	Notes	Additional Notes
Clindamycin (Cleocin®)	Oral streptococci Staphylococci Anaerobes **Resistant:** Enteric flora *Eikenella corrodens*	150–600 mg qid Children: 15–30 mg/kg/day	Bactericidal or bacteriostatic. Interferes with protein synthesis.	Common cause of antibiotic-associated colitis.	Colitis is due to *C. difficile* – treatable with oral metronidazole. Does **not** cross blood–brain barrier.
Cephalexin (Keflex—1st generation cephalosporin)	Staphylococci Oral streptococci **Resistant:** Oral anaerobes Enteric flora *B. fragilis*	500 mg qid Children: 25–50 mg/kg/day	Bactericidal. Interferes with cell wall synthesis of bacteria in their growth phase.	Allergy cross-reacts with those that have had an anaphylactoid reaction to penicillins.	Does not cross blood–brain barrier in a predictable fashion.
Metronidazole (Flagyl)	Obligate anaerobes only All *Bacteroides* spp. **Resistant:** All facultative and aerobic bacteria	500 mg qid **Children: DO NOT USE**	Bactericidal. Interferes with folic acid metabolism.	Metallic taste. Antabuse-like effect. Carcinogenic in rats, in pregnancy. May aggravate candidiasis.	Crosses blood–brain barrier well. Can be used with other antibiotics, esp. penicillin.
Moxifloxacin (Avelox)	Oral streps and anaerobes, *E. corrodens* Actinomyces, *B. fragilis*, Staph, incl. some MRSA, most enteric flora **Resistant:** Enterococci, *P. aeruginosa*	400 mg qid **Children: DO NOT USE** **Pregnancy: DO NOT USE**	Bactericidal. Interferes with DNA synthesis (DNA gyrase).	Possible ↑QT interval if used with quinidine, procainamide, amiodarone, sotalol, or if hypokalemic.	Chondrotoxic in pregnancy and children. May cause Achilles tendon rupture. Mental clouding and decreased energy common.

drainage, or other signs of infection, yet malaise is a quite reliable indicator of the patient's progress. If malaise is improving and the drainage has diminished significantly, drains may be removed. The incision is left open to allow further drainage to occur if needed. The patient may be instructed to irrigate the oral wound with a plastic-tipped syringe using saline solution. Healing is by secondary intention.

A second follow-up visit is made approximately 7 days after incision and drainage, assuming that a sooner follow-up visit is not indicated. In uncomplicated cases, the swelling will be markedly decreased, the pain level will be minimal, and the oral wound will be healing without further drainage. Continued pain, drainage, or swelling may indicate a treatment failure, which may require evaluation by an oral and maxillofacial surgeon.

The potential causes of treatment failure are shown in Table 14.12. Inadequate surgery is the first cause of treatment failure that should be ruled out. Surgical treatment may be inadequate if the cause of the infection, such as an additional tooth, has not been completely removed; if there is an undrained loculation of pus; or if a foreign body, such as a dental implant, is providing a microenvironment for bacteria that is sheltered from antibiotics and physical debridement.

Another potential cause of treatment failure may concern compliance with the prescribed the antibiotic regimen. The patient may not be taking the antibiotic correctly due to misunderstanding or may not be taking the antibiotic at all because he or she cannot afford to buy it. A patient also may not comply with the prescribed regimen because of tolerance issues, such as nausea, allergic reaction, or another unpleasant side effect. Such issues may be elucidated by thoughtful, considerate questioning.

Table 14.12 Causes of treatment failure

Inadequate surgery
Incomplete removal of cause of infection
Remaining loculations of abscess/cellulitis
Blocked surgical drainage pathway
Postoperative spread of infection
Retained foreign body
Oroantral fistula
Lack of compliance with antibiotic regimen
Insufficient time for antibiotic effect
Antibiotic resistance
Osteomyelitis
Underlying tumor, especially malignancy

After inadequate surgery and antibiotic compliance issues have been ruled out, the clinician may consider bacterial resistance to the antibiotic. First, the dentist should allow at least 3 days for the antibiotic to achieve a noticeable clinical effect. With many antibiotics, including the penicillins, the blood level that can be achieved by the oral administration route is only a fraction of what can be achieved intravenously. Therefore, given appropriate surgical therapy, in the absence of clear clinical deterioration, the antibiotic should not be changed before adequate time has passed for its effect to become clinically apparent.

If resistant bacteria are suspected, it is wise to sample the site of infection with both aerobic and anaerobic cultures as early as possible. The oral pathogens grow slowly in the laboratory, which may delay useful antibiotic sensitivity results for as much as 2 weeks after sampling.

When orofacial infection persists for more than 4 weeks after the initiation of treatment, osteomyelitis may be suspected. A clinical sign highly suggestive of osteomyelitis is the onset of paresthesia of the lower lip and/or chin during the treatment course for orofacial infection. Paresthesia that develops immediately after surgery suggests surgical trauma to the inferior alveolar nerve, but if the paresthesia is not closely related temporally to a surgical insult, then it is likely that the infection is causing inflammation along the sheath of the inferior alveolar nerve. Because the inferior alveolar nerve canal is deep within the mandible, bone infection may be present. Confirming a diagnosis of osteomyelitis can be difficult as radiographic changes occur late, and radionuclide bone scans are often falsely positive in an area that has undergone recent surgery. Suspected osteomyelitis is an indication for consultation with an oral and maxillofacial surgeon.

Less commonly, infection will not resolve if there is an underlying oroantral fistula, with repeated contamination of the site by retained food, fluids, and infection in the maxillary sinus. An infected tumor, especially a malignancy, has limited blood supply and little potential for healing, which will promote persistent infection.

Prophylactic antibiotics

There are three types of infection following dental procedures which prophylactic antibiotics have been used to prevent: endocarditis, late prosthetic joint infection, and surgical wound infection. For ethical reasons, it is impossible to do definitive clinical trials of the effectiveness of prophylactic antibiotics in preventing post-procedure endocarditis and late prosthetic joint infection. Therefore, the available research is primarily descriptive and only able to identify correlations among dental procedures, pre-existing dental disease, and the outcomes of endocarditis or infection of prosthetic joints; it cannot identify causation. Therefore, dentists must use published guidelines, leavened with clinical judgment.

Endocarditis

The American Dental Association and the American Heart Association have long collaborated to develop guidelines for dentists to prevent post-procedural endocarditis; there have been a series of revisions to these guidelines over the past several decades. The dentist must remain abreast of each successive revision. According to the current guidelines, all dental procedures that involve manipulation of gingival tissue or the periapical region of teeth or perforation of the oral mucosa (other than local anesthetic injections through uninfected tissue) require antibiotic prophylaxis. The latest guidelines were published in 2007 and are summarized in Tables 14.13 and 14.14.[10]

Late prosthetic joint infection

In 1997 and in 2003, the American Dental Association and the American Academy of Orthopaedic Surgeons published joint guidelines on the prevention of infection of prosthetic joint implants following dental procedures. The revised 2003 guidelines recommended antibiotic prophylaxis for dental procedures likely to cause bacteremia in prosthetic joints placed 2 years or less previously, and in certain comorbidities, such as insulin-dependent diabetes.

In 2009, the American Academy of Orthopaedic Surgeons unilaterally published a statement saying that all patients with prosthetic joints should receive antibiotic prophylaxis for dental procedures likely to cause bleeding, regardless of the time of initial placement of the joint prosthesis.

In 2012, the American Dental Association and the American Academy of Orthopaedic Surgeons jointly published an evidence-based guideline and report that critically evaluated the scientific evidence concerning the causation of late prosthetic joint infection by dental procedures and the potential benefit of antibiotic

Table 14.13 Indications for antibiotic prophylaxis of endocarditis following dental procedures

Prosthetic cardiac valve or prosthetic material used for cardiac valve repair
Previous infective endocarditis
Congenital heart disease (CHD)*
Unrepaired cyanotic CHD, including palliative shunts and conduits
Completely repaired congenital heart defect with prosthetic material or device, whether placed by surgery or by catheter intervention, during the first 6 months after the procedure[†]
Repaired CHD with residual defects at the site or adjacent to the site of a prosthetic patch or prosthetic device (which inhibit endothelialization)
Cardiac transplantation recipients who develop cardiac valvulopathy

*Except for the conditions listed above, antibiotic prophylaxis is no longer recommended for any other form of CHD.
†Prophylaxis is reasonable because endothelialization of prosthetic material occurs within 6 months after the procedure.
Source: Wilson W, Taubert KA, Gewitz M, Lockhart PB. Prevention of Infective Endocarditis: Guidelines from the American Heart Association: A Guideline from the American Heart Association Rheumatic Fever, Endocarditis, and Kawasaki Disease Committee, Council on Cardiovascular Disease in the Young, and the Council on Clinical Cardiology, Council on Cardiovascular Surgery and Anesthesia, and the Quality of Care and Outcomes Research Interdisciplinary Working Group. *Circulation.* 2007;116:1736–54; originally published online April 19, 2007.

prophylaxis for dental procedures in patients with prosthetic joints. Their three recommendations are:[11]

1. The practitioner might consider discontinuing the practice of routinely prescribing prophylactic antibiotics for patients with hip and knee prosthetic joint implants who are undergoing dental procedures. (Strength of Recommendation: Limited)

2. We are unable to recommend for or against the use of topical oral antimicrobials in patients with prosthetic joint implants or other orthopedic implants who are undergoing dental procedures. (Strength of Recommendation: Inconclusive)

3. In the absence of reliable evidence linking poor oral health to prosthetic joint infection, it is the opinion of the working group that patients with prosthetic joint implants or other orthopedic implants should maintain appropriate oral hygiene. (Strength of Recommendation: Consensus)

The lack of strength of these recommendations reflects the lack of determinative scientific information about this question. The report states, "Practitioners should be cautious in deciding whether to follow a recommendation

Table 14.14 Prophylactic antibiotic regimens for prevention of endocarditis following dental procedures

Situation	Agent	Single dose: 30–60 minutes before procedure
Oral	Amoxicillin	Adults: 2 g; Children: 50 mg/kg
Unable to take oral medications	Ampicillin	Adults: 2 g IM or IV; Children: 50 mg/kg IM or IV
	OR	
	Cefazolin	Adults: 1 g IM or IV; Children: 50 mg/kg IM or IV
	OR	
	Ceftriaxone	Adults: 1 g IM or IV; Children: 50 mg/kg IM or IV
Allergic to penicillin	Clindamycin	Adults: 600 mg; Children: 20 mg/kg
	OR	
	Cephalexin[†]	Adults: 2 g; Children: 50 mg/kg
	OR	
	Azithromycin or clarithromycin	Adults: 500 mg; Children: 15 mg/kg
Allergic to penicillin and unable to take oral medications	Clindamycin	Adults: 600 mg; Children: 20 mg/kg IV
	OR	
	Cefazolin[†] or ceftriaxone[†]	Adults: 1 g IM or IV; Children: 50 mg/kg IM or IV

Total children's dose should not exceed adult dose.
[†]Cephalosporins should not be used in an individual with a history of anaphylaxis, angioedema, or urticaria with penicillins or ampicillin.
IM = intramuscular; IV = intravenous.
Adapted from: Wilson W, Taubert KA, Gewitz M, Lockhart PB. Prevention of Infective Endocarditis: Guidelines from the American Heart Association: A Guideline from the American Heart Association Rheumatic Fever, Endocarditis, and Kawasaki Disease Committee, Council on Cardiovascular Disease in the Young, and the Council on Clinical Cardiology, Council on Cardiovascular Surgery and Anesthesia, and the Quality of Care and Outcomes Research Interdisciplinary Working Group. *Circulation*. 2007;116:1736–54; originally published online April 19, 2007.

classified as Limited, and should exercise judgment and be alert to emerging publications that report evidence. Patient preference should have a substantial influencing role."[11]

Two recently published case series have not found any association between late prosthetic joint infection and dental procedures, whether antibiotic prophylaxis was used or not. The weakness of these studies is that they were not able to differentiate between prosthetic joint infections caused by oral pathogens and those caused by other bacteria, such as *Staphylococcus aureus*.[12,13] In one of these studies, there were no microbiologic data available for consideration,[12] and, in the other, there was not a large enough subset of cases caused by oral pathogens to allow for statistically valid conclusions to be drawn.[13]

The risks of allergic reaction to antibiotics and the development of antibiotic resistance, in addition to the cost of antibiotic prophylaxis, may outweigh the potential benefit of preventing late prosthetic joint infection. Scientific evidence is insufficient on this question. Therefore, the clinician must use clinical judgment to decide whether to use antibiotic prophylaxis in the patient with a prosthetic joint.

Wound infection

Fortunately, there is evidence to support the benefit of antibiotic prophylaxis in prevention of postoperative wound infection for certain dental procedures.

In 2007, two reliable studies were published that provided evidence that antibiotic prophylaxis does reduce the risk of infection following removal of impacted mandibular third molars. Ren *et al.* performed a systematic review and meta-analysis of the available randomized clinical trials of antibiotic prophylaxis for impacted mandibular third molar removal. After combining all the available studies, their statistical method demonstrated a benefit of antibiotic prophylaxis for third molar removal only when the antibiotic was started 30 to 90 minutes before the surgery. There was a small additional benefit when the antibiotic was continued for 3 to 5 days after

Table 14.15 Recommendations about antibiotic prophylaxis for dental procedures

Medical condition	Prophylaxis recommended?	Antibiotic regimen
High risk of endocarditis*	Yes	AHA regimen**
Mitral valve prolapse	No	
Heart murmurs	No	
Cardiac pacemaker	No	
Implanted defibrillator	No	
Coronary artery bypass graft	No	
Coronary artery stents	No	
Prosthetic joints	No	
Cancer chemotherapy	Yes, although definite evidence is lacking	AHA regimen**
Renal hemodialysis	Yes, although definite evidence is lacking	AHA regimen**
Poorly controlled diabetes mellitus	Yes, although definite evidence is lacking	AHA regimen**
Ventriculoatrial shunts for hydrocephalus	Yes	AHA regimen**
Ventriculoperitoneal shunts for hydrocephalus	No	
Immune system compromise	Yes, only for invasive dental procedures	AHA regimen**
Impacted mandibular third molar removal	Yes	Preoperative dose before procedure, with possible 3–5 day postoperative course
Dental implant placement	Yes	AHA regimen**
Extraction of erupted teeth	No	

*See Table 14.13 for conditions with high risk of endocarditis.
**See Table 14.14 for American Heart Association recommended prophylactic antibiotic regimens.

surgery. There was no additional benefit when the antibiotic was started postoperatively.[14]

Halpern *et al.* performed a randomized clinical trial comparing an intravenous antibiotic started just before impacted mandibular third molar removal with no antibiotic. They found a significant benefit of the antibiotic in reducing postoperative infection.[15]

Thus, it appears evident that preoperative, not postoperative antibiotic administration is of benefit in preventing infection following impacted mandibular third molar removal. The antibiotic may be continued for 3 to 5 days postoperatively. However, starting the antibiotic after surgery is of no benefit.

The short-term survival of dental implants is significantly increased when antibiotic prophylaxis is used, at least in most of the available studies.[16] Some studies, however, show no benefit of the antibiotic. All of the studies used a preoperative antibiotic dose. The available evidence is thus not definitive but suggests that antibiotic prophylaxis may be indicated for dental implant placement.

For immunocompromised patients, there are expert recommendations for antibiotic prophylaxis for dental procedures in patients undergoing cancer chemotherapy, hemodialysis (because of the surgically constructed arteriovenous shunt), organ transplantation, and in patients who have ventriculoatrial shunts used to treat hydrocephalus.[17]

There is no scientific evidence or expert recommendation to support antibiotic prophylaxis for removal of erupted teeth in otherwise healthy patients.

Table 14.15 summarizes the current recommendations about the use of prophylactic antibiotics in dentistry.

Summary

This chapter has discussed several principles that general dentists may use in the management and prevention of orofacial infections. These are now summarized and may represent a revision of long-held beliefs that have not withstood the scrutiny of scientific investigation.

1. The primary treatment of dental infections is surgery, not antibiotics. Appropriate surgery includes but is not limited to root canal therapy, periodontal debridement, tooth extraction, and incision and drainage.

2. Within the first few minutes of the clinical encounter with a patient suffering from an orofacial infection, the decision to treat or refer the patient to an oral

and maxillofacial surgeon has a determinative effect on the outcome.

3. Incision and drainage of an infected site in the cellulitis stage appears to abort the spread of infection into deeper spaces.

4. The choice of supportive antibiotic therapy, among those commonly used for orofacial infection, is determined by the individual patient's medical history, pharmacologic safety, and cost. No one of these antibiotics has demonstrated therapeutic superiority over the others.

5. Treatment failure in orofacial infections is managed by re-evaluation of the need for additional surgical procedures, compliance with the supportive antibiotic regimen, the time necessary for clinical effect of the antibiotic, and the need for culture and sensitivity testing. When these potential causes are ruled out, a change of antibiotic therapy may be considered.

6. Antibiotic prophylaxis may be effective in dentistry. Published guidelines and available scientific evidence should guide the use of antibiotic prophylaxis. Currently, antibiotic prophylaxis may be of benefit in prevention of endocarditis, in impacted mandibular third molar surgery, in dental implant surgery, and in immunocompromised conditions.

References

1. Flynn TR, Shanti RM, Levy M, Adamo AK, Kraut RA, Trieger N. Severe odontogenic infections, Part one: prospective report. *Journal of Oral and Maxillofacial Surgery.* 2006; 64: 1093–103.
2. Flynn TR, Shanti RM, Hayes C. Severe odontogenic infections, Part two: prospective outcomes study. *Journal of Oral and Maxillofacial Surgery.* 2006; 64: 1104–13.
3. Williams AC. Ludwig's angina. *Surgery for Gynecology and Obstetrics.* 1940; 70: 140.
4. Williams AC, Guralnick WC. The diagnosis and treatment of Ludwig's angina: a report of twenty cases. *New England Journal of Medicine.* 1943; 228: 443.
5. Flynn TR. What are the antibiotics of choice for odontogenic infections, and how long should the treatment course last? *Oral and Maxillofacial Surgical Clinics of North America.* 2011; 23: 519–36.
6. Runyon MS, Brennan MT, Batts JJ, Glaser TE, Fox PC, Norton HJ, et al. Efficacy of Penicillin for dental pain without overt infection. *Academic Emergency Medicine.* 2004; 11: 1268–71.
7. ADA Council on Scientific Affairs: Combating antibiotic resistance. *Journal of the American Dental Association.* 2004; 135: 484–7.
8. Lewis MA, McGowan DA, MacFarlane TW. Short-course high-dosage amoxycillin in the treatment of acute dentoalveolar abscess. *British Dental Journal.* 1986; 161(8): 299–302.
9. Chardin H, Yasukawa K, Nouacer N, et al. Reduced susceptibility to amoxicillin of oral streptococci following amoxicillin exposure. *Journal of Medical Microbiology.* 2009; 58(Pt 8): 1092–7.
10. Wilson W, Taubert KA, Gewitz M, Lockhart PB, Baddour LM, Levison MD, et al. Prevention of infective endocarditis: Guidelines from the American Heart Association: A Guideline from the American Heart Association Rheumatic Fever, Endocarditis, and Kawasaki Disease Committee, Council on Cardiovascular Disease in the Young, and the Council on Clinical Cardiology, Council on Cardiovascular Surgery and Anesthesia, and the Quality of Care and Outcomes Research Interdisciplinary Working Group. *Circulation.* 2007; 116: 1736–54; originally published online April 19, 2007.
11. American Academy of Orthopaedic Surgeons, American Dental Association. Prevention of orthopaedic implant infection in patients undergoing dental procedures: Evidence-based guideline and evidence report. Available from http://www.ada.org/sections/professionalResources/pdfs/PUDP_guideline.pdf (accessed 16 January 2015).
12. Skaar DD, O'Connor H, Hodges JS, Michalowicz BS. Dental procedures and subsequent prosthetic joint infections: Findings from the Medicare current beneficiary survey. *Journal of the American Dental Association.* 2011; 142: 1343–51.
13. Berbari EF, Osmon DR, Carr A, Hanssen AD, Baddour LM, Greene D, et al. Dental procedures as risk factors for prosthetic hip or knee infection: a hospital-based prospective case-control study. *Clinical Infectious Diseases.* 2010; 50: 8–16.
14. Ren Y-F, Malmstrom HS. Effectiveness of antibiotic prophylaxis in third molar surgery: A meta-analysis of randomized controlled clinical trials. *Journal of Oral and Maxillofacial Surgery.* 2007; 65: 1909–21.
15. Halpern LR, Dodson TB. Does prophylactic administration of systemic antibiotics prevent postoperative inflammatory complications after third molar surgery? *Journal of Oral and Maxillofacial Surgery* 2007; 65: 177–85.
16. Sharaf B, Dodson TB. Does the use of prophylactic antibiotics decrease implant failure? *Oral and Maxillofacial Surgical Clinics of North America.* 2011; 23(4): 547–50.
17. Tong DC, Rothwell BR. Antibiotic prophylaxis in dentistry: A review and practice recommendations. *Journal of the American Dental Association.* 2000; 131: 366–74.
18. Gilmore WC, Jacobus NV, Gorbach SL, Doku HC, Tally FP. A prospective double-blind evaluation of penicillin versus clindamycin in the treatment of odontogenic infections. *Journal of Oral and Maxillofacial Surgery* 1986; 46: 1065–70.
19. von Konow L, Nord CE. Ornidazole compared to phenoxymethylpenicillin in the treatment of orofacial infections. *Journal of Antimicrobial Chemotherapy.* 1983; 11: 207–15.

20. Mangundjaja S, Hardjawinata K. Clindamycin versus ampicillin in the treatment of odontogenic infections. *Clinical Therapy.* 1990; 12: 242–9.

21. Lewis MA, Carmichael F, MacFarlane TW, Milligan SG. A randomised trial of co-amoxiclav (Augmentin) versus penicillin V in the treatment of acute dentoalveolar abscess. *British Dental Journal.* 1993; 175: 169–74.

22. Davis WM Jr, Balcom JH 3rd. Lincomycin studies of drug absorption and efficacy. An evaluation by double-blind technique in treatment of odontogenic infections. *Oral Surgery, Oral Medicine and Oral Pathology.* 1969; 27: 688–96.

23. Matijević S, Lazić Z, Kuljić-Kapulica N, Nonković Z. Empirical antimicrobial therapy of acute dentoalveolar abscess. *Vojnosanit Pregl.* 2009; 66: 544–50.

24. Ingham HR, Hood FJ, Bradnum P, Tharagonnet D, Selkon JB. Metronidazole compared with penicillin in the treatment of acute dental infections. *British Journal of Oral Surgery.* 1977; 14: 264–9.

25. Al-Nawas B, Walter C, Morbach T, Seitner N, Siegel E, Maeurer M, et al. Clinical and microbiological efficacy of moxifloxacin versus amoxicillin/clavulanic acid in severe odontogenic abscesses: a pilot study. *European Journal of Clinical Microbiology and Infectious Diseases.* 2009; 28: 75–82.

26. Brook I, Frazier EH, Gher ME. Aerobic and anaerobic microbiology of periapical abscess. *Oral Microbiology and Immunology.* 1991; 6: 123–5.

27. von Konow L, Köndell PA, Nord CE, Heimdahl A. Clindamycin versus phenoxymethylpenicillin in the treatment of acute orofacial infections. *European Journal of Clinical Microbiology and Infectious Diseases.* 1992; 11: 1129–35.

28. Lewis MA, Parkhurst CL, Douglas CW, Martin MV, Absi EG, Bishop PA, et al. Prevalence of penicillin resistant bacteria in acute suppurative oral infection. *Journal of Antimicrobial Chemotherapy.* 1995; 35: 785–91.

CHAPTER 15

Complications of Dentoalveolar Surgery

Patrick J. Louis

Department of Oral and Maxillofacial Surgery, University of Alabama at Birmingham, Birmingham, AL, USA

Introduction

Dentoalveolar procedures are among the most common procedures performed by the oral and maxillofacial surgeon (OMS). The OMS must be familiar with the complications associated with dentoalveolar procedures and how to prevent and manage them.

Many complications are avoidable. Certainly, surgical skills and knowledge of the anatomy play an important role in the prevention of complications. It is also important for the OMS to be familiar with the patient and to know why the patient is seeking treatment. This starts with a detailed history and physical examination (H&P). Although not the focus of this chapter, risk assessment must be performed before treating any patient. Without a proper H&P, the clinician is unable to assess the risks of giving anesthesia to and performing surgery on each patient. Systemic risk assessment will be discussed elsewhere in this text. This chapter will focus on local complications associated with dentoalveolar surgery and how to prevent and manage them. The following complications will be discussed: non-healing wound, hemorrhage, postoperative edema, trismus, tooth and root displacement, oroantral communication, alveolar osteitis, nerve damage, and fracture.

Non-healing wound

Background

Failure of a wound to heal can be caused by local and systemic disorders.[1-5] In developed countries, nutritional deficiencies are uncommon but can occur.

Two conditions that have an effect on healing and that are frequently encountered by the OMS and must be considered include radiation-induced osteonecrosis (ORN) and medication related osteonecrosis of the jaw (MRONJ). ORN is defined as an area of exposed, devitalized irradiated bone that fails to heal over a period of 3 to 6 months in the absence of local neoplastic disease.[6,7] Radiation results in a hypovascular, hypocellular, and hypoxic tissue bed with poor healing capabilities.[8] The radiation-induced fibroatrophic theory has been more recently proposed due to further research.[9] It suggests that the key event in the progression of ORN is the activation and deregulation of fibroblastic activity, which leads to atrophic tissue within a previously radiated area. The mechanism of cellular injury caused by radiation is well described.[4] Radiation interaction is both direct and indirect. Interactions with H_2O molecules create secondary particles that interact with cellular DNA. Ionizing radiation induces a variety of DNA lesions, including oxidized base damage, abasic sites, and single-strand breaks as well as double-strand breaks. Areas that receive higher doses of radiation Gy (Gy = one joule of absorbed dose per kilogram) are at risk for ORN if undergoing surgical procedures such as extraction (Figure 15.1).[10]

Medication related osteonecrosis of the jaw (MRONJ) is defined as necrotic exposed bone or bone that can be probed through an intraoral or extraoral fistula(e) in the maxillofacial region that persists for more than 8 weeks in a patient on current or previous antiresorptive or antiangiogenic agents in the absence of previous radiation without obvious metastatic disease. ONJ has been a growing concern for the dental and medical community. Many patients are on bisphosphonates for multiple

Manual of Minor Oral Surgery for the General Dentist, Second Edition. Edited by Pushkar Mehra and Richard D'Innocenzo.
© 2016 John Wiley & Sons, Inc. Published 2016 by John Wiley & Sons, Inc.

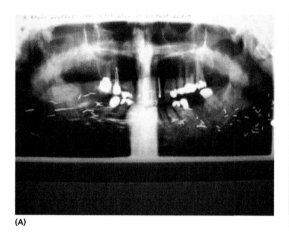
(A)

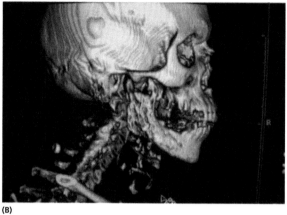
(B)

Figure 15.1 (A) Panoramic radiograph of a patient with osteonecrosis of the mandible secondary to previous radiation therapy (ORN). (B) Three-dimensional CT scan of the patient with ORN.

Table 15.1 Antiresorptive preparations commonly used in the US

	Primary Indication	Nitrogen Containing	Dose	Route
Alendronate (Fosamax®)	Osteoporosis	Yes	10 mg/day 70 mg/week	Oral
Risedronate (Actonel®)	Osteoporosis	Yes	5 mg/day 35 mg/week	Oral
Ibandronate (Boniva®)	Osteoporosis	Yes	2.5 mg/day 150 mg/month 3 mg every 3 months	Oral IV
Pamidronate (Aredia®)	Bone metastases	Yes	90 mg/3 weeks	IV
Zolendronate (Zometa®)	Bone metastases	Yes	4 mg/3 weeks	IV
(Reclast®)	Osteoporosis		5 mg/year	IV
Denosumab (Xgeva®)	Bone metastases	No	120 mg/4 weeks	SQ
(Prolia®)	Osteoporosis	Humanized monoclonal antibody	60 mg/6 months	SQ

Adapted from Ruggiero et al.[23] With permission from Elsevier.

reasons.[11–13] Bisphosphonates (BPs) are used to treat osteopenia, osteoporosis, and metastatic bone disease.[14–18] The mechanism of action is as follows: The potent groups of BPs (amino-BPs) are inhibitors of the mevalonate pathway, a biosynthetic pathway for isoprenoid proteins such as farsenyldiphosphate and geranylgeranyldiphosphate.[13] The Rho and Rac groups of proteins are responsible for cytoskeleton organization and cell membrane ruffling and are activated through geranylgeranylation.[19–21] The cytoskeleton is essential to maintain the "ruffled border," the area with which the osteoclast makes contact with bone and breaks down bone tissue. With the ruffled border compromised, the osteoclast initiates apoptosis, netting a decrease in bone turnover.

Patients undergoing treatment with oral bisphosphonates are considered to be at low risk for developing MRONJ when compared to patients undergoing therapy with intravenous (IV) bisphosphonates. The relative potency of the available bisphosphonates is listed in Table 15.1. Increased length of treatment and drug potency increase the risk of developing MRONJ.[22,23] Estimates of the cumulative incidence for developing ONJ in patients receiving IV bisphosphonate therapy range from 0.8 to 12%.[22–26] Patients receiving long-term oral BP therapy have an estimated incidence of developing MRONJ between 0.02 and 0.06%[23,27] (Figure 15.2). Two other agents have been implicated in causing MRONJ. These include denosumab, a RANKL

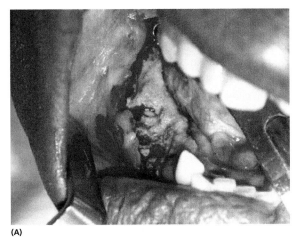
(A)

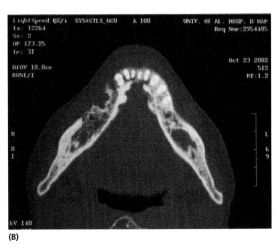
(B)

Figure 15.2 (A) Intraoral view of a mandible with ONJ. The patient has a history of multiple myeloma. (B) CT showing ONJ of the mandible.

ligand inhibitor, with similar indications as the bisphosphonates and antiangeogenic agents that interfere with the angiogenesis-signaling cascade and is used to treat certain types of tumors. The RANKL ligand inhibitors do not bind to the bone. The effects on bone are significantly diminished in 6 months once discontinued.

Prevention

Prevention of osteonecrosis is difficult for multiple reasons. Many cases of osteonecrosis are related to dental extraction, which is usually not an elective procedure. It is difficult for the clinician to determine a true risk for the development of osteonecrosis (ORN and MRONJ) in each patient. This makes it difficult to give clear recommendations to each patient. Also, evidence regarding preventive measures is difficult to interpret, may not be effective, and may not always be possible to implement.

Before radiation, the following is recommended:

- Patients should undergo a comprehensive dental evaluation including a detailed head and neck evaluation, radiographs, and detailed evaluation of the teeth for dental caries and periodontal disease.
- Teeth with poor or questionable prognoses must be extracted.
  - The optimal time for extraction of teeth is 21 days before initiating radiation therapy, and no less than 2 weeks before starting therapy.
  - Less optimally, extractions can be performed within 4 months of completion of therapy.[28]
- Dental treatment to optimize oral health should be performed:

  - Dental cleaning and fluoride treatment
  - Dental restorations (e.g., fillings) to eliminate dental caries
  - Removal of large- to moderate-sized tori
- Meticulous oral hygiene instructions are given:
  - Brush and floss twice daily.
  - Interproximal brushes should be used.
  - Avoid mouth rinses that contain alcohol.
  - Use an oral hygiene rinse formulated for xerostomia (e.g., Biotene).
- Custom dental trays are fabricated for the application of daily fluoride treatments.
- Weekly dental evaluation should occur during radiation therapy.
- Monthly dental evaluations should occur for the first 6 months following radiation.
- Post-radiation patients should be on 4-month recall appointments:
  - Perform dental and periodontal evaluation
  - Perform dental cleaning and fluoride treatment
  - Reinforce meticulous oral hygiene and the daily application of topical fluoride
  - Repair dental caries
  - Manage xerostomia (repair root caries and prescribe pilocarpine and other mouth moisturizing agents, as indicated).

There are several strategies that can be used for patients who have previously undergone radiation therapy. Identifying the degree of risk entails obtaining the patient's radiation dosimetry map to determine the amount of radiation exposure to the area that requires treatment. The incidence of ORN in the mandible following radiation treatment ranges from 2.6 to 18%. Dental extraction, before or after radiation, is reported as the most common cause of ORN in the irradiated maxilla or mandible.[28,29] Mandibular surgery, the use of cobalt radiation, and radiation doses greater than the biologically equivalent dose (BED) values of 102.6 Gy were significantly associated with the development of ORN.[10] A systematic review of the literature in another study reported that a radiation dose greater than 60 Gy resulted in a 12% risk of developing ORN, while doses of less than 60 Gy resulted in no patients developing ORN.[30] Advances in the delivery of radiation therapy, such as intensity-modulated radiation therapy (IMRT) have reduced the risk to 6% or less.[31,32]

Hyperbaric oxygen therapy (HBOT) is controversial but may have some benefit in the prevention and management of ORN. A pentoxifylline-tocopherol-clodronate combination (Pentoclo) may be beneficial in the management and prevention of ORN. Pentoxifylline, a methylxanthine derivative, exerts an anti-tumor necrosis factor (TNF)-alpha effect, vasodilates, and inhibits inflammatory reactions. Tocopherol (vitamin E) scavenges the reactive oxygen species (ROS) generated during oxidative stress. These two drugs work synergistically as potent antifibrotic agents. Clodronate is a BP that inhibits osteoclastic bone destruction and osteolysis.[33] With the cost of HBOT and the difficulty in obtaining insurance approval for prophylactic use, many clinicians have adopted the use of pentoxifylline and vitamin E, both before and after dental extractions until the wound has healed.

Before initiating antiresorptive or antiangiogenic therapy:

- Patients should undergo a comprehensive dental evaluation including a detailed head and neck evaluation, radiographs, and detailed evaluation of the teeth for dental caries and periodontal disease.
- Teeth with poor or questionable prognoses should be extracted.
  ○ The optimal time is before initiating IV therapy or before 4 years of oral therapy.
- Dental treatment to optimize oral health should be performed:
  ○ Dental cleaning and fluoride treatment
  ○ Dental restorations (e.g., fillings) to eliminate dental caries
  ○ Removal of large- to moderate-sized tori

- Meticulous oral hygiene instructions are given:
  ○ Brush and floss twice daily.
  ○ Interproximal brushes should be used.
- Custom dental trays are fabricated for the application of daily fluoride treatments.
- After initiating therapy, patients should be on 4-month recall appointments:
  ○ Perform dental and periodontal evaluation
  ○ Perform dental cleaning and fluoride treatment
  ○ Reinforce meticulous oral hygiene and the daily application of topical fluoride
  ○ Perform dental restorations, perform endodontic therapy, and eliminate irritational foci from restorations or dentures
  ○ The risks associated with oral surgical procedures such as dental implants, extractions, and extensive periodontal surgeries must be discussed with the patient and weighted against the benefits.

For individuals on IV BP therapy:

- Procedures that involve direct osseous injury should be avoided.
- Non-restorable teeth may be treated with endodontic therapy.
- Placement of dental implants in patients on the potent IV form of BPs and who have other risk factors should be avoided.

For individuals on oral BP therapy:

- Elective dentoalveolar surgery is not contraindicated.
- Patients should be adequately informed about the risk of compromised bone healing.
- Alteration in surgical planning is not necessary for patients who have taken oral BPs for less than 4 years and who have no other risk factors.
- For a patient who has taken oral BPs and corticosteroids and antiangiogenic agents for less than 4 years, consider discontinuing the oral BP therapy for 2 months. Treatment may be resumed after bone healing is completed. This decision should be made after consulting the treating physician and only if systemic conditions permit. The same strategy applies for patients who have taken oral BPs and steroids for more than 4 years.

There is some evidence to suggest that discontinuing oral BP therapy for 2 months before dentoalveolar surgery, and until osseous healing occurs, reduces the risk of developing MRONJ.[34,35] Zoledronate once yearly for the management of osteoporosis appears to be associated with a low risk for developing ONJ over a 3-year period.[36]

Management

According to one study, patients with higher-stage tumors, patients who continued to smoke or consume alcohol, and patients who had received a radiation dose >60 Gy had a poor response to conservative management of ORN and often required surgical resection.[37] A recent systematic review did not identify any reliable evidence to either support or refute the efficacy of HBOT in the prevention of post-extraction ORN in irradiated patients.[38] In cohort and observational studies, the occurrence rate of ORN in patients undergoing prophylactic HBOT ranged from 0 to 11% (median: 4.1%), whereas in the non-HBOT patients the range was from 0 to 29.9% (median: 7.1%).[38] Marx showed, in a randomized, prospective study, that patients undergoing HBOT had a lower incidence of ORN compared with an antibiotic group (5.4% vs. 29.9%).[39]

The treatment of ORN is based on the clinical stage. Jacobson *et al.* recommended the following protocol to manage ORN:

- Stage I disease represents small, superficial, localized bone resorption with cutaneous or mucosal dehiscence. This is treated with local wound care (oral rinses), HBOT for 20 dives, and antibiotic therapy to quell the superinfection that is often present. Patients who show improvement undergo an additional 10 dives of HBOT. Patients who do not show signs of healing undergo trans-oral debridement and additional HBOT.
- Stage II disease represents larger and deeper areas of bone resorption. Cortical and medullary bone is involved, and the mucosal or cutaneous areas of breakdown are moderate in size. This disease is treated with antibiotics, trans-oral debridement or sequestrectomy, and HBOT (20 dives preoperatively and 10 postoperative dives). Debridement is to bleeding bone, and a primary mucosal closure is achieved. If the mucosa is unable to be closed primarily, flap coverage is recommended. All wound problems or repeat bone exposures are treated with aggressive surgical extirpation of all diseased hard and soft tissue and an immediate reconstruction with vascularized free-tissue transfer.
- Stage III ORN is defined by full-thickness devitalization of bone, resorption of the inferior border of the mandible, fistula, or a pathological fracture. These patients are treated with an aggressive surgical

extirpation of all diseased hard and soft tissue, and then immediate reconstruction is performed using a free-tissue transfer. This aggressive surgical treatment is often performed without using HBOT (pre- or postoperatively) or debridement. HBOT may not be helpful in the management of these cases.[40]

In patients with MRONJ, treatment is directed at pain control, reducing the risk of infection, and extension of bone exposure and necrosis.[23] Because all of the patient's bone has been exposed to BP, surgical resection may not be effective. Mobile necrotic bone segments should be removed without exposing uninvolved bone. When possible, in consultation with the prescribing physician, BP therapy should be stopped or modified. Discontinuation of oral BP therapy in patients with bisphosphonate-related osteonecrosis of the jaw (BRONJ) has been associated with gradual improvement in clinical disease.[41]

In patients who have been diagnosed with MRONJ, management of the disease is based on staging (Table 15.2). The following list is based on the American Association of Oral and Maxillofacial Surgeons' position paper on Medication related ONJ—2014 update (Table 15.3).[23]

- Stage 0 is defined as patients who show no clinical evidence of necrotic bone but who present with nonspecific symptoms or clinical and radiographic findings. Provide symptomatic treatment, and manage conservatively. Systemic management can include the use of medication for chronic pain and the control of infection with antibiotics, when indicated.
- Stage 1 is defined as exposed and necrotic bone in patients who are asymptomatic and have no evidence of infection. These patients benefit from the use of oral antimicrobial rinses, such as chlorhexidine 0.12%. No surgical treatment is indicated.
- Stage 2 is defined as exposed and necrotic bone in patients who have pain and who show clinical evidence of infection. These patients benefit from the use of oral antimicrobial rinses combined with antibiotic therapy. Debridement may be indicated.
- Stage 3 is defined as exposed and necrotic bone in patients who have pain, infection, and one or more of the following: exposed necrotic bone extending beyond the region of alveolar bone (i.e., inferior border and ramus in the mandible, maxillary sinus, and zygoma in the maxilla), pathologic fracture, extraoral fistula, oral antral/oral nasal communication,

Table 15.2 Clinical staging of osteoradionecrosis

Stage		Description	Treatment
I		Superficial involvement, only cortical bone exposed Minimal soft tissue ulceration	Majority improve with conservative management
II	a: Minimal soft tissue ulceration b: Soft-tissue necrosis	Localized involvement of mandible, exposed cortical and medullary bone are necrotic Possible orocutaneous fistula	Majority improve with conservative management, surgical procedures, or hyperbaric oxygen therapy
III	a: Minimal soft tissue ulceration b: Soft tissue necrosis	Diffuse involvement of the mandible, including the lower border. Pathologic fracture may occur Possible orocutaneous fistula	Require surgical intervention, resection, and reconstruction

Source: Schwartz HC, Kagan AR. Osteoradionecrosis of the mandible: scientific basis for clinical staging. *Am J Clin Oncol.* 2002;25(2):168–9. Reproduced with permission of Lippincott Williams & Wilkins.

Table 15.3 Staging and treatment strategies

MRONJ[†] Staging	Treatment Strategies[‡]
At risk category No apparent necrotic bone in patients who have been treated with either oral or IV bisphosphonates	• No treatment indicated • Patient education
Stage 0 No clinical evidence of necrotic bone, but non-specific clinical findings, radiographic changes and symptoms	• Systemic management, including the use of pain medication and antibiotics
Stage 1 Exposed and necrotic bone, or fistulae that probes to bone, in patients who are asymptomatic and have no evidence of infection	• Antibacterial mouth rinse • Clinical follow-up on a quarterly basis • Patient education and review of indications for continued bisphosphonate therapy
Stage 2 Exposed and necrotic bone, or fistulae that probes to bone, associated with infection as evidenced by pain and erythema in the region of the exposed bone with or without purulent drainage	• Symptomatic treatment with oral antibiotics • Oral antibacterial mouth rinse • Pain control • Debridement to relieve soft tissue irritation and infection control
Stage 3 Exposed and necrotic bone or a fistula that probes to bone in patients with pain, infection, and one or more of the following: exposed and necrotic bone extending beyond the region of alveolar bone (i.e., inferior border and ramus in the mandible, maxillary sinus and zygoma in the maxilla) resulting in pathologic fracture, extra-oral fistula, oral antral/oral nasal communication, or osteolysis extending to the inferior border of the mandible of sinus floor	• Antibacterial mouth rinse • Antibiotic therapy and pain control • Surgical debridement/resection for longer term palliation of infection and pain

[†]Exposed or probable bone in the maxillofacial region without resolution for greater than 8 weeks in patients treated with an antiresorptive and/or an antiangiogenic agent who have not received radiation therapy to the jaws.
[‡]Regardless of the disease stage, mobile segments of bony sequestrum should be removed without exposing uninvolved bone.
The extraction of symptomatic teeth within exposed, necrotic bone should be considered since it is unlikely that the extraction will exacerbate the established necrotic process.

and osteolysis extending to the inferior border of the mandible or sinus floor. These patients benefit from debridement, including resection, combined with antibiotic therapy, which might offer long-term palliation with resolution of acute infection and pain.

Hemorrhage

Background

Bleeding during and/or after a dentoalveolar procedure is a significant concern for the clinician. Left untreated, this bleeding can result in the patient's death.[42] The risk of hemorrhage associated with third molar removal is estimated to be 0.2 to 1.4%.[43] Bleeding during surgery can be caused by local and systemic factors. Local causes include normal anatomic structures and pathologic lesions.[44,45] Systemic causes include hereditary coagulopathies and medications.[46,47]

Injury to any major vessel (arterial or venous) can result in significant bleeding. Life-threatening hemorrhage and airway compromise has been reported during dental implant placement in the mandible.[48,49] However, there is little risk of injury to vessels when performing most dentoalveolar surgical procedures. Knowledge of the general location of the vessels is helpful in planning surgery. Vessels that may be encountered include the lingual, facial, inferior alveolar, sublingual, submental, mental, buccal and greater palatine, arteries and veins.[45] The lingual and facial arteries arise directly from the external carotid. The terminal branches of many of these vessels in the head and neck anastomose with the vessel from the opposite side or with other vessels in the region, which allows for excellent collateral blood flow. The facial artery is close to the dentoalveolar region as it crosses the inferior border of the mandible anterior to the masseter muscle. The sublingual artery, which is a branch of the lingual artery, courses between the genioglossus and mylohyoid muscles and continues on to supply the sublingual salivary gland, the mylohyoid and surrounding muscles, and the mucous membranes and gingiva of the lingual surface of the mandible. The inferior alveolar artery (IAA) arises from the maxillary artery, the larger of the two terminal branches of the external carotid artery. The mylohyoid artery is a branch of the IAA, which travels in a groove along the lingual surface of the mandible. The mental artery is one of two terminal branches of the IAA that exits the mental foramen to supply blood to the chin and lip. The buccal artery is a branch of the maxillary artery that supplies the posterior aspect of the buccinator muscle. It is at risk for injury as it crosses the anterior aspect of the ramus of the mandible. The greater palatine artery originates from the descending palatine artery in the pterygopalatine fossa and descends into the pterygopalatine canal to emerge from the greater palatine foramen. It is the main artery supplying the tissues of the hard palate.

Pathologic lesions that can bleed if encountered during dentoalveolar procedures include arteriovenous malformations (AVMs), hemangiomas, giant cell tumors (GCTs), and aneurysmal bone cysts (ABCs) (Figure 15.3).[50-52] AVMs occur due to a lack of differentiation of arteries, veins, and capillaries during development, which results in direct communication between the arteries and veins. AVMs grow throughout life and are characterized according to the main vessel type and the flow. The character of the bleeding caused by an AVM is significantly different compared to the other lesions. Bleeding from an AVM is significant due to the high pressure and high flow associated with these lesions. Hemangiomas are present at birth, even if not clinically apparent. They typically appear during the first 2 years of life. Classically, a rapid proliferative phase occurs that outpaces body growth. Approximately 50% of hemangiomas involute by age 5 and about 70% by age 7.[53-55] ABCs are reactive lesions and can be associated with other bony lesions.[56] The histological exam reveals sinusoidal blood spaces devoid of endothelial lining.[57] GCTs predominately affect children and young adults. The histology is characterized by a proliferation of fibroblasts with various amounts of collagen with multinucleated giant cells dispersed throughout. A recent hypothesis is that these lesions should be considered proliferative vascular in origin or angiogenesis-dependent (Figure 15.4).[58,59]

Systemic disorders associated with an increased risk of bleeding are termed coagulopathies. They can be divided into hereditary and acquired causes. Hereditary coagulopathies include hemophilia A and B and von Willebrand disease (vWD). These are X-linked recessive diseases. Hemophilia A is due to missing or deficient normal factor VIII, and hemophilia B is due to missing or deficient normal factor IX production. In the general population, the incidence of these disorders are 1:5,000–10,000 male births for hemophilia A, and 1:20,000–34,000 male births for hemophilia B. Hemophilia can further be classified into mild, moderate, and severe depending on the amount of normal factor produced. Mild disease is characterized by 5 to 35% factor level, moderate disease has 1 to 5% factor level, and severe disease has less than 1% factor level. This impairs the capacity of the blood to coagulate and increases the risk of bleeding. If inadequately treated, hemophilia causes painful bleeding in joints and leads to disability. Intracranial bleeding can be fatal. von Willebrand disease (vWD) was first described in 1926 by Finnish physician Dr. Erik von Willebrand. vWD is caused by deficient or defective plasma von Willebrand factor (vWF), which is a large multimeric glycoprotein that plays a pivotal role in hemostasis by mediating platelet hemostatic function and stabilizing blood coagulation factor VIII. This disease affects 0.16 to 1% of the population (approximately 1 in 10,000).[60-62] It is divided into three subtypes: Type 1

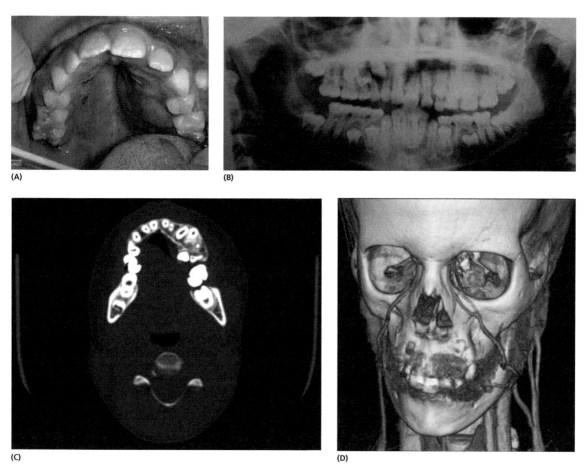

Figure 15.3 (A) Clinical photo of central capillary hemangioma involving the left maxilla. (B) Panoramic radiograph of the patient with central capillary hemangioma of the left maxilla showing asymmetry. (C) CT scan showing that the lesion is low-flow. (D) Three-dimensional CT reconstruction showing no significant increase in vascularity to the left maxilla.

vWD is a partial quantitative deficiency of essentially normal vWF. Type 2 vWD is characterized by a qualitative deficiency and defective vWF (further subdivided into types 2A, 2B, 2M, and 2N). Type 3 vWD is a virtually complete quantitative deficiency of vWF.[63] Acquired vWD has been described from multiple causes.[64–66]

Thrombocytopenia is defined as a platelet count below the 2.5th lower percentile of the normal platelet count distribution. However, the adoption of a cutoff value of 100×10^9/L may be more appropriate to identify a pathologic condition.[67,68] The major mechanisms for a reduced platelet count are decreased production (e.g., aplastic anemia, myelodysplastic syndromes, and chemotherapy-induced thrombocytopenia) and increased destruction of platelets (e.g., disseminated intravascular coagulation and the thrombotic micro-angiopathies). Less common mechanisms are platelet sequestration (congestive splenomegaly) and hemodilution (massive blood transfusion).[69,70] Other platelet disorders include adhesion defects, aggregation defects, and granular defects.[71,72]

Some medications that are known to prolong bleeding include antiplatelet drugs (aspirin, clopidogrel) and drugs that interfere with the clotting cascade (warfarin, enoxaparin, dabigatran etexilate).

- Aspirin: Low-dose (75–81 mg) aspirin inhibits cycloxygenase-1 (COX-1) in such a way that only thromboxane A2 (TXA_2) production is inhibited and not that of prostaglandin I2 (PGI_2).
- Clopidogrel: irreversibly binds to the P2Y12 adenosine diphosphate receptors, reducing platelet aggregation and adhesion. The half-life is 8 hours. The antiplatelet effects are irreversible and last for the life of the platelet (7 to 10 days).[73]

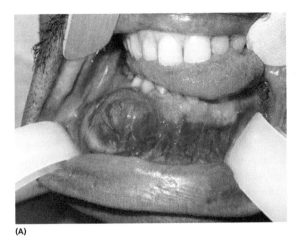
(A)

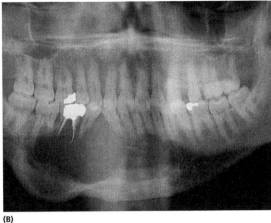
(B)

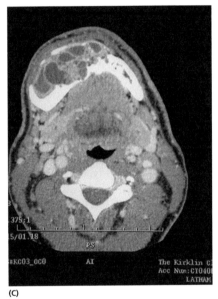
(C)

Figure 15.4 (A) Clinical photo of a patient with a pathologic lesion of the mandible. Needle aspiration should be performed before biopsy to rule out a vascular lesion that may cause bleeding. (B) Panoramic radiograph showing a large radiolucent lesion. (C) CT scan showing a large lesion in the anterior mandible.

- Warfarin: inhibits vitamin K-dependent coagulation factors; its effect is dose dependent. The half-life is 36 hours, and its full effect takes 72 to 96 hours.
- Enoxaparin: binds to antithrombin III and accelerates activity, inhibiting thrombin and factor Xa. The half-life is 4.5 to 7 hours.
- Dabigatran etexilate: directly and reversibly inhibits thrombin by interfering with the conversion of fibrinogen to fibrin. The half-life is 12 to 17 hours.[74]
- Rivaroxaban and apixaban: direct factor Xa inhibitors that bind to factor Xa.[74] The half-life is 5 to 9 hours for rivaroxaban and 12 hours for apixaban.

Prevention

Avoiding vessels that can cause significant bleeding during dentoalveolar surgery is usually not difficult because most of the structures that cause significant bleeding are distant from the surgical field. A structure that may be encountered during dentoalveolar surgery in the maxilla is the greater palatine artery (GPA). This encounter may occur during tori removal or soft-tissue graft harvest. Damage to this vessel can be avoided by placing full-thickness incisions in the midline or along the palatal gingival crevice. A subperiosteal dissection can proceed to and around the foramen with care not to disrupt the neurovascular bundle. Partial-thickness incisions can be used when harvesting epithelial grafts. When harvesting connective tissue grafts, the incisions are generally placed in the premolar region and anteriorly to avoid the GPA. In a recent study, the greater palatine foramen was located adjacent to the second molar (35.7%) or adjacent to the interproximal region of the second and third molars (35.7%) in women. In men, it was usually adjacent to the second molar (65%). The GPA branches most frequently at the level of the first premolar (38%) and the first and second molar region (43%) in women. In men, branching was commonly observed at the level of the first and second premolar region (56%) and the second and third molar region (32%).[75] In the mandible, the sublingual artery and vein, the IAA and inferior alveolar vein, and the mental artery and vein would be more commonly encountered due to their proximity to the surgical field for commonly performed dentoalveolar procedures. The sublingual artery can be avoided by performing a subperiosteal dissection along the lingual aspect of the mandible. The clinician should avoid perforation of the lingual cortex during dentoalveolar procedures. There have been reports of life-threatening hemorrhage during implant placement secondary to lingual cortical perforation.[48,49] The IAA and inferior alveolar vein could be encountered during removal of impacted wisdom teeth, removal of mandibular root fragments, and placement of a dental implant. In a recent study of the inferior neurovascular bundle, the vein was superior to the nerve, and there were often multiple veins. The artery was solitary and lingual to the nerve, slightly above the horizontal position. This position appeared to be consistent in all cases.[76] Thus, it is possible to have injury to the vessels without injury to the nerves.

Vascular lesions can be encountered during dentoalveolar procedures. These lesions may appear to be a periapical granuloma or abscess on plain films. A detailed history and exam may inform the clinician about the nature of lesion. Many patients will give a history of previous episodes of bleeding from the area. When a radiolucent the lesion is encountered, it is recommended that a needle be inserted into the lesion and aspirated to determine if the lesion is vascular. The lesion should be aspirated and the quality and quantity of the fluid assessed. When the aspirate is blood under pressure, the lesion is considered to be an AVM until proven otherwise. Bleeding from these lesions is life threatening, thus

additional work up is indicated, including a computerized tomography (CT) scan with contrast. If the aspirate is blood but with low flow, then other lesions should be considered, such as ABCs or GCTs. Three-dimensional imaging with contrast is recommended. The goal of this process is to avoid opening the lesion or performing surgery in this location until the threat of significant bleeding has been further elucidated.

Many patients with systemic coagulopathies will have a diagnosis before the visit with the oral and maxillofacial surgeon, but this is not always the case. This fact again underscores the need for a detailed H&P, including a review of systems (ROS), before any procedure is performed. The patient may complain of prolonged bleeding after a cut or minor surgery. Patients with this history should undergo further evaluation before surgery. The two main treatments for vWD are desmopressin (1-deamino-8-D-arginine vasopressin [DDAVP]) and clotting factor concentrates containing both vWF and FVIII (vWF/FVIII concentrate). Many hemophiliacs will have access to replacement factor and are aware of how much medication they require in order to achieve their therapeutic goal. For surgical procedures in which significant bleeding is anticipated, the goal is to achieve a factor level between 60 and 100%, depending on the type of hemophilia. The use of epsilon aminocaproic acid can help with clot stabilization and reduce the need for additional factor after tooth extraction.[77]

Thrombocytopenia can be managed by transfusion with platelets. Patients with platelet counts less than 30,000 to 50,000 are usually transfused when undergoing invasive procedures.[78,79] Patients with end-stage liver disease must also be thoroughly evaluated to determine the risk of bleeding; an international normalized ratio (INR) close to a normal range is recommended in these patients due to a significant risk of bleeding.

Some medications that are known to prolong bleeding include antiplatelet drugs (aspirin, clopidogrel) and drugs that interfere with the clotting cascade (warfarin, enoxaparin, dabigatran etexilate). When discontinuing these therapies, it is important to consult the prescribing physician to determine whether "bridging therapy" with enoxaparin or heparin is indicated. This procedure is always indicated for high-risk patients to shorten the time they are at risk for a thrombotic event. It is considered safe to proceed with minor dentoalveolar procedures such as dental extractions when the patient's INR is between 2 and 4.[80–82] Surgical extractions and dentoalveolar procedures in which significant bleeding is anticipated requires an INR of less than 2.

Low risk for thrombotic event

1. When indicated, consult the prescribing physician regarding discontinuing anticoagulant therapy.
2. Stop anticoagulant therapy 3 to 5 days before surgery.
3. If the INR is in a safe range, then proceed with the surgery. If the INR is elevated, then delay the surgical procedure.

High risk for thrombotic event

1. Evaluate the patient's risk of a thrombotic event.
2. When indicated, consult the prescribing physician regarding discontinuing anticoagulant therapy.
3. Stop anticoagulant therapy 3 to 5 days before surgery.
4. Begin enoxaparin the day after discontinuing warfarin.
5. Discontinue enoxaparin on the morning of the surgery (approximately 8 to 12 hours before surgery).
6. Check the INR on the morning of the surgery. If the INR is in a safe range, then proceed with the surgery. If the INR is elevated, then delay the surgical procedure. Restart enoxaparin until the INR is in a safe range.
7. After surgery, restart enoxaparin (usually 6 to 12 hours after completion of surgery).
8. Restart warfarin the evening after the surgery.
9. Check the INR beginning day 3 after the surgery. When in the therapeutic range, discontinue the enoxaparin.

Ecarin clotting time (ECT) is the most sensitive assay for monitoring dabigatran, but it is not readily available.[83] Thrombin time (TT) has been reported to be inaccurate at high concentrations of dabigatran. Although rivaroxaban and apixaban inhibit factor Xa levels, ECT or TT are not affected. Activated partial thromboplastin time (aPTT) is the best test for monitoring dabigatran, but sensitivity is reduced at higher concentrations. Although aPTT also may be prolonged by rivaroxaban, the aPTT is less reliable than PT at high concentrations of rivaroxaban.[74,83]

Management

Management of bleeding must take into account the etiology and character of the bleeding as well as the type of surgery. A tooth extraction is handled differently than a

procedure in which extensive soft-tissue dissection has been performed, such as a vestibuloplasty or floor of mouth lowering procedure.

When acute hemorrhage is encountered from an extraction site, digital pressure is used. The socket should be packed tight with a hemostatic agent such as a gelatin sponge or oxidized cellulose. The socket can also be sutured in a figure-eight fashion. Pressure with gauze is held for 20 to 30 minutes.

With soft-tissue bleeding or bone sources that are not as easily packed as an extraction site, other techniques must be used. Digital pressure is applied while supplies are gathered. Electrocautery is used for small vessels. Larger vessels and vessels that are not controlled with cautery should be ligated. If this procedure is unsuccessful, additional pressure with gauze should be applied.

If the bleeding is not controlled by the above actions, then call for help and transport the patient to the hospital. IV access must be established if it is not already in place. Fluid resuscitation must be started with lactated ringer or normal saline. If the airway is compromised secondary to the amount of bleeding or airway swelling, then placement of a laryngeal mask or endotracheal tube must be considered. In some cases, a surgical airway must be established. Once in the hospital, consider blood transfusion with O-negative or typed and cross-matched blood. The restrictive transfusion strategy is a threshold for transfusion of red blood cells for a hemoglobin level of 7 g/dl, with a target of 7 to 9 g/dl (70 to 90 g/L) in adults and most children.[79,84,85] A more liberal transfusion strategy is recommended for preterm infants or children with cyanotic heart disease, severe hypoxemia, active blood loss, or hemodynamic instability (a trigger of 9.5 g/dl, target 11 to 12 g/dl).[79,84,85] Additional diagnostic tests should be performed to determine the etiology of the bleeding. Laboratory tests should include PT (INR), PTT, and complete blood count (CBC) with platelets. A CT scan with contrast can be beneficial in evaluating pathology (neoplasm or hematoma).

When normal structures are the source of the bleeding or when a pathologic lesion is the source of the hemorrhage, ligation or embolization is the treatment of choice. The treatment is determined by the accessibility to the bleeding source and the potential complexity of the surgery. According to one study, ligation close to the source of bleeding is more effective than external carotid ligation due to the rich anastomosis of vessels in the head and neck. Selective embolization is recommended for AVMs and bleeding sources that are difficult to access and/or have failed to respond to previous surgery.

When a coagulopathy is suspected as the etiology of the bleeding, it must be corrected. An additional laboratory test that may be helpful is a clotting factor assay. This test takes valuable time, however, and treatment cannot be delayed while waiting for the results. Acute correction of a coagulopathy can be performed with the use of fresh frozen plasma (FFP) or prothrombin complex concentrates (PCCs). Plasma transfusion is recommended in patients with active bleeding and an INR greater than 1.6 or before an invasive procedure or surgery if a patient has been anticoagulated.[78] Platelet transfusion is indicated for the management of thrombocytopenia with platelet counts of less than 20,000 or between 20,000 and 30,000 when there is active bleeding.

PCCs are concentrated pooled plasma products that typically contain three (factors II, IX, and X) or four (factors II, VII, IX, and X) clotting factors.[74] PCCs have been reported to have advantages over FFP.[86] PCCs correct the INR more rapidly than FFP in patients taking warfarin who develop non-traumatic intracerebral hemorrhage (ICH).[87] Preparation time for PCCs is shorter than for FFP, which must be thawed before use.[88] PCCs also contain a higher concentration of clotting factors than FFP; thus, smaller infusion volumes are required.[74,88]

Delayed bleeding must be taken seriously. Often the clinician is made aware of this via a phone call or return to the office. When the patient calls with a concern about postoperative bleeding, the clinician must determine the amount and intensity of the bleeding. Even slow bleeding can be problematic if left untreated. If the bleeding is slow, then pressure with gauze over the site may be helpful. If this is unsuccessful or in cases where bleeding is moderate to severe or has occurred over a long period, the patient should return to the office or go to a hospital emergency room. In some cases, the bleeding is internal and presents as an expanding hematoma. Management of a rapidly expanding hematoma should proceed using the protocol noted above. Pressure over the suspected source, airway management, CT scan with contrast, and laboratory data should be part of

the initial management. The definitive management will require embolization and/or surgery, and correction of any coagulopathy.

Swelling and trismus

Background

Postoperative edema is expected after surgical procedures. It is usually not considered a complication of surgery unless it is excessive. Concerns associated with postoperative edema include wound dehiscence, increased pain, decreased function, and delay in return to daily activities such as work or social activities. When performing third molar surgery, older age (greater than 30 years), deeply impacted teeth, and long operation times (greater than 10 minutes) are associated with significantly greater amounts of swelling.[89] Deeply impacted teeth and longer operation times are also associated with higher postoperative pain scores.

Trismus is defined as limited opening of the jaw secondary to spasm of the closing muscles of the mandible. This is usually temporary, and it will commonly resolve after the inflammation has subsided. The overriding etiology is inflammation of the closing muscles of the mandible or the temporomandibular joint (TMJ). Causes associated with dentoalveolar surgery trismus include local anesthetic injection, deep space infection, hematoma or bleeding in the masticatory muscles, muscle reflection for surgical access, muscle or TMJ trauma secondary to forceful dental extraction, and prolonged opening. In one study involving impacted mandibular third molars, the incidence of reduced mouth opening greater than 10 mm at 1 day postoperative was 18.3% and was significantly associated with the depth of impaction.[89]

Prevention

Multiple treatments have been recommended to reduce swelling associated with dentoalveolar procedures, especially third molar removal and bone-grafting procedures. Preventive measures currently employed include the use of ice and corticosteroids. There are multiple studies showing the benefits of perioperative steroid use. In a systematic review and meta-analysis of the literature, subjects receiving corticosteroids had significantly less edema during both early and late periods after surgery and less trismus than controls during the early and late postoperative periods.[90] Additionally, steroids have been reported to decrease postoperative nausea and vomiting (PONV).[91,92]

Strategies to reduce the risk of postoperative trismus include preoperative antimicrobial mouth rinse, perioperative steroids, perioperative non-steroidal anti-inflammatory drugs (NSAIDs), proper injection techniques for local anesthesia administration (sharp needle, avoid contaminating the local anesthetic capsule, atraumatic injection technique, etc.), avoiding excessive force on the mandible, limiting surgical access when possible, using a bite block for mandibular extractions, and avoiding excessive mouth opening.

Management

The management of postoperative swelling is based on degree and etiology. Swelling related to other causes such as hemorrhage and infection are addressed in other sections of this chapter or elsewhere in this text. Intubation secondary to postoperative edema alone should be rare; thus, the clinician should explore other causes. Corticosteroid administration may aid in swelling reduction.

When a patient initially presents with postoperative trismus, it may be difficult to determine the cause.[93] A careful examination, including radiographs, is important to determine the etiology. In the absence of fracture, the treatment should include physical therapy (jaw stretching exercises, ice/heat, and ultrasound), a soft diet, and medications (NSAIDs. corticosteroids, muscle relaxants, and possibly antibiotics).

Displacement

Background

The frequency of displacement of teeth or root fragments or needles used for local anesthesia is difficult to estimate but is considered low. Because these displacements occur in an office setting, there are no reporting mechanisms in place to ascertain the true incidence. Displaced teeth should be addressed to prevent infection. Maxillary teeth and roots can be displaced into the maxillary sinus, the buccal space, and the infratemporal fossa. Mandibular teeth and roots can be displaced into the sublingual space, the submandibular space, the lateral pharyngeal space, and the inferior alveolar canal (IAC).[94] They may

also be displaced into the airway or gastrointestinal tract. The underlying etiology for displacement of root fragments into the maxillary sinus or the submandibular space and the IAC is that the bone is thin and/or excessive or misdirected force is applied which can result in displacement. Teeth or root fragments displaced into the buccal or infratemporal fossa are usually the result of improper flap design, inadequate soft-tissue reflection, or loss of control of the flap during tooth delivery.

Prevention

Displacement of root fragments and teeth is sometimes preventable if proper surgical techniques are used. Proper imaging is important in order to plan the surgical procedure. Plain film radiographs (periapical and panoramic) and three-dimensional (cone beam) CT (CBCT) are both appropriate.

In a conscious or moderately sedated patient, placing an oropharyngeal screen at the level between the posterior tongue and anterior soft palate prevents a tooth or tooth fragment from entering the airway. This is generally achieved with a dry 4×4-inch piece of gauze with a long segment of umbilical tape or floss attached. Dry gauze is preferred because it is difficult to swallow. This gauze should be constantly checked throughout the surgery and replaced as necessary. In patients undergoing general anesthesia (GA), a throat pack is placed before beginning the procedure. It is usually a 4×8-inch piece of gauze with a radiographic marker embedded within it. Umbilical tape is attached to the throat pack for ease of removal and to remind the surgeon to remove it at the end of the operation.

Flap design and elevation helps with visualization and surgical access to the tooth or root. Use of a broad retractor that rest on the bone above the level of the tooth or root can prevent displacement into the buccal or infratemporal space. Prevention of displacement of a root into the sinus is based on direction of force. Placement of the dental elevator must be between the root and the bone socket. The clinician must avoid using excessive force or force directly on the root towards the apex. The same is true for mandibular root fragments.

In the case of residual root fragments that are close to the maxillary sinus, a flap can be reflected to expose the bone above the level of the apex. A window is created at the apex in order to gain access to the residual root fragment. This procedure preserves the crestal bone, which is important for reconstruction with dental implants. The root fragment can be removed with an elevator placed through the window with a downward force, thus helping to prevent displacement into the sinus.

Management

When a root or tooth is displaced, the initial management will depend on the location of displacement. Some surgeons advocate delaying removal to allow for fibrosis, but others advocate immediate removal to decrease the risk of infection.[95]

The tooth can usually be palpated if it is displaced into the buccal space. The clinician should attempt to trap the tooth between his or her finger and the bone. The tooth can then be gently pushed toward the occlusal edge of the flap and removed with a large hemostat or Kelly clamp.

A tooth or root fragment that is displaced into the maxillary sinus is managed by first attempting to place a suction tip into the sinus through the extraction socket, to see if the tooth or root fragment can be removed. This is usually unsuccessful, and the tooth or root fragment must be removed through a small window placed in the canine fossa. This window often gives the best line of sight, and the tooth or root fragment can usually be removed with a suction tip placed through the window. An endoscope may help the clinician to visualize and retrieve the tooth or root fragment.[96,97] The hole created by pushing the tooth or tooth root into the maxillary sinus should be closed at this time. This will be addressed in the section on oroantral communication.

Displacement of the root fragment into the submandibular space can sometimes be managed be trapping the fragment between the clinician's finger and the bone. It can sometimes be pushed back through the defect. When this is not successful, the tooth or root fragment can be approached in one of two ways. The traditional method is to remove the root fragment through an incision made in the lingual gingival crevice extending posteriorly and laterally toward the buccal area in the third molar region, to avoid injury to the lingual nerve. The flap is reflected while holding digital pressure on the fragment to avoid further displacement. After the fragment or tooth is located, it is removed with a large hemostat. However, this approach can result in injury to the lingual nerve or further displacement of the tooth or root. An approach that has been recently described is to create an osteotomy along the lingual aspect of the third molar tooth socket, leaving it attached to the lingual

mucosa.[98] The rest of the lingual envelope is elevated along the gingival crevice. The lingual aspect of the socket is then out-fractured, allowing more direct visual access to the fragment than the traditional approach. The author has performed seven procedures using this technique to retrieve a mandibular third molar root fragment with no reported lingual nerve injuries.

Removal of fragments that have been displaced into the IAC entails obtaining access through a buccal flap. Buccal bone removal is usually required for better access to the area. The IAC is exposed with a small- to medium-sized round burr or pieziotome. The fragment can commonly be removed with a root-tip pick.

When the above maneuvers are unsuccessful or when the clinician is unsure which space the root fragment or tooth has been displaced into, three-dimensional imaging, or films at right angles to each other, are used to determine the location.[99] If the tooth or root fragment is in the maxillary sinus, additional tools are usually not needed to remove it. If it is in another space, the surgeon should consider the use of navigation to help locate the tooth or root fragment intraoperatively.[99] A "thin-cut" maxillofacial CT scan is obtained just before surgery. It is recommended, in the case of a mandibular tooth or root fragment displacement, that the CT scan is performed with a bite-block in place to accurately reflect the position that the mandible will be in at the time of surgery. The scan is fed into a computer in the operating room (OR) that contains navigational software that will be used at the time of the surgery. Once in the OR, after GA is given, the patient is properly positioned before prepping and draping is done. Infrared sensors are used to register where the patient is in space. The navigational system can help locate the tooth or root fragment and can shorten the surgical time (Figure 15.5). In cases where the tooth or root fragment has been displaced into the infratemporal fossa, a coronal flap may be needed for access.

If the tooth or tooth fragment is displaced into the airway, it could be aspirated or swallowed. Aspiration in an awake or moderately sedated patient will usually result in violent coughing. If this fails to bring the tooth up, then transfer the patient to the hospital for retrieval via bronchoscopy. In a case when the tooth is swallowed, it may not elicit any response in the patient although an awake patient will realize that the tooth has been swallowed. A chest radiograph is indicated to verify that the tooth is not in the bronchus.

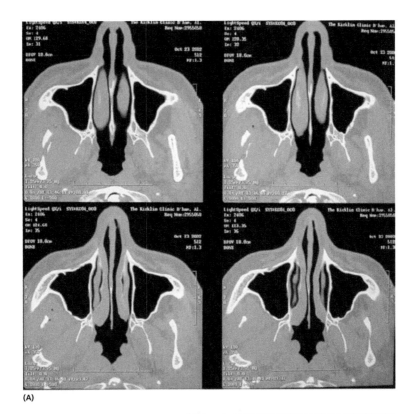

(A)

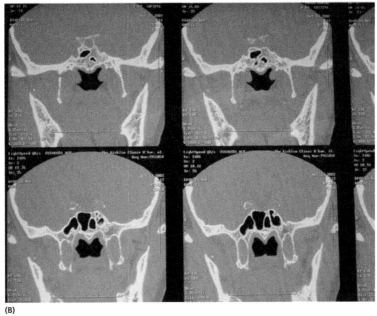

(B)

Figure 15.5 (A) Axil CT showing a broken needle in the right pterygomandibular space. (B) Coronal CT showing a broken needle in the right pterygomandibular space. (C) Registration of the patient using a navigation system. (D) Screenshot localizing the needle to facilitate its removal. (E) Wand used intraoperatively to help localize the broken needle. (F) Retrieved needle.

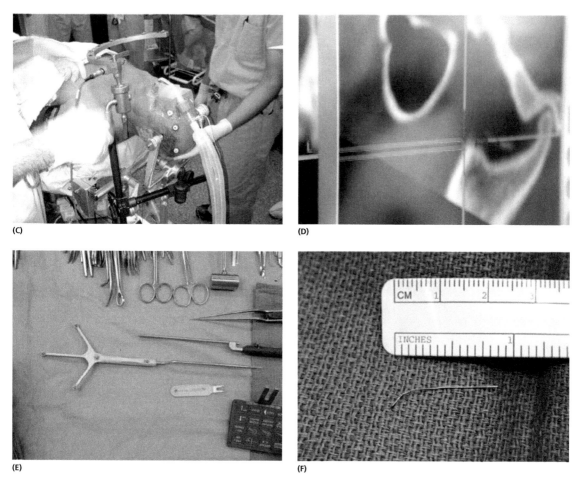

(C)   (D)

(E)   (F)

Figure 15.5 *(Continued)*

Oroantral communication

Background

Oroantral communications (OAC) can be the result of extracting erupted or impacted teeth, alveloplasty, tuberosity reduction, and removal of a pathologic lesion or sinus lift procedure. Conditions that predispose patients to developing an OAC include increased pneumatization of the sinus, proximity of the roots to the sinus, widely divergent roots, periapical pathology, excessive force, posterior maxillary pathology, and maxillary sinusitis. The relative incidence of developing an OAC during tooth extraction is reported to be around 5%.[100,101] When removing maxillary third molars, the incidence is reported to be between 11 and 13%.[102,103] Intraoperative fracture of the root, a higher degree of impaction, and greater age of the patient were associated with a greater

likelihood of OAC. Dental extractions are reported as the most common cause of OAC (73.3%), followed by maxillofacial pathology removal.[104] In a study that reviewed the etiology of OAC and oronasal communications in a case series of 27 patients, the underlying factors were tooth extraction in 13 patients (48%), tumor in 5 (18.5%), osteomyelitis in 3 (11%), Caldwell–Luc procedure in 2 (7.5%), trauma in 2 (7.5%), dentigerous cyst in 1 (3.7%), and correction of septal perforation in 1 (3.7%). Among the fistulas, 23 were oroantral, 3 were oroantronasal, and 1 was oronasal (Figure 15.6).[105]

Prevention

The thickness of the bone between the maxillary sinus and the molar and premolar roots has been reported to have a wide range (1 to 7 mm).[106] The clinician should exercise more caution when removing teeth where

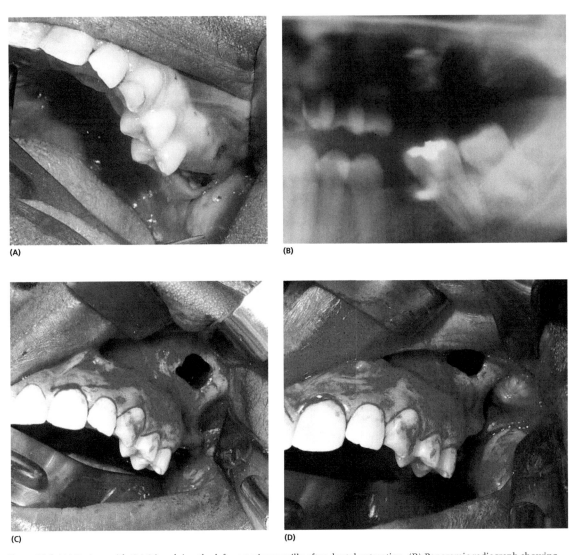

Figure 15.6 (A) Patient with OAC involving the left posterior maxilla after dental extraction. (B) Panoramic radiograph showing the extraction site in the left posterior maxilla. (C) Maxillary sinus window to remove diseased tissue in the left maxillary sinus. (D) Mobilization of the buccal fat pad to cover the OAC.

the bone is thin and the roots are widely divergent. The bone within the furcation may be removed with the roots. A surgical extraction, removing each root separately, may be helpful in these situations. Avoiding an OAC during tooth or root removal has also been addressed in the section on displacement. The mechanism is different and sometimes unavoidable when excising a pathologic lesion. This may result in a large defect that requires a large flap for closure. When performing a tuberosity reduction, radiographs are helpful in planning surgery. When a hard-tissue

tuberosity reduction is indicated and there is a small amount of crestal bone present, a segmental osteotomy should be considered to reduce the bone height.

Management

The management of an OAC varies with the timing of the defect. If an OAC occurs at the time of dental extraction, then a simple closure is usually sufficient. Size of the defect has also been reported to be a factor in determining whether the clinician should achieve primary closure at the time of the initial development of an OAC. Although spontaneous healing of defects of less than 5 mm have been reported, randomized clinical trials evaluating this topic do not exist in the literature.[107] Thus, OAC should be closed immediately or within 24 to 48 hours, before an infection develops.[108] Chronic defects require the exploration of the sinus through a window in the canine fossa, removal of only diseased mucosa (usually with a suction tip), removal of foreign bodies, excision of the fistulous tract, and a two-layered closure. In patients with a patent ostium, a nasal antrostomy is not required to establish drainage for the sinus. In a retrospective report of 50 patients who underwent a Caldwell–Luc operation without a nasal antrostomy for management of odontogenic disease of the maxillary sinus, all operations were successful. Forty-four percent of the patients in this group were treated for OAC with chronic maxillary sinusitis.[109] If the ostium for the maxillary sinus is blocked, then consider functional endoscopic sinus surgery to establish long-lasting sinus drainage. Teeth without bone along the root surface that are adjacent to the OAC must be extracted; otherwise, this condition will result in failure to achieve closure.

One of the most common surgical treatments for an OAC is the buccal advancement flap procedure designed by Rehrmann in 1936 and Berger in 1939. In this procedure, a broad-based trapezoid mucoperiosteal flap is created from the buccal side of the alveolus and sutured over the defect. The periosteum of the flap must be released in order to advance the flap. Its broad base assures an adequate blood supply. This flap has been reported to have a high success rate (93%).[110] Disadvantages of the buccal flap include the risk of reduction of the buccal sulcus depth.

The buccal fat pad is readily available and versatile, and it is an axial pattern flap. Its use as the first layer of closure of an OAC is well documented in the literature.[111] It can also be used alone as a single-layer closure (Figure 15.7).[112] It has been reported to undergo complete epithelialization in 6 to 8 weeks and is slowly replaced by fibrous tissue.[113] The buccal fat pad flap had been successfully employed in the coverage of 7 × 4 × 3-cm defects in one study and a 6.1 × 1.5-cm defect in another study.[114] When employed as a single layer, it has the advantage of not obliterating the buccal vestibule. After the sinus has been addressed and the fistulous tract excised, the buccal fat pad is mobilized by an incision through the periosteum high in the vestibule, underneath the flap. The fat pad is mobilized via blunt dissection. It should not be

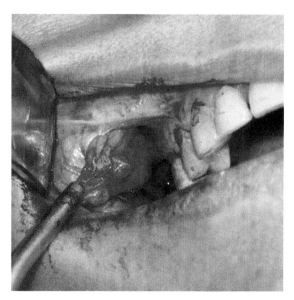

Figure 15.7 Right buccal fat pad that has been mobilized to cover an OAC.

forced or pulled out with forceps as this will only tear it. After the flap is mobilized, it is secured to the undersurface of the palatal mucosa with interrupted horizontal mattress sutures. Alternatively, the buccal fat pad flap can be secured to holes placed in the palatal bone with a wire-passing burr. Using the buccal flap in combination with the buccal fat pad flap may offer the advantage of improved predictability in case of large defects or when there is a hole or tear in the fat pad flap.[111,115]

Full-thickness mucoperiosteal palatal flaps can be used to close an OAC.[116] They have reported a success rate of 76% when used as random palatal flaps.[117] An appropriate length–width ratio is the most important factor in determining the clinical outcome of random palatal flaps. Many clinicians will use an axial pattern flap to close an OAC based on the greater palatine artery (GPA) with a higher expected success rate. Modification of the palatal flap used for closure of the cleft palate has be advocated for a large OAC.[118] However, elevation of a palatal flap is associated with significant postoperative pain and with prolonged healing. The submucosal palatal flap has been advocated to avoid denuded areas of the palate and minimize postoperative morbidity.[119] When using the palatal flap, it is important to make sure it is long and wide enough to cover the defect. This can be done by using a template and estimating the pivot point. When needed, a small back-cut can be made to aid in rotating the flap over the defect. Interrupted horizontal mattress sutures are used to secure the flap in position.

Other flaps and the use of bone grafts have been reported to aid in reconstruction for dental implants, but this topic will not be covered in this section.

The patient is placed on antibiotics, nasal decongestants, and saline nasal spray postoperatively. Sinus precaution instructions (no nose blowing and sneezing with the mouth open for the first 2 weeks, to decrease the force on the repair) are recommended.

Alveolar osteitis

Background

Alveolar osteitis (AO) is a common postoperative complication associated with dental extractions. This disorder is commonly known as a "dry socket" because the socket is often devoid of a blood clot, with exposed bone. The disorder is defined as increased fibrinolytic activity within the early postextraction tooth socket, probably secondary to a subclinical infection. It is reported to occur in approximately 2% (1 to 3%) of routine extractions and 20% (0.5 to 37.5%) of impacted mandibular third molar extractions.[120-126] It usually occurs on the third or fourth day postextraction, although it can occur earlier.[125] The classic triad of AO is (1) clot lysis, (2) fetor oris, and (3) intense pain. Smoking, oral contraceptives, an inexperienced surgeon, poor oral hygiene, increased age, female gender, partial impaction, and periodontal disease have all been reported to increase the risk of AO.[124,127-129]

Prevention

Multiple treatments have been recommended to prevent AO. The risk of AO has been reported to be reduced with the use of various agents; however, due to varying levels of evidence, especially in many of the earlier papers, the use of some agents remains controversial. Agents that have been used include systemic antibiotics,[125,130] topical antibiotics, steroids, NSAIDs, clot stabilizers (gelfoam, surgicel, avitene), chlorhexidine antimicrobial mouth rinses, antifibrinolytic agents, antiseptics, and aloe vera.

Two meta-analyses in the literature that investigated the efficacy of prophylactic systemic antibiotic use found a positive effect in reducing the incidence of AO. Hedstrom *et al.* determined that tetracycline was the most effective antibiotic, while penicillin, amoxicillin, and clindamycin yielded inconsistent results.[131]

Ren and Malmstrom also concluded that both broad- and narrow-spectrum antibiotics were effective.[132] In a recent contribution to the Cochrane Database of Systematic Reviews, the authors reported that there is evidence that antibiotics may reduce the risk of dry socket by 38% following extraction of impacted wisdom teeth.[133] Even with this evidence, there is still controversy regarding the routine uses of systemic antibiotics following third molar extraction due to the risk of antibiotic-associated complications.[134]

Multiple topical agents with and without antibiotics, especially tetracycline, have been used with varying degrees of success.[135-139] Topical antibiotic on a gelatin sponge was effective, but a gelatin sponge alone was not effective in reducing the incidence of AO.[139] Topical antibiotics can cause delayed healing, giant cell reaction, nerve injury, and myospherulosis from petroleum-based carriers.[135,140-142] Their routine use following third molar removal has been brought into question by these potential reactions. A seldom-mentioned study is one that compared the records of 587 patients (1,031 sockets) whose extraction sites had been treated with clindamycin-soaked gelatin sponges with a prospective trial of 607 patients (1,064 sockets) treated with SaliCept Patches (Carrington Laboratories, Inc., Irving, TX) placed immediately after extraction.[143] A SaliCept Patch is a freeze-dried product that contains Acemannan Hydrogel, a mixture of naturally occurring substances with the primary component being acemannan, a beta-(1,4)-acetylated mannan obtained from the clear inner gel of Aloe vera L. Analysis restricted to mandibular third molar sites showed that 78 of 975 sites (8.0%) in the clindamycin-soaked gelatin group developed AO, whereas only 11 of 958 sites (1.1%) in the SaliCept group developed AO, which was statistically significant. Despite the limitations of the study, the SaliCept Patch shows some promise as a preventative material for AO.

Due to a low risk of side effects and high efficacy, routine use of a chlorhexidine rinse, 1 week preoperatively and for 1 week postoperatively, is recommended to prevent AO. This regimen resulted in an 8% incidence (38 to 60% reduction) of AO following third molar removal.[124,144]

Management

Management of AO is directed toward pain relief. After a diagnosis is made, the wound is irrigated with saline solution or mouthwash. When the pain is severe, local anesthesia may be required. A dry socket dressing is placed in the socket. Common ingredients include eugenol, benzocaine, and balsam of Peru. The dressing is changed every other day for 3 to 6 days. Another recommended treatment is socket curettage. This requires reflection of a flap, removal of bone particles, curettage, and removal of granulation tissue with irrigation.[121] Reportedly, this method has the benefits of not interfering with healing and not requiring the patient to return for a dressing change. Low-level laser therapy (LLLT) may radically change how we manage AO in the future. Irradiation of the socket after irrigation and curettage with a 808 nm, 100 mW continuous mode gallium aluminum arsenide diode laser resulted in a more rapid resolution of signs and symptoms when compared to the use of SaliCept patches and dry socket dressings.[145]

After the resolution of symptoms, the socket will usually heal uneventfully.

Nerve injury

Background

The proximity of some of the sensory branches of the trigeminal nerve to the dentoalveolar structures makes it vulnerable to injury during certain dentoalveolar procedures, especially in the mandible. The main branches of the trigeminal nerve that are at risk for injury during dentoalveolar procedures include the inferior alveolar nerve (IAN), the lingual nerve (LN), the mental nerve (MN), the buccal nerve (BN), and the infraorbital nerve (IFN). The procedure with the highest incidence of nerve injury is the removal of impacted mandibular third molars.

The incidence of IAN injury after mandibular third molar extraction has been reported to be between 0.4 and 8.4%, with less than 1% reporting permanent numbness (Figure 15.8).[146,147] Other procedures with a lower frequency of injury to branches of the trigeminal nerve include bone graft harvest for alveolar ridge reconstruction, dental implant placement, surgical extractions, vestibuloplasty, and the maxillary sinus lift procedure. The incidence of implant-related IAN injuries has been reported to vary widely from 0 to 33.2%.[148]

The LN is also most commonly injured by third molar removal. This is due to the proximity of the lingual nerve to the lingual aspect of the mandible in the third molar region (Figure 15.9).[149] The lingual nerve is affected 0.06 to 11.5% of the time following third molar removal.[150] However, permanent injury to the LN from third molar surgery has ranged from 0.04 to 0.6%.[150–154]

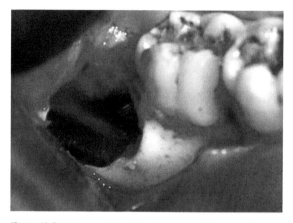

Figure 15.8 IAN seen at the inferior aspect of the extraction site after third molar removal.

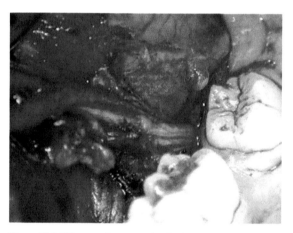

Figure 15.9 LN seen adjacent to the third molar region after sublingual gland removal. Note the relationship to the submandibular duct.

Based on anatomic dissection, the mean distance from the lingual nerve to the lingual cortical plate in the molar and retromolar pad region ranges from 0.58 to 3.45 mm.[149,155] Based on a small sample of volunteers and the use of magnetic resonance imaging (MRI), the distances of the lingual nerve to the lingual crest and lingual plate of the mandible were determined in the third molar region. The mean vertical distance was 2.75 mm (range, 1.52 to 4.61 mm) and the horizontal distance was 2.53 mm (range, 0 to 4.35 mm).

The motor nerves in the region are usually not injured during dentoalveolar procedures due to the types of procedures and lack of proximity to the surgical field. Injury to the buccal branch of the facial nerve could occur with a vestibuloplasty procedure and creation of a buccal fat pad flap. In one study, the buccal branches of the facial nerve were reported to pass through the buccal extension of the buccal fat pad 26.3% of the time.[156]

Prevention

Injury to branches of the trigeminal nerve during dentoalveolar surgery has decreased with newer techniques that have been designed to minimize morbidity. The use of cone beam CT (CBCT) in the clinician's office has improved risk assessment for potential IAN injury, especially during mandibular third molar removal and implant placement in the posterior mandible.

Reducing the risk of injury to the IAN starts with a detailed evaluation and treatment plan. Preoperative evaluation should include assessing the patient for preoperative nerve deficits. Older patients must be made aware that increasing age is associated with increased risk. Radiographic evaluation must be performed before surgery. The panoramic radiograph is an excellent screening tool for many surgical procedures. Many studies have evaluated radiographic findings on panoramic radiograph and the risk of IAN injury.

Depth of impaction is a significant risk factor for injury to the inferior alveolar canal (IAC). Darkening of the roots, deflection of the roots, narrowing of the roots, dark and bifid apexes of the roots, and narrowing of the canal have also been reported to be significant risk factors when the roots of the mandibular third molar overlap the IAC.[157] However, the relatively low positive predictive value (0.7 to 6.9%) of superimposition signs on panoramic radiographs has called into question the use of plain films alone when assessing the risk of IAN injury. CBCT is recommended when the above findings are present. In the absence of the above radiographic signs, the risk of injury to the IAN is negligible.[157]

Coronectomy of the mandibular third molar has been reported to successfully prevent IAN injuries (Figure 15.10). Patients must be informed of the potential risks associated with this procedure and the possible need for a second surgery due to migration of the root or infectious complications.

Prevention of injury to the lingual nerve is through avoidance of surgery along the lingual aspect of the mandible. Lingual nerve retraction has been used to protect the nerve. The incidence of altered sensation using lingual nerve retraction has been reported to be between 1.6 and 9.1%. This is usually a neuropraxia and resolves with time.[158,159]

Management

The vast majority of sensory symptoms associated with IAN injury resolve within 6 months to 1 year. It is important to evaluate the patient regarding the extent of the injury, the duration of symptoms, and whether symptoms have improved. The initial exam should include a detailed neurologic exam assessing light touch, pinprick, sharp-blunt discrimination, brushstroke direction, and two-point discrimination thresholds. The detailed exam should be documented over time to determine if there is improvement. Microneural repair is recommended for the LN if there is no improvement in 1 to 3 months and for IAN if there is no improvement in 3 to 6 months. The indications for repair include complete postoperative anesthesia; less than 50 precent residual sensation in Sunderland III, IV, or V; and 50% residual sensation in a Sunderland I or II if it is unacceptable to the patient (Table 15.4).

Timing has a significant effect on outcomes of lingual nerve repair. One study reported that 93% of subjects who underwent "early" repair (less than 90 days after injury) achieved functional sensory recovery within 1 year compared with 62.9% of subjects who underwent "late" repair (more than 90 days after injury).[160] In a similar study, 125 patients (94%) treated early (within 6 months) demonstrated functional sensory recovery compared to patients (85.4%) who underwent late treatment (after 6 months).[161]

Nerve repair

Various types of repair to the branches of the trigeminal nerve have been described based on the extent of the injury. The details of repair are beyond the scope of this chapter.

Fracture

Background

The reported incidence of an iatrogenic mandibular fracture associated with the removal of teeth ranges from 0.0034 to 0.0075%.[162] These fractures can occur during the procedure or within the first 4 weeks postoperatively. Factors affecting the incidence and etiology of iatrogenic mandibular fractures include the depth of impaction, type of tooth angulation, length of roots, patient age, age and experience of the surgeon, presence of a cyst or tumor around an impacted third molar,

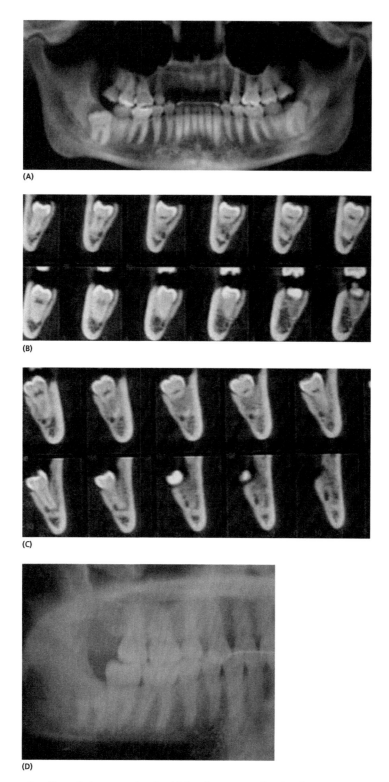

Figure 15.10 (A) Panoramic radiograph demonstrating the third molar roots overlapping the IAN canal. (B) Cone beam CT of the right mandible showing the third molar root and the IAN canal in intimate contact. (C) Cone beam CT of the left side of the mandible showing less contact between the nerve and root surface. (D) Postoperative radiograph showing that coronectomy was performed on the right side. A coronectomy was also planned for the left side, but, during removal of the crown, the roots were noted to be mobile and were removed without injury to the IAN.

Table 15.4 Comparison of Seddon's and Sunderland's classification of peripheral nerve injuries as applied to the trigeminal nerve

Seddon	Neurapraxia	Axonotmesis	Neurotmesis
Sunderland	I	II, III, IV	V[a]
Nerve sheath	Intact	Intact	Interrupted
Axons	Intact	Some interrupted	All interrupted
Wallerian degeneration	None	Yes, some distal axons	Yes, all distal axons
Conduction failure	Transitory	Prolonged	Permanent
Potential for spontaneous recovery	Complete	Partial	Little or none
Time to spontaneous recovery	Within 4 wk	Begins at 5–12 wk; may take months	None, if not begun by 12 wk

Seddon's classification is most helpful to clinicians in making timely decisions regarding surgical intervention.
[a] Sunderland also has a class VI (complex) injury, which is a combination of classes I–V within the same injured nerve.
Source: Meyer RA, Bagheri SC. Microsurgical reconstruction of the trigeminal nerve. Oral Maxillofac Surg Clin North Am. 2013; 25: 287–302. Reproduced with permission of Elsevier.

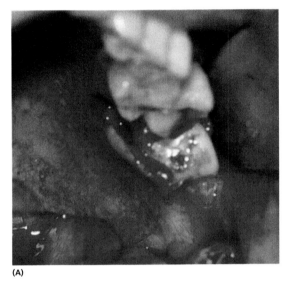

(A)

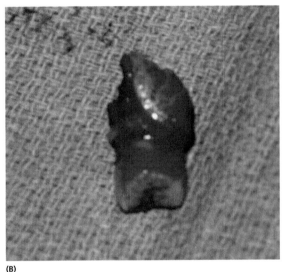

(B)

Figure 15.11 (A) The tuberosity fracture noted will elevate the erupted maxillary third molar distally. (B) The maxillary third molar was removed, and most of the tuberosity was salvaged by leaving it attached to the overlying mucosa and separating the tooth from the bone.

systemic disease or medications that may impair bone strength, preoperative infections in the third molar site, and inadequate preoperative examination.[163–168]

Mandibular fractures have also been reported with implant placement in the atrophic mandible. These fractures are rare and are most commonly reported in the symphysis region followed by the body of the mandible.[169–172] The timing of implant-related mandibular fractures is extremely variable, with most fractures occurring either 3 to 6 weeks or 3 months after implant placement, although some cases have been reported immediately after surgery, before and after loading.[169,173]

Tuberosity and alveolar segment fractures can occur during dental extractions. These fractures may interfere with planned dental implant placement. Tuberosity fractures are probably more common than is reported, and they are occasionally associated with significant hemorrhage (Figure 15.11).[174]

Prevention

Deeply impacted third molars have a greater risk of associated mandibular fractures secondary to the need for more bone removal. The inexperienced surgeon may be fooled by the radiographic appearance of some third molars or partially impacted or erupted teeth, thinking they may be simple to remove. Inadequate bone removal and improper or lack of sectioning can result in the need for large amounts of force, which could result in fracture of the mandible. It is advisable to perform adequate bone removal and tooth sectioning to reduce the amount of removed bone and decrease the amount of force required to remove the tooth.[175–178] A recent literature review reported that 74% of fractures occurred postoperatively and 26% of pathological mandibular fractures were observed intraoperatively.[173] A soft diet is recommended for 4 weeks postoperatively, especially in patients with full dentition who have risk factors for mandibular fracture.[162,179–181]

In the severely atrophic mandible, the clinician should avoid wide-diameter implants and penetration of the inferior border of the mandible, which can significantly weaken the jaw.[172] Good oral hygiene and proper maintenance of implants to avoid marginal bone loss in the atrophic mandible can help to prevent fractures.[169] Proper biomechanics of the restoration can prevent late fractures.[169] Nerve repositioning procedures can also result in fracture of the body of the mandible in atrophic cases.[169,182] Minimal bone removal is recommended in these cases.

Management

Fractures of the mandible can be treated via open or closed reduction. Principles of fracture management must be followed.[183–185]

Implants in the line of fracture were left in place when they were osseointegrated, not mobile, not infected, and did not present with nearby areas of osteomyelitis.[170]

References

1. Akintoye SO, Hersh EV. Risks for jaw osteonecrosis drastically increases after 2 years of bisphosphonate therapy. *Journal of Evidence-Based Dental Practice*. 2012; 12(3 Suppl): 251–3.
2. Allen MR, Burr DB. The pathogenesis of bisphosphonate-related osteonecrosis of the jaw: so many hypotheses, so few data. *Journal of Oral and Maxillofacial Surgery*. 2009; 67(5 Suppl): 61–70.
3. Lambade PN, Lambade D, Goel M. Osteoradionecrosis of the mandible: a review. *Oral and Maxillofacial Surgery*. 2013; 17(4): 243–9.
4. Carlson ER. The radiobiology, treatment, and prevention of osteoradionecrosis of the mandible. *Recent Results in Cancer Research*. 1994; 134: 191–9.
5. Sisson R, Lang S, Serkes K, Pareira MD. Comparison of wound healing in various nutritional deficiency states. *Surgery*. 1958; 44(4): 613–8.
6. Beumer J, Harrison R, Sanders B, Kurrasch M. Osteoradionecrosis: predisposing factors and outcomes of therapy. *Head and Neck Surgery*. 1984; 6(4): 819–27.
7. Epstein JB, Rea G, Wong FL, Spinelli J, Stevenson-Moore P. Osteonecrosis: study of the relationship of dental extractions in patients receiving radiotherapy. *Head and Neck Surgery*. 1987; 10(1): 48–54.
8. Marx RE. Osteoradionecrosis: a new concept of its pathophysiology. *Journal of Oral and Maxillofacial Surgery*. 1983; 41(5): 283–8.
9. Delanian S, Lefaix JL. The radiation-induced fibroatrophic process: therapeutic perspective via the antioxidant pathway. *Radiotherapy in Oncology*. 2004; 73(2): 119–31.
10. Lee IJ, Koom WS, Lee CG, Kim YB, Yoo SW, Keum KC, et al. Risk factors and dose-effect relationship for mandibular osteoradionecrosis in oral and oropharyngeal cancer patients. *International Journal of Radiation Oncology, Biology, Physics*. 2009; 75(4): 1084–91.
11. Nussbaum SR, Younger J, Vandepol CJ, Gagel RF, Zubler MA, Chapman R, et al. Single-dose intravenous therapy with pamidronate for the treatment of hypercalcemia of malignancy: comparison of 30-, 60-, and 90-mg dosages. *American Journal of Medicine*. 1993; 95(3): 297–304.
12. Major P, Lortholary A, Hon J, Abdi E, Mills G, Menssen HD, et al. Zoledronic acid is superior to pamidronate in the treatment of hypercalcemia of malignancy: a pooled analysis of two randomized, controlled clinical trials. *Journal of Clinical Oncology*. 2001; 19(2): 558–67.
13. Delmas PD, Meunier PJ. The management of Paget's disease of bone. *New England Journal of Medicine*. 1997; 336(8): 558–66.
14. Delmas PD. The use of bisphosphonates in the treatment of osteoporosis. *Current Opinion in Rheumatology*. 2005; 17(4): 462–6.
15. Berenson JR. Treatment of hypercalcemia of malignancy with bisphosphonates. *Seminars in Oncology*. 2002; 29(6 Suppl 21): 12–8.
16. Berenson JR. Advances in the biology and treatment of myeloma bone disease. *Seminars in Oncology*. 2002; 29(6 Suppl 17): 11–6.
17. Berenson JR, Hillner BE, Kyle RA, Anderson K, Lipton A, Yee GC, et al. American Society of Clinical Oncology clinical practice guidelines: the role of bisphosphonates in multiple myeloma. *Journal of Clinical Oncology*. 2002; 20(17): 3719–36.
18. Bone HG, Hosking D, Devogelaer JP, Tucci JR, Emkey RD, Tonino RP, et al. Ten years' experience with alendronate for osteoporosis in postmenopausal women. *New England Journal of Medicine*. 2004; 350(12): 1189–99.
19. Murakami H, Takahashi N, Sasaki T, Udagawa N, Tanaka S, Nakamura I, et al. A possible mechanism of the specific action of bisphosphonates on osteoclasts: tiludronate preferentially affects polarized osteoclasts having ruffled borders. *Bone*. 1995; 17(2): 137–44.

20. Hall A. Rho GTPases and the actin cytoskeleton. *Science.* 1998; 279(5350): 509–14.

21. Sato M, Grasser W, Endo N, Akins R, Simmons H, Thompson DD, *et al.* Bisphosphonate action. *Alendronate localization in rat bone and effects on osteoclast ultrastructure. Journal of Clinical Investigation.* 1991; 88(6): 2095–105.

22. Bamias A, Kastritis E, Bamia C, Moulopoulos LA, Melakopoulos I, Bozas G, *et al.* Osteonecrosis of the jaw in cancer after treatment with bisphosphonates: incidence and risk factors. *Journal of Clinical Oncology.* 2005; 23(34): 8580–7.

23. Ruggiero SL, Dodson TB, Fantasia J, Goodday R, Aghaloo T, Mehrotra B, O'Ryan F; American Association of Oral and Maxillofacial Surgeons. American Association of Oral and Maxillofacial Surgeons position paper on medication-related osteonecrosis of the jaw–2014 update. *Journal of Oral and Maxillofacial Surgery.* 2014; 72(10): 1938–56.

24. Durie BG, Katz M, Crowley J. Osteonecrosis of the jaw and bisphosphonates. *New England Journal of Medicine.* 2005; 353(1): 99–102; discussion 99–102.

25. Dimopoulos MA, Kastritis E, Anagnostopoulos A, Melakopoulos I, Gika D, Moulopoulos LA, *et al.* Osteonecrosis of the jaw in patients with multiple myeloma treated with bisphosphonates: evidence of increased risk after treatment with zoledronic acid. *Haematologica.* 2006; 91(7): 968–71.

26. Zavras AI, Zhu S. Bisphosphonates are associated with increased risk for jaw surgery in medical claims data: is it osteonecrosis? *Journal of Oral and Maxillofacial Surgery.* 2006; 64(6): 917–23.

27. Mavrokokki T, Cheng A, Stein B, Goss A. Nature and frequency of bisphosphonate-associated osteonecrosis of the jaws in Australia. *Journal of Oral and Maxillofacial Surgery.* 2007; 65(3): 415–23.

28. Marx RE, Johnson RP. Studies in the radiobiology of osteoradionecrosis and their clinical significance. *Oral Surgery, Oral Medicine, and Oral Pathology.* 1987; 64(4): 379–90.

29. Thorn JJ, Hansen HS, Specht L, Bastholt L. Osteoradionecrosis of the jaws: clinical characteristics and relation to the field of irradiation. *Journal of Oral and Maxillofacial Surgery.* 2000; 58(10): 1088–93; discussion 93–5.

30. Nabil S, Samman N. Incidence and prevention of osteoradionecrosis after dental extraction in irradiated patients: a systematic review. *International Journal of Oral and Maxillofacial Surgery.* 2011; 40(3): 229–43.

31. Studer G, Gratz KW, Glanzmann C. Osteoradionecrosis of the mandibula in patients treated with different fractionations. *Strahlentherapie und Onkologie.* 2004; 180(4): 233–40.

32. Vissink A, Jansma J, Spijkervet FK, Burlage FR, Coppes RP. Oral sequelae of head and neck radiotherapy. *Critical Reviews in Oral Biological Medicine.* 2003; 14(3): 199–212.

33. Delanian S, Chatel C, Porcher R, Depondt J, Lefaix JL. Complete restoration of refractory mandibular osteoradionecrosis by prolonged treatment with a pentoxifylline-tocopherol-clodronate combination (PENTOCLO): a phase II trial. *International Journal of Radiation Oncology, Biology, Physics.* 2011; 80(3): 832–9.

34. Dimopoulos MA, Kastritis E, Bamia C, Melakopoulos I, Gika D, Roussou M, *et al.* Reduction of osteonecrosis of the jaw (ONJ) after implementation of preventive measures in patients with multiple myeloma treated with zoledronic acid. *Annals of Oncology.* 2009; 20(1): 117–20.

35. Ripamonti CI, Maniezzo M, Campa T, Fagnoni E, Brunelli C, Saibene G, *et al.* Decreased occurrence of osteonecrosis of the jaw after implementation of dental preventive measures in solid tumour patients with bone metastases treated with bisphosphonates. *The experience of the National Cancer Institute of Milan. Annals of Oncology.* 2009; 20(1): 137–45.

36. Black DM, Delmas PD, Eastell R, Reid IR, Boonen S, Cauley JA, *et al.* Once-yearly zoledronic acid for treatment of postmenopausal osteoporosis. *New England Journal of Medicine.* 2007; 356(18): 1809–22.

37. Oh HK, Chambers MS, Martin JW, Lim HJ, Park HJ. Osteoradionecrosis of the mandible: treatment outcomes and factors influencing the progress of osteoradionecrosis. *Journal of Oral and Maxillofacial Surgery.* 2009; 67(7): 1378–86.

38. Chuang SK. Limited evidence to demonstrate that the use of hyperbaric oxygen (HBO) therapy reduces the incidence of osteoradionecrosis in irradiated patients requiring tooth extraction. *Journal of Evidence-Based Dental Practice.* 2012; 12(3 Suppl): 248–50.

39. Marx RE, Johnson RP, Kline SN. Prevention of osteoradionecrosis: a randomized prospective clinical trial of hyperbaric oxygen versus penicillin. *Journal of the American Dental Association.* 1985; 111(1): 49–54.

40. Gal TJ, Yueh B, Futran ND. Influence of prior hyperbaric oxygen therapy in complications following microvascular reconstruction for advanced osteoradionecrosis. *Archives of Otolaryngology, Head and Neck Surgery.* 2003; 129(1): 72–6.

41. Marx RE, Cillo JE Jr., Ulloa JJ. Oral bisphosphonate-induced osteonecrosis: risk factors, prediction of risk using serum CTX testing, prevention, and treatment. *Journal of Oral and Maxillofacial Surgery.* 2007; 65(12): 2397–410.

42. Wasson M, Ghodke B, Dillon JK. Exsanguinating hemorrhage following third molar extraction: report of a case and discussion of materials and methods in selective embolization. *Journal of Oral and Maxillofacial Surgery.* 2012; 70(10): 2271–5.

43. Moghadam HG, Caminiti MF. Life-threatening hemorrhage after extraction of third molars: case report and management protocol. *Journal of the Canadian Dental Association.* 2002; 68(11): 670–4.

44. Lamberg MA, Tasanen A, Jaaskelainen J. Fatality from central hemangioma of the mandible. *Journal of Oral Surgery.* 1979; 37(8): 578–84.

45. Flanagan D. Important arterial supply of the mandible, control of an arterial hemorrhage, and report of a hemorrhagic incident. *Journal of Oral Implantology.* 2003; 29(4): 165–73.

46. Orlian AI, Karmel R. Postoperative bleeding in an undiagnosed hemophilia A patient: report of case. *Journal of the American Dental Association.* 1989; 118(5): 583–4.

47. Hong C, Napenas JJ, Brennan M, Furney S, Lockhart P. Risk of postoperative bleeding after dental procedures in patients on warfarin: a retrospective study. *Oral Surgery, Oral Medicine, Oral Pathology, Oral Radiology.* 2012; 114(4): 464–8.

48. Givol N, Chaushu G, Halamish-Shani T, Taicher S. Emergency tracheostomy following life-threatening hemorrhage in the floor of the mouth during immediate implant placement in the mandibular canine region. *Journal of Periodontology.* 2000; 71(12): 1893–5.

49. Mason ME, Triplett RG, Alfonso WF. Life-threatening hemorrhage from placement of a dental implant. *Journal of Oral and Maxillofacial Surgery.* 1990; 48(2): 201–4.

50. Ennis JT, Bateson EM, Moule NJ. Uncommon arteriovenous fistulae. *Clinical Radiology.* 1972; 23(3): 392–8.

51. Hassard AD, Byrne BD. Arteriovenous malformations and vascular anatomy of the upper lip and soft palate. *Laryngoscope.* 1985; 95(7 Pt 1): 829–32.

52. Darlow LD, Murphy JB, Berrios RJ, Park Y, Feldman RS. Arteriovenous malformation of the maxillary sinus: an unusual clinical presentation. *Oral Surgery, Oral Medicine, Oral Pathology.* 1988; 66(1): 21–3.

53. Mulliken JB, Glowacki J. Classification of pediatric vascular lesions. *Plastic and Reconstructive Surgery.* 1982; 70(1): 120–1.

54. Mulliken JB, Glowacki J. Hemangiomas and vascular malformations in infants and children: a classification based on endothelial characteristics. *Plastic and Reconstructive Surgery.* 1982; 69(3): 412–22.

55. Buckmiller LM. Update on hemangiomas and vascular malformations. *Current Opinion in Otolaryngology, Head and Neck Surgery.* 2004; 12(6): 476–87.

56. Padwa BL, Denhart BC, Kaban LB. Aneurysmal bone cyst-"plus": a report of three cases. *Journal of Oral and Maxillofacial Surgery.* 1997; 55(10): 1144–52.

57. Vollmer E, Roessner A, Lipecki KH, *et al.* Biologic characterization of human bone tumors. VI. The aneurysmal bone cyst: an enzyme histochemical, electron microscopical, and immunohistological study. *Virchows Archiv B Cell Pathology Including Molecular Pathology.* 1987; 53(1): 58–65.

58. O'Malley M, Pogrel MA, Stewart JC, Silva RG, Regezi JA. Central giant cell granulomas of the jaws: phenotype and proliferation-associated markers. *Journal of Oral Pathology and Medicine.* 1997; 26(4): 159–63.

59. Kaban LB, Dodson TB. Management of giant cell lesions. *International Journal of Oral and Maxillofacial Surgery.* 2006; 35(11): 1074–5; author reply 76.

60. Rodeghiero F, Castaman G, Dini E. Epidemiological investigation of the prevalence of von Willebrand's disease. *Blood.* 1987; 69(2): 454–9.

61. Werner EJ, Broxson EH, Tucker EL, *et al.* Prevalence of von Willebrand disease in children: a multiethnic study. *Journal of Pediatrics.* 1993; 123(6): 893–8.

62. Bloom AL. von Willebrand factor: clinical features of inherited and acquired disorders. *Mayo Clinic Proceedings.* 1991; 66(7): 743–51.

63. Sadler JE, Budde U, Eikenboom JC, *et al.* Update on the pathophysiology and classification of von Willebrand disease: a report of the Subcommittee on von Willebrand Factor. *Journal of Thrombosis and Haemostasis.* 2006; 4(10): 2103–14.

64. Sucker C, Michiels JJ, Zotz RB. Causes, etiology and diagnosis of acquired von Willebrand disease: a prospective diagnostic workup to establish the most effective therapeutic strategies. *Acta Haematologica.* 2009; 121(2–3): 177–82.

65. Federici AB. Acquired von Willebrand syndrome: an underdiagnosed and misdiagnosed bleeding complication in patients with lymphoproliferative and myeloproliferative disorders. *Seminars in Hematology.* 2006; 43(1 Suppl 1): S48–58.

66. James PD, Goodeve AC. von Willebrand disease. *Genetics in Medicine.* 2011; 13(5): 365–76.

67. Cheng CK, Chan J, Cembrowski GS, van Assendelft OW. Complete blood count reference interval diagrams derived from NHANES III: stratification by age, sex, and race. *Laboratory Hematology.* 2004; 10(1): 42–53.

68. Rodeghiero F, Stasi R, Gernsheimer T, Michel M, Provan D, Arnold DM, *et al.* Standardization of terminology, definitions and outcome criteria in immune thrombocytopenic purpura of adults and children: report from an international working group. *Blood.* 2009; 113(11): 2386–93.

69. Stasi R. How to approach thrombocytopenia. *Hematology American Society of Hematologists Education Program.* 2012; 2012: 191–7.

70 Aster RH. Pooling of platelets in the spleen: role in the pathogenesis of "hypersplenic" thrombocytopenia. *Journal of Clinical Investigation.* 1966; 45(5): 645–57.

71. Clemetson KJ. Platelet glycoproteins and their role in diseases. *Transfusion Clinical Biology.* 2001; 8(3): 155–62.

72. Cattaneo M. Inherited platelet-based bleeding disorders. *Journal of Thrombosis and Haemostasis.* 2003; 1(7): 1628–36.

73. CAPRIE Steering Committee. A randomised, blinded, trial of clopidogrel versus aspirin in patients at risk of ischaemic events (CAPRIE). *Lancet.* 1996; 348(9038): 1329–39.

74. Nitzki-George D, Wozniak I, Caprini JA. Current state of knowledge on oral anticoagulant reversal using procoagulant factors. *Annals of Pharmacotherapy.* 2013; 47(6): 841–55.

75. Klosek SK, Rungruang T. Anatomical study of the greater palatine artery and related structures of the palatal vault: considerations for palate as the subepithelial connective tissue graft donor site. *Surgical Radiology and Anatomy.* 2009; 31(4): 245–50.

76. Pogrel MA, Dorfman D, Fallah H. The anatomic structure of the inferior alveolar neurovascular bundle in the third

molar region. *Journal of Oral and Maxillofacial Surgery.* 2009; 67(11): 2452–4.

77. Needleman HL, Kaban LB, Kevy SV. The use of epsilon-aminocaproic acid for the management of hemophilia in dental and oral surgery patients. *Journal of the American Dental Association.* 1976; 93(3): 586–90.

78. Holland LL, Brooks JP. Toward rational fresh frozen plasma transfusion: The effect of plasma transfusion on coagulation test results. *American Journal of Clinical Pathology.* 2006; 126(1): 133–9.

79. Sharma S, Sharma P, Tyler LN. Transfusion of blood and blood products: indications and complications. *American Family Physician.* 2011; 83(6): 719–24.

80. Beirne OR. Evidence to continue oral anticoagulant therapy for ambulatory oral surgery. *Journal of Oral and Maxillofacial Surgery.* 2005; 63(4): 540–5.

81. Evans IL, Sayers MS, Gibbons AJ, Price G, Snooks H, Sugar AW. Can warfarin be continued during dental extraction? Results of a randomized controlled trial. *British Journal of Oral and Maxillofacial Surgery.* 2002; 40(3): 248–52.

82. Dodson TB. Strategies for managing anticoagulated patients requiring dental extractions: an exercise in evidence-based clinical practice. *Journal of the Massachusetts Dental Society.* 2002; 50(4): 44–50.

83. Favaloro EJ, Lippi G, Koutts J. Laboratory testing of anticoagulants: the present and the future. *Pathology.* 2011; 43(7): 682–92.

84. Hebert PC, Wells G, Blajchman MA, *et al.* A multicenter, randomized, controlled clinical trial of transfusion requirements in critical care. Transfusion Requirements in Critical Care Investigators, Canadian Critical Care Trials Group. *New England Journal of Medicine.* 1999; 340(6): 409–17.

85. Carless PA, Henry DA, Carson JL, Hebert PP, McClelland B, Ker K. Transfusion thresholds and other strategies for guiding allogeneic red blood cell transfusion. *Cochrane Database Systematic Reviews.* 2010(10): CD002042.

86. Bershad EM, Suarez JI. Prothrombin complex concentrates for oral anticoagulant therapy-related intracranial hemorrhage: a review of the literature. *Neurocritical Care.* 2010; 12(3): 403–13.

87. Fredriksson K, Norrving B, Stromblad LG. Emergency reversal of anticoagulation after intracerebral hemorrhage. *Stroke.* 1992; 23(7): 972–7.

88. Lemon SJ Jr., Crannage AJ. Pharmacologic anticoagulation reversal in the emergency department. *Advances in Emergency Nursing Journal.* 2011; 33(3): 212–23; quiz 24–5.

89. Kim JC, Choi SS, Wang SJ, Kim SG. Minor complications after mandibular third molar surgery: type, incidence, and possible prevention. *Oral Surgery, Oral Medicine, Oral Pathology, Oral Radiology and Endodontics.* 2006; 102(2): e4–11.

90. Markiewicz MR, Brady MF, Ding EL, Dodson TB. Corticosteroids reduce postoperative morbidity after third molar surgery: a systematic review and meta-analysis. *Journal of Oral and Maxillofacial Surgery.* 2008; 66(9): 1881–94.

91. Tolver MA, Strandfelt P, Bryld EB, Rosenberg J, Bisgaard T. Randomized clinical trial of dexamethasone versus placebo in laparoscopic inguinal hernia repair. *British Journal of Surgery.* 2012; 99(10): 1374–80.

92. Mataruski MR, Keis NA, Smouse DJ, Workman ML. Effects of steroids on postoperative nausea and vomiting. *Nurse Anesthesia.* 1990; 1(4): 183–8.

93. Osunde OD, Adebola RA, Omeje UK. Management of inflammatory complications in third molar surgery: a review of the literature. *African Health Sciences.* 2011; 11(3): 530–7.

94. Esen E, Aydogan LB, Akcali MC. Accidental displacement of an impacted mandibular third molar into the lateral pharyngeal space. *Journal of Oral and Maxillofacial Surgery.* 2000; 58(1): 96–7.

95. Gay-Escoda C, Berini-Aytes L, Pinera-Penalva M. Accidental displacement of a lower third molar. Report of a case in the lateral cervical position. *Oral Surgery, Oral Medicine, Oral Pathology.* 1993; 76(2): 159–60.

96. Iwai T, Matsui Y, Hirota M, Tohnai I. Endoscopic removal of a maxillary third molar displaced into the maxillary sinus via the socket. *Journal of Craniofacial Surgery.* 2012; 23(4): e295–6.

97. Iwai T, Chikumaru H, Shibasaki M, Tohnai I. Safe method of extraction to prevent a deeply-impacted maxillary third molar being displaced into the maxillary sinus. *British Journal of Oral and Maxillofacial Surgery.* 2013; 51(5): e75-6.

98. Huang IY, Wu CW, Worthington P. The displaced lower third molar: a literature review and suggestions for management. *Journal of Oral and Maxillofacial Surgery.* 2007; 65(6): 1186–90.

99. Campbell A, Costello BJ. Retrieval of a displaced third molar using navigation and active image guidance. *Journal of Oral and Maxillofacial Surgery.* 2010; 68(2): 480–5.

100. del Rey-Santamaria M, Valmaseda Castellon E, Berini Aytes L, Gay Escoda C. Incidence of oral sinus communications in 389 upper thirmolar extraction. *Medicina Oral Patologia Oral y Cirugia Bucal.* 2006; 11(4): E334–8.

101. Bodner L, Gatot A, Bar-Ziv J. Technical note: oroantral fistula: improved imaging with a dental computed tomography software program. *British Journal of Radiology.* 1995; 68(815): 1249–50.

102. Wachter R, Stoll P. [Complications of surgical wisdom tooth removal of the maxilla. A clinical and roentgenologic study of 1,013 patients with statistical evaluation]. *Fortschr Kiefer Gesichtschir.* 1995; 40: 128–33.

103. Rothamel D, Wahl G, d'Hoedt B, *et al.* Incidence and predictive factors for perforation of the maxillary antrum in operations to remove upper wisdom teeth: prospective multicentre study. *British Journal of Oral and Maxillofacial Surgery.* 2007; 45(5): 387–91.

104. Jain MK, Ramesh C, Sankar K, Lokesh Babu KT. Pedicled buccal fat pad in the management of oroantral fistula: a clinical study of 15 cases. *International Journal of Oral and Maxillofacial Surgery.* 2012; 41(8): 1025–9.

105. Yilmaz T, Suslu AE, Gursel B. Treatment of oroantral fistula: experience with 27 cases. *American Journal of Otolaryngology.* 2003; 24(4): 221–3.

106. Skoglund LA, Pedersen SS, Holst E. Surgical management of 85 perforations to the maxillary sinus. *International Journal of Oral Surgery.* 1983; 12(1): 1–5.

107. von Wowern N. Correlation between the development of an oroantral fistula and the size of the corresponding bony defect. *Journal of Oral Surgery.* 1973; 31(2): 98–102.

108. Schulz D, Bührmann K. [Pathological changes in the maxillary sinus—important secondary findings in orthodontic x-ray diagnosis]. *Fortschr Kieferorthop.* 1987; 48(4): 298–312.

109. Huang YC, Chen WH. Caldwell–Luc operation without inferior meatal antrostomy: a retrospective study of 50 cases. *Journal of Oral and Maxillofacial Surgery.* 2012; 70(9): 2080–4.

110. Killey HC, Kay LW. Observations based on the surgical closure of 362 oro-antral fistulas. *International Surgery.* 1972; 57(7): 545–9.

111. Candamourty R, Jain MK, Sankar K, Babu MR. Double-layered closure of oroantral fistula using buccal fat pad and buccal advancement flap. *Journal of Natural Sciences Biology Medicine.* 2012; 3(2): 203–5.

112. Poeschl PW, Baumann A, Russmueller G, *et al.* Closure of oroantral communications with Bichat's buccal fat pad. *Journal of Oral and Maxillofacial Surgery.* 2009; 67(7): 1460–6.

113. Fan L, Chen G, Zhao S, Hu J. Clinical application and histological observation of pedicled buccal fat pad grafting. *Chinese Medical Journal (English).* 2002; 115(10): 1556–9.

114. Rapidis AD, Alexandridis CA, Eleftheriadis E, Angelopoulos AP. The use of the buccal fat pad for reconstruction of oral defects: review of the literature and report of 15 cases. *Journal of Oral and Maxillofacial Surgery.* 2000; 58(2): 158–63.

115. Samman N, Cheung LK, Tideman H. The buccal fat pad in oral reconstruction. *International Journal of Oral and Maxillofacial Surgery.* 1993; 22(1): 2–6.

116. Ehrl PA. Oroantral communication. Epicritical study of 175 patients, with special concern to secondary operative closure. *International Journal of Oral Surgery.* 1980; 9(5): 351–8.

117. Lee JJ, Kok SH, Chang HH, *et al.* Repair of oroantral communications in the third molar region by random palatal flap. *International Journal of Oral and Maxillofacial Surgery.* 2002; 31(6): 677–80.

118. James RB. Surgical closure of large oroantral fistulas using a palatal island flap. *Journal of Oral Surgery.* 1980; 38(8): 591–5.

119. Yamazaki Y, Yamaoka M, Hirayama M, Shimada H. The submucosal island flap in the closure of oro-antral fistula. *British Journal of Oral and Maxillofacial Surgery.* 1985; 23(4): 259–63.

120. Field EA, Speechley JA, Rotter E, Scott J. Dry socket incidence compared after a 12 year interval. *British Journal of Oral and Maxillofacial Surgery.* 1985; 23(6): 419–27.

121. Turner PS. A clinical study of "dry socket." *International Journal of Oral Surgery.* 1982; 11(4): 226–31.

122. Osborn TP, Frederickson G Jr., Small IA, Torgerson TS. A prospective study of complications related to mandibular third molar surgery. *Journal of Oral and Maxillofacial Surgery.* 1985; 43(10): 767–9.

123. Kolokythas A, Olech E, Miloro M. Alveolar osteitis: a comprehensive review of concepts and controversies. *International Journal of Dentistry.* 2010; 2010: 249073.

124. Larsen PE. Alveolar osteitis after surgical removal of impacted mandibular third molars. *Identification of the patient at risk. Oral Surgery Oral Medicine Oral Pathology.* 1992; 73(4): 393–7.

125. Blum IR. Contemporary views on dry socket (alveolar osteitis): a clinical appraisal of standardization, aetiopathogenesis and management: a critical review. *International Journal of Oral and Maxillofacial Surgery.* 2002; 31(3): 309–17.

126. Heasman PA, Jacobs DJ. A clinical investigation into the incidence of dry socket. *British Journal of Oral and Maxillofacial Surgery.* 1984; 22(2): 115–22.

127. Nitzan DW. On the genesis of "dry socket." *Journal of Oral and Maxillofacial Surgery.* 1983; 41(11): 706–10.

128. Rood JP, Murgatroyd J. Metronidazole in the prevention of 'dry socket'. *British Journal of Oral Surgery.* 1979; 17(1): 62–70.

129. Catellani JE, Harvey S, Erickson SH, Cherkin D. Effect of oral contraceptive cycle on dry socket (localized alveolar osteitis). *Journal of the American Dental Association.* 1980; 101(5): 777–80.

130. Bergdahl M, Hedstrom L. Metronidazole for the prevention of dry socket after removal of partially impacted mandibular third molar: a randomised controlled trial. *British Journal of Oral and Maxillofacial Surgery.* 2004; 42(6): 555–8.

131. Hedstrom L, Sjogren P. Effect estimates and methodological quality of randomized controlled trials about prevention of alveolar osteitis following tooth extraction: a systematic review. *Oral Surgery Oral Medicine Oral Pathology Oral Radiology and Endodontics.* 2007; 103(1): 8–15.

132. Ren YF, Malmstrom HS. Effectiveness of antibiotic prophylaxis in third molar surgery: a meta-analysis of randomized controlled clinical trials. *Journal of Oral and Maxillofacial Surgery.* 2007; 65(10): 1909–21.

133. Lodi G, Figini L, Sardella A, *et al.* Antibiotics to prevent complications following tooth extractions. *Cochrane Database of Systematic Reviews.* 2012; 11: CD003811.

134. Ataoglu H, Oz GY, Candirli C, Kiziloglu D. Routine antibiotic prophylaxis is not necessary during operations to remove third molars. *British Journal of Oral and Maxillofacial Surgery.* 2008; 46(2): 133–5.

135. Swanson AE. A double-blind study on the effectiveness of tetracycline in reducing the incidence of fibrinolytic alveolitis. *Journal of Oral and Maxillofacial Surgery*. 1989; 47(2): 165–7.

136. Davis WM Jr., Buchs AU, Davis WM. The use of granular gelatin-tetracycline compound after third molar removal. *Journal of Oral Surgery*. 1981; 39(6): 466–7.

137. Sorensen DC, Preisch JW. The effect of tetracycline on the incidence of postextraction alveolar osteitis. *Journal of Oral and Maxillofacial Surgery*. 1987; 45(12): 1029–33.

138. Akota I, Alvsaker B, Bjornland T. The effect of locally applied gauze drain impregnated with chlortetracycline ointment in mandibular third-molar surgery. *Acta Odontologica Scandinavica*. 1998; 56(1): 25–9.

139. Fridrich KL, Olson RA. Alveolar osteitis following surgical removal of mandibular third molars. *Anesthesia Progress*. 1990; 37(1): 32–41.

140. Schow SR. Evaluation of postoperative localized osteitis in mandibular third molar surgery. *Oral Surgery Oral Medicine Oral Pathology*. 1974; 38(3): 352–8.

141. Zuniga JR, Leist JC. Topical tetracycline-induced neuritis: a case report. *Journal of Oral and Maxillofacial Surgery*. 1995; 53(2): 196–9.

142. Lynch DP, Newland JR, McClendon JL. Myospherulosis of the oral hard and soft tissues. *Journal of Oral and Maxillofacial Surgery*. 1984; 42(6): 349–55.

143. Poor MR, Hall JE, Poor AS. Reduction in the incidence of alveolar osteitis in patients treated with the SaliCept patch, containing Acemannan hydrogel. *Journal of Oral and Maxillofacial Surgery*. 2002; 60(4): 374–9; discussion 79.

144. Hermesch CB, Hilton TJ, Biesbrock AR, *et al.* Perioperative use of 0.12% chlorhexidine gluconate for the prevention of alveolar osteitis: efficacy and risk factor analysis. *Oral Surgery Oral Medicine Oral Pathology Oral Radiology and Endodontics*. 1998; 85(4): 381–7.

145. Kaya GS, Yapici G, Savas Z, Gungormus M. Comparison of alvogyl, SaliCept patch, and low-level laser therapy in the management of alveolar osteitis. *Journal of Oral and Maxillofacial Surgery*. 2011; 69(6): 1571–7.

146. Sisk AL, Hammer WB, Shelton DW, Joy ED Jr. Complications following removal of impacted third molars: the role of the experience of the surgeon. *Journal of Oral and Maxillofacial Surgery*. 1986; 44(11): 855–9.

147. Lopes V, Mumenya R, Feinmann C, Harris M. Third molar surgery: an audit of the indications for surgery, post-operative complaints and patient satisfaction. *British Journal of Oral and Maxillofacial Surgery*. 1995; 33(1): 33–5.

148. Renton T, Dawood A, Shah A, Searson L, Yilmaz Z. Post-implant neuropathy of the trigeminal nerve. A case series. *British Dental Journal*. 2012; 212(11): E17.

149. Pogrel MA, Renaut A, Schmidt B, Ammar A. The relationship of the lingual nerve to the mandibular third molar region: an anatomic study. *Journal of Oral and Maxillofacial Surgery*. 1995; 53(10): 1178–81.

150. Valmaseda-Castellon E, Berini-Aytes L, Gay-Escoda C. Lingual nerve damage after third lower molar surgical extraction. *Oral Surgery Oral Medicine Oral Pathology Oral Radiology and Endodontics*. 2000; 90(5): 567–73.

151. Blackburn CW, Bramley PA. Lingual nerve damage associated with the removal of lower third molars. *British Dental Journal*. 1989; 167(3): 103–7.

152. Mason DA. Lingual nerve damage following lower third molar surgery. *International Journal of Oral and Maxillofacial Surgery*. 1988; 17(5): 290–4.

153. Robert RC, Bacchetti P, Pogrel MA. Frequency of trigeminal nerve injuries following third molar removal. *Journal of Oral and Maxillofacial Surgery*. 2005; 63(6): 732–5; discussion 36.

154. Hillerup S, Stoltze K. Lingual nerve injury in third molar surgery I. *Observations on recovery of sensation with spontaneous healing. International Journal of Oral and Maxillofacial Surgery*. 2007; 36(10): 884–9.

155. Kiesselbach JE, Chamberlain JG. Clinical and anatomic observations on the relationship of the lingual nerve to the mandibular third molar region. *Journal of Oral and Maxillofacial Surgery*. 1984; 42(9): 565–7.

156. Hwang K, Cho HJ, Battuvshin D, Chung IH, Hwang SH. Interrelated buccal fat pad with facial buccal branches and parotid duct. *Journal of Craniofacial Surgery*. 2005; 16(4): 658–60.

157. Kim JW, Cha IH, Kim SJ, Kim MR. Which risk factors are associated with neurosensory deficits of inferior alveolar nerve after mandibular third molar extraction? *Journal of Oral and Maxillofacial Surgery*. 2012; 70(11): 2508–14.

158. Pogrel MA, Goldman KE. Lingual flap retraction for third molar removal. *Journal of Oral and Maxillofacial Surgery*. 2004; 62(9): 1125–30.

159. Gomes AC, Vasconcelos BC, de Oliveira e Silva ED, da Silva LC. *Lingual nerve damage after mandibular third molar surgery: a randomized clinical trial. Journal of Oral and Maxillofacial Surgery*. 2005; 63(10): 1443–6.

160. Susarla SM, Kaban LB, Donoff RB, Dodson TB. Does early repair of lingual nerve injuries improve functional sensory recovery? *Journal of Oral and Maxillofacial Surgery*. 2007; 65(6): 1070–6.

161. Bagheri SC, Meyer RA, Khan HA, Kuhmichel A, Steed MB. Retrospective review of microsurgical repair of 222 lingual nerve injuries. *Journal of Oral and Maxillofacial Surgery*. 2010; 68(4): 715–23.

162. Libersa P, Roze D, Cachart T, Libersa JC. Immediate and late mandibular fractures after third molar removal. *Journal of Oral and Maxillofacial Surgery*. 2002; 60(2): 163–5; discussion 65–6.

163. Sakr K, Farag IA, Zeitoun IM. Review of 509 mandibular fractures treated at the University Hospital, Alexandria, Egypt. *British Journal of Oral and Maxillofacial Surgery*. 2006; 44(2): 107–11.

164. Yamaoka M, Furusawa K, Iguchi K, Tanaka M, Okuda D. The assessment of fracture of the mandibular condyle by use of computerized tomography. Incidence of sagittal

split fracture. *British Journal of Oral and Maxillofacial Surgery.* 1994; 32(2): 77–9.

165. Thorn JJ, Mogeltoft M, Hansen PK. Incidence and aetiological pattern of jaw fractures in Greenland. *International Journal of Oral and Maxillofacial Surgery.* 1986; 15(4): 372–9.

166. Cankaya AB, Erdem MA, Cakarer S, Cifter M, Oral CK. Iatrogenic mandibular fracture associated with third molar removal. *International Journal of Medical Science.* 2011; 8(7): 547–53.

167. Dunstan SP, Sugar AW. Fractures after removal of wisdom teeth. *British Journal of Oral and Maxillofacial Surgery.* 1997; 35(6): 396–7.

168. Krimmel M, Reinert S. Mandibular fracture after third molar removal. *Journal of Oral and Maxillofacial Surgery.* 2000; 58(10): 1110–2.

169. Chrcanovic BR, Custodio AL. Mandibular fractures associated with endosteal implants. *Oral and Maxillofacial Surgery.* 2009; 13(4): 231–8.

170. Mason ME, Triplett RG, Van Sickels JE, Parel SM. Mandibular fractures through endosseous cylinder implants: report of cases and review. *Journal of Oral and Maxillofacial Surgery.* 1990; 48(3): 311–7.

171. Raghoebar GM, Stellingsma K, Batenburg RH, Vissink A. Etiology and management of mandibular fractures associated with endosteal implants in the atrophic mandible. *Oral Surgery Oral Medicine Oral Pathology Oral Radiology and Endodontics.* 2000; 89(5): 553–9.

172. Oh WS, Roumanas ED, Beumer J 3rd. Mandibular fracture in conjunction with bicortical penetration, using wide-diameter endosseous dental implants. *Journal of Prosthodontics.* 2010; 19(8): 625–9.

173. Boffano P, Roccia F, Gallesio C, Berrone S. Pathological mandibular fractures: a review of the literature of the last two decades. *Dental Traumatology.* 2013; 29(3): 185–96.

174. Bertram AR, Rao AC, Akbiyik KM, Haddad S, Zoud K. Maxillary tuberosity fracture: a life-threatening haemorrhage following simple exodontia. *Australian Dental Journal.* 2011; 56(2): 212–5.

175. Coletti D, Ord RA. Treatment rationale for pathological fractures of the mandible: a series of 44 fractures. *International Journal of Oral and Maxillofacial Surgery.* 2008; 37(3): 215–22.

176. Grau-Manclus V, Gargallo-Albiol J, Almendros-Marques N, Gay-Escoda C. Mandibular fractures related to the surgical extraction of impacted lower third molars: a report of 11 cases. *Journal of Oral and Maxillofacial Surgery.* 2011; 69(5): 1286–90.

177. Bodner L, Brennan PA, McLeod NM. Characteristics of iatrogenic mandibular fractures associated with tooth removal: review and analysis of 189 cases. *British Journal of Oral and Maxillofacial Surgery.* 2011; 49(7): 567–72.

178. Al-Belasy FA, Tozoglu S, Ertas U. Mastication and late mandibular fracture after surgery of impacted third molars associated with no gross pathology. *Journal of Oral and Maxillofacial Surgery.* 2009; 67(4): 856–61.

179. Perry PA, Goldberg MH. Late mandibular fracture after third molar surgery: a survey of Connecticut oral and maxillofacial surgeons. *Journal of Oral and Maxillofacial Surgery.* 2000; 58(8): 858–61.

180. Komerik N, Karaduman AI. Mandibular fracture 2 weeks after third molar extraction. *Dental Traumatology.* 2006; 22(1): 53–5.

181. Kao YH, Huang IY, Chen CM, *et al.* Late mandibular fracture after lower third molar extraction in a patient with Stafne bone cavity: a case report. *Journal of Oral and Maxillofacial Surgery.* 2010; 68(7): 1698–700.

182. Karlis V, Bae RD, Glickman RS. Mandibular fracture as a complication of inferior alveolar nerve transposition and placement of endosseous implants: a case report. *Implant Dentistry.* 2003; 12(3): 211–6.

183. Moreno JC, Fernandez A, Ortiz JA, Montalvo JJ. Complication rates associated with different treatments for mandibular fractures. *Journal of Oral and Maxillofacial Surgery.* 2000; 58(3): 273–80; discussion 80–1.

184. Ellis E 3rd, Walker LR. Treatment of mandibular angle fractures using one noncompression miniplate. *Journal of Oral and Maxillofacial Surgery.* 1996; 54(7): 864–71; discussion 71–2.

185. Ellis E 3rd. Treatment methods for fractures of the mandibular angle. *Journal of Craniomaxillofacial Trauma.* 1996; 2(1): 28–36.

Index

Note: Pages numbers in *italics* refer to Figures; page numbers in **bold** refer to Tables

Manual of Minor Oral Surgery for the General Dentist, Second Edition. Edited by Pushkar Mehra and Richard D'Innocenzo.
© 2016 John Wiley & Sons, Inc. Published 2016 by John Wiley & Sons, Inc.

Printed and bound by CPI Group (UK) Ltd, Croydon, CR0 4YY

16/04/2025

14658464-0002